# ARTHRITIS RESEARCH: TREATMENT AND MANAGEMENT

# ARTHRITIS RESEARCH: TREATMENT AND MANAGEMENT

**FRANK COLUMBUS**
**(EDITOR)**

**Nova Biomedical Books**
*New York*

For permission to use material from this book please contact us:
Telephone 631-231-7269; Fax 631-231-8175
Web Site: http://www.novapublishers.com



Library of Congress Cataloging-in-Publication Data
*Availible Upon Request*

ISBN: 1-59033-984-3.

*Published by Nova Science Publishers, Inc. ✣ New York*

# Content

# Preface

The aetiopathogenetic mechanism of this disease involves an interaction between genetic and environmental/microbial factors. Extensive genetic analyses have shown that HLA-DR4/1 genes in chromosome 6 are most likely to have a role in RA. Various independent molecular, microbiological and immunological studies have shown that the main microbial trigger in the initiation and/or perpetuation of the disease in RA is *Proteus mirabilis* infection of the upper urinary tract. The most likely mechanism explaining this microbial-disease association is molecular mimicry or cross-reactivity. Chapter 1 explores new diagnostic criteria involving a combination of clinical, genetic and immuno-microbiological features are proposed to identify RA patients, especially in the early stages of the disease, so that therapy involving anti-microbial and other measures can be started before irreversible arthritic damage has occurred.

The spondyloarthropathies can be difficult to diagnose and resistant to treatment. Diagnosis has primarily been based upon clinical characteristics and plain radiographic changes; however, radiographic changes are slow to progress. Similarly, treatment has been largely empiric with minimal impact on disease progression and disability. Chapter 2 reviews the diagnosis and treatment of spondyloarthropathies with special emphasis on more recent advances.

As presented in Chapter 3, medical researchers are reporting new applications for an old medicine. Over the centuries colchicine has been used preponderantly to treat and prevent gout, but an astonishing array of therapeutic properties is now being ascribed to this age-old substance. Besides its stabilizing effect on the cytoskeleton and cell membranes, colchicine has anti-inflammatory and antifibrotic properties. Responses have been especially favorable in fibrotic and inflammatory systemic diseases. The outlook for further therapeutic possibilities is promising and due to the virtual absence of side effects when properly applied, a significant new phase in low-dose colchicine therapy can be predicted if controlled studies succeed in demonstrating its multiplicity and its benefits.

Rheumatoid arthritis is a chronic inflammatory disease affecting the joint, and as the disease develops it may cause severe disability. The disease shows periods of active inflammation and periods of no inflammation. Apart from treatment of the inflammatory condition, it is important to keep the patients at the best obtainable functional level, both during inflammation and in the periods with no inflammation. Chapter 4 examines aquatic exercise, also known as pool therapy, hydrotherapy, and sometimes in earlier literature even balneotherapy, which is treatment in water involving, for the patient specially designed, aquatic exercises.

In the first part of Chapter 5, the physical fitness levels of children with Juvenile Arthritis (JA) are reviewed. The majority of the studies indicate that JA patients do have an impaired physical fitness (for example muscle strength, muscle bulk, anaerobic and aerobic fitness) compared to healthy children. These results will be discussed in the light of the paradigm of *rheumatoid cachexia*. In the second part of Chapter 5, the available clinical trials on exercise training for juvenile arthritis patients are reviewed. These observations from the literature indicate a need for a randomized controlled trial with adequate sample size and objective measures of functional ability and quality of life. As presented in Chapter 6, pediatric rheumatic diseases with predominantly arthritic involvement such as juvenile idiopathic arthritis (JIA) can cause considerable physical functional impairment and significantly affect the children's quality of life (QOL). Physical function, QOL, health-related QOL (HRQOL) and health status are personal constructs used as outcomes to estimate the impact of these diseases and often used as proxies for each other. The chronic, fluctuating nature of these diseases differs within and between patients, and complicates the measurement of these outcomes. In children, additional dimensions such as their growing needs and expectations, limited use of age-specific questionnaires, and the use of proxy respondents further obscure this evaluation. This chapter will briefly review the different constructs inclusive of and related to physical function, and the different scales used for measuring them.

Osteoarthritis (OA) is the most prevalent form of arthritis, and represents a major burden on individuals, health systems and societies. Chapter 7 discusses the issues relating to the successful management of OA are discussed, these include epidemiology, diagnosis, treatment and service provision. OA is a complex condition with a number of factors influencing disease progression and so need for treatment and services. Treatment is split between non-surgical patient self-managed treatment and surgical health professional managed treatment. The one area that appears to be lacking in the research literature is identifying which packages of care are most effective on which patients. However, successful management of OA is possible.

As presented in Chapter 8, degenerative joint disease which results in deterioration of joint structure and function is the most common cause of long-term disability and has significant economic impact. It affects people in all geographic locations. There is a strong association between joint degeneration and age. Etiology of degenerative joint disease is still not clearly understood and there is no specific management for this group of diseases. Various pathological conditions cause damage of the articular cartilage and lead to clinically and radiographically recognized impairment of the patients. Biomechanical, metabolic, genetic factors, inflammation and other risk factors contribute to the development of osteoarthrosis.

In: Arthritis Research: Treatment and Management
Editor: F. Columbus, pp. 1-25
ISBN 1-59033-984-3


*Chapter I*

# Triggering Aetiological Factors and Proposal for Early Treatment

***Taha Rashid, Clyde Wilson, Lucy Hughes and Alan Ebringer[1*]***
Division of Life Sciences, Infection and Immunity Group, King's College London
[1]Department of Rheumatology, Middlesex Hospital, University College London

## Abstract

Rheumatoid arthritis (RA) is the most common inflammatory arthritic condition, causing severe disabilities in many patients. The disease has a worldwide distribution and affects mainly females of middle age groups.

The aetiopathogenetic mechanism of this disease involves an interaction between genetic and environmental/microbial factors. Extensive genetic analyses have shown that HLA-DR4/1 genes in chromosome 6 are most likely to have a role in RA. Various independent molecular, microbiological and immunological studies have shown that the main microbial trigger in the initiation and/or perpetuation of the disease in RA is *Proteus mirabilis* infection of the upper urinary tract. The most likely mechanism explaining this microbial-disease association is molecular mimicry or cross-reactivity.

New diagnostic criteria involving a combination of clinical, genetic and immuno-microbiological features are proposed to identify RA patients, especially in the early stages of the disease, so that therapy involving anti-microbial and other measures can be started before irreversible arthritic damage has occurred.

---

* Correspondence to: Prof. Alan Ebringer, Division of Life Sciences, Infection and Immunity Group, King's College London, 150 Stamford Street, London SE1 8WA, U.K. E-mail: alan.ebringer@kcl.ac.uk or taha.rashid@kcl.ac.uk

# Introduction

Rheumatoid arthritis (RA) is a chronic systemic inflammatory disease, predominantly affecting females of middle age. So far no curative treatment, which could possibly halt or prevent the destructive pathological lesions, is available for this disease. In the long term, up to 50% of patients with RA are unable to work and the life expectancy is reduced by between 5-10 years (Pincus and Callahan, 1993).

The typical clinical presentation of RA is characterized by insidious onset of pain, stiffness and symmetrical swellings of the small joints of the hands and feet, although no joint in the body is immune to this disease. Apart from the musculo-skeletal system, other organs are also involved either as an inter-related association or as a complication of the disease (Turesson et al, 2003).

The diagnosis of RA is made through assessment of a collection of characteristic clinical presentations with or without the results of certain laboratory and radiological investigations. The American College of Rheumatology (ACR) diagnostic criteria for RA (Arnett et al, 1988) are still commonly used among clinical scientists for the selection of RA patients for the purpose of research studies.

# Historical Background

A historical review indicates that the idea of considering RA as a separate disease entity and distinct from other rheumatic diseases such as gout and rheumatic fever has emerged since the 18th century. The main problem in the $19^{th}$ and $20^{th}$ centuries was how to differentiate between RA and a group of related inflammatory arthritic diseases, collectively termed spondyloarthropathies. These include; ankylosing spondylitis (AS), reactive arthritis and Reiter's syndrome, enteropathic arthritis, psoriatic arthritis, Behcet's disease, and Whipple's disease. The separation of RA from this latter group of diseases began to emerge in the early 1970s, where in contradistinction to RA these disorders were found to be frequently associated with HLA-B27 genetic markers, had spinal involvement and were negative for rheumatoid factors. (Calin A, 1998).

# Epidemiological Background

RA is a relatively common disease affecting millions of people throughout the world. The prevalence rate ranges from 0.2% and 5.3% (Spector, 1990). The high prevalence rate in the North American Pima Indians could be attributed to the effect of genetic and/or environmental factors. However, the decreased incidence of RA among this population over a long period (Jacobsson et al, 1994) favours the possibility that the triggering environmental factors might have been eradicated by means of improved hygienic health status. Similar findings in the decreased incidence rate among RA patients have also been reported among other populations of both American (Doran et al, 2002) and European origin (Silman, 2002).

In a review of data collected from various studies to assess the incidence of RA between 1950 and 1990 in different populations, the overall annual incidence seems to be 0.5/1000 in females and 0.2/1000 in males (MacGregor and Silman, 1998). There is an increased incidence with age, which continues into the seventh decade. The female rate is higher than male rate at all ages with the greater female excess occurring in those with childbearing age, and this could possibly be attributed to the higher incidence of urinary tract infections (UTIs) occurring in women of this age group. The greater incidence of RA in women throughout the world is an important feature, which bears directly on the aetiological factors of this disease. Any theory trying to explain the cause of RA must adequately account for the link to women in middle and old age.

# Aetiopathogenesis

## Evidence from Genetic Factors

Familial distribution of RA among first-degree relatives (Deighton et al, 1992a) and twins (MacGregor et al, 2000), indicates that RA runs in some families, basically supporting the concept of genetic contribution, but at the same time arguing against the proposition that RA could be considered as a purely genetic disorder.

Attempts to identify the genes involved in susceptibility to RA started in mid 1970s, when in two consecutive studies by Stastny's group from USA, it was discovered that the HLA-DR4/Dw4 genetic marker could be found in around 70 percent of patients with RA using both mixed lymphocyte culture assay (Stastny, 1976) and serological methods (Stastny, 1978). This genetic marker was found to be significantly correlated with the disease severity in RA (Valenzuela et al, 1999), raising the possibility that it could be involved directly or indirectly in the pathogenesis of this condition. Increased frequency of HLA-DR4 was found in Caucasians, but not in an Indian immigrant community in the United Kingdom (Woodrow et al, 1981), or in Israelis (Schiff et al, 1982), among whom increased frequency of HLA-DR1 was observed. Molecular characterization of the HLA genes in RA, however, has resolved this difference in the distribution of RA-associated genetic markers among various ethnic groups.

The third hypervariable region of all RA-associated HLA-DRβ1 alleles (HLA-DR4 subtypes, DRβ1*0401, 0404, 0405 and 0408; HLA-DR1 subtypes, DRβ1*0101 and *0102; HLA-DR6, DRβ1*0402 and HLA-DR10, DRβ1*1001) (Nepom and Nepom, 1998) were found to share a hexameric amino acid sequence homology, except for few conserved amino acid substitutions, involving positions 69-74 and consisting of glutamic acid, glutamine, lysine or arginine, arginine, alanine and alanine "EQK/RRAA". However, this particular amino acid motif, which has been given the name of "shared epitope" (SE) (Gregerson et al,

1987) was not found in those HLA-DR molecules which are not associated with RA, such as HLA-DR4 subtypes, DRβ1*0402 and DRβ1*0403.

## Evidence from Environmental Factors

A great deal of evidence exists which supports the proposition that RA is mainly triggered and possibly perpetuated by certain environmental factor(s) in genetically predisposed individuals.

1. The occurrence of RA among 15% (Silman et al, 1993) or even less than 10% (Svendsen et al, 2002) of monozygotic twins supports the notion that a substantial part in the aetiology of this disease lies in the role of non-genetic environmental factors.
2. Repeated bouts of remissions and exacerbations, which is characteristic in most cases with RA, usually suggests that a temporary change in the appearance or disappearance of the inciting or triggering factor could possibly occur in this disease.
3. Although the vast majority of cases with RA occur sporadically, identification of three clusters of patients among which five unrelated cases with inflammatory polyarthritis (possibly including RA) developed over a five year period (Silman et al, 2000). This observation along with the mild increase in the incidence of this disease among spouses of RA patients (Dalakos et al, 1968), may suggest that a common environmental or infectious triggering factor exists in the environment.

### *Links between Proteus Microbes and RA*

There is substantial evidence, which assigns to the *Proteus* microbe, the role of the main triggering bacterial factor in RA. These observations are based on the results of various molecular, immunological and microbiological studies, which have been carried out by different independent groups.

### *Molecular* Associations

Computer database search studies were carried out to identify amino acid sequences possessed by various microorganisms, which are homologous with self-antigens, particularly the sequence present in RA-associated HLA-DR molecules comprising the "SE" motif. In these studies the putatively triggering microbe, such as *Proteus,* or other related enterobacterial microbes, were analysed. In a preliminary study in 1992, a molecular similarity was observed between the "EQK/RRAA" sequences and the "ESRRAL" amino acid motif present in *P. mirabilis* haemolysins (Ebringer et al, 1992). Subsequently, another molecular homology was discovered between the 5-mer "IRRET" amino acid sequences present in *Proteus* urease and the "LRREI" sequences found in type XI collagen (Wilson et al, 1995), which is a component of hyaline cartilage found predominantly in the small joints of the hands and feet (Figure 1).

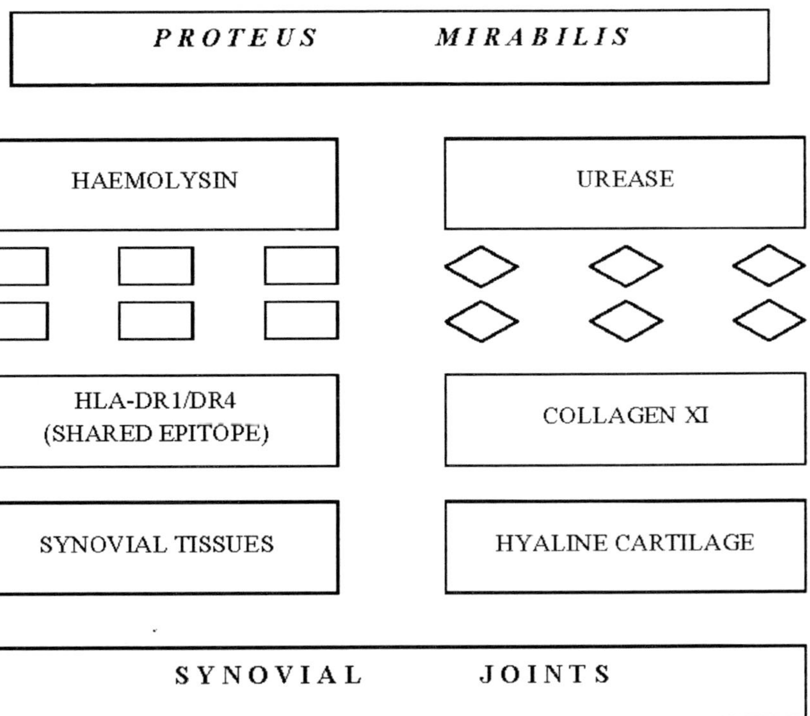


Figure 1. Schematic molecular similarity between Proteus haemolysin or urease enzymes and the HLA-DR1/DR4 or collagen XI auto-antigens respectively.

Although other bacteria and viruses, such as *E. coli*, *Serratia marcescens* and Epstein Barr virus possess sequences similar or homologous to the "EQK/RRAA" amino acid motif, significantly elevated antibodies against *Proteus* only but not against *Serratia* or *Escherichia* microbes have been found in RA patients (Tiwana et al, 1996). Furthermore, significant correlation between anti-bacterial and anti-peptide antibodies to *Proteus* but not to *E. coli* and *Serratia* was detected among RA patients from Finland and Japan (Rashid et al, 2004).

## Immunological Associations

During the last two decades extensive studies have been carried out by different independent groups on the humoral immune response against *Proteus* microorganisms in RA. From these data, it appears that antibodies against *P. mirabilis* were significantly elevated among a total of 1375 RA patients but not in diseased or healthy subject controls from more than 14 different countries (Ebringer et al, 2003).

The specificity of these findings followed from the results of various studies, which showed elevated antibodies to *Proteus* only but not against other microbes, such as *E. coli, Pseudomonas, Salmonella, Yersinia, Chlamydia, Shigella, Serratia, Campylobacter*, parvovirus as well as three anaerobic bowel-inhabitant bacteria (Fielder et al, 1995a; Subair et al, 1995; Tiwana et al, 1996; Goldbach-Mansky et al, 2000). In one particular study carried out earlier by Deighton and colleagues, active RA patients were found to have significantly elevated antibodies against *P. mirabilis* only, but not to four viruses; influenza A, adenovirus, rubella and parvovirus. Furthermore, there was no correlation between anti-*Proteus* antibodies and the levels of antibodies against these viruses or eight different auto-antigens (Deighton et al, 1992b).

The idea of carrying out these immunological and serological experiments has emerged from the results of a preliminary cross-reactivity study where sera from rabbits immunized with HLA-DR4 positive lymphocytes were binding only to *Proteus* species in comparison to 18 other microbes (Ebringer et al, 1985). HLA-DR4 allogeneic tissue typing sera were also binding more significantly to *P. mirabilis* than to *E. coli* microbes, when compared to non-DR4 tissue typing sera (Khalafpour and Ebringer, 1987). This cross-reactivity observation was extended further by using peptide-binding assay (Tiwana et al, 1999), where antiserum against the RA susceptibility sequence "EQKRAA" was shown to bind to a homologous "ESRRAL" peptide present in the haemolysin of the *P. mirabilis*, and vice versa, anti-ESRRAL serum reacted with "EQKRAA" peptides. However, there was no reactivity of either anti-EQKRAA or anti-ESRRAL immune sera to a peptide containing the "EDERAA" sequence which is present in HLA-DRB1*0402, an allele not associated with RA. Moreover, the "EQKRAA" and "ESRRAL" antisera were found to bind to a mouse fibroblast transfectant cell line (Dap.3) expressing HLA-DRB1*0401 but not DRB1*0402.

In a recent in vitro study these cross-reactive epitopes were shown to be cytotoxic and putatively pathogenic in patients with RA (Wilson et al, 2003), where the percentage lysis for sheep red blood cell (SRBC) coated with a 16-mer amino acid peptide containing "EQRRAA" was found to be significantly higher with RA sera compared to sera from AS patients ($P<0.0001$) and healthy controls ($P<0.0001$). Similar results were also observed when sera from RA, AS and healthy controls were tested against SRBCs coated with peptides containing "LRREI" sequence which are present in type XI collagen and homologous to "IRRET" amino acid sequence present in the *Proteus* urease enzyme. There was a significant correlation between anti-ESRRAL and anti-IRRET antibody levels and the percentage lysis of SRBC coated with "EQRRAA" ($P<0.0001$) or "LRREI" ($P<0.0001$) peptides respectively.

## Microbiological Associations

*Proteus mirabilis* is a motile Gram-negative bacillus. It is the second most common infectious agent, after *E. coli*, that causes urinary tract infections (UTI) (Sussman, 1998). The majority of *Proteus* UTIs show kidney involvement (Fairley et al, 1971). This bacterial characteristic is due to increased adherence to uro-epithelium within the genito-urinary tract, which is apparently helped by the possessions by this microbe of epithelial receptors ligands and various virulence factors. For example, *Proteus* microorganisms apart from possessing flagella and fimbriae, also produce many enzymes such as; haemolysins, urease, IgA and IgG proteases, deaminases and endotoxins (Rozalski et al, 1997). Although most of *Proteus* virulent factors help the bacteria to reach the upper parts of the urinary system, some of these, also produce damaging and cytotoxic effects on the urinary epithelium (Mobley et al, 1991).

The incidence of UTIs is increased in patients with RA (Tishler et al, 1992), but this association is not always observed (Vandenbroucke et al, 1987). This discrepancy in the results with an apparent lack of the epidemiological link between urinary infections and RA could be due to the occurrence of sub-clinical or occult infections, which are merely characterized by bacteriuria. This was recognised through the results of two independent studies, in which RA patients were found to have asymptomatic *Proteus* bacteriuria more frequently than healthy controls (Ebringer et al, 1993; Senior et al, 1999). Further supportive evidence emerges from another study where a significant correlation was detected between increased urinary isolation rate of this microbe and serum levels of antibodies to *P. mirabilis* in patients with RA (Wilson et al, 1997).

## Molecular Mimicry and Autoimmunity as the Main Pathogenetic Mechanism in RA

Among all rheumatic diseases, RA is the second most common, after systemic lupus erythematosus, to be considered as having an autoimmune pathology. The discovery of IgM rheumatic factor (RF), an antibody that binds to the heavy chain portion of immunoglobulins, in RA patients was the principal reason behind its inclusion in the group of autoimmune disorders. Apart from RF, many other autoantibodies are frequently found to be elevated in patients with RA, such as antibodies against collagens, keratins, cytoplasmic and nuclear products to name a few (Fox, 2001). The appearance of these autoantibodies in patients with RA is generally considered to be related to the advanced or late stages of the disease. However, other researchers have claimed that these autoantibodies could also be observed and even exploited as prognostic markers in early cases with RA (Vencovsky et al, 2003).

There is much evidence, which tends to implicate that the occurrence of these autoantibodies, especially RFs, is a secondary phenomenon resulting from preceding microbial infections. For example, RF response is transiently associated with many bacterial, viral and parasitic infectious diseases (Newkirk, 2002). RFs can be produced experimentally by polyclonal B cell activation with lipopolysaccharides in mice (Hara et al, 1996) and the Epstein Barr virus and cytomegalovirus infections in humans (Ferraro and Newkirk, 1993). Furthermore, the increased RFs in subacute bacterial endocarditis were reported to be cleared out when the offending agents, *Streptococci*, were eradicated by use of antibiotics (Williams and Kunkel, 1962). Interestingly, only certain components, such as LPS, of some bacteria can stimulate production of RF (Newkirk, 2002), which may explain why around 30% of RA patients have no associated RFs.

In an earlier experimental study carried out by a Dutch group, it was observed that initiation of autoimmunity in the form of splenic lympho-proliferation as well as increased levels of autoantibodies and circulating immune complexes was produced following intraperitoneal injection of mice with *E. coli* and *S. typhimurium*. It was also concluded that the induction of more prominent autoimmune reactivity by these microbes must be ascribed to a longer survival time in vivo (Hol et al, 1993).

The existence of a relationship between RA and *Proteus* infections on one hand and RA and autoimmunity on the other could raise the proposition that the "cross-reactivity or molecular mimicry" hypothesis is the main aetiopathogenetic mechanism in the development of RA. The basic pathological sequence, which is presumed to occur in RA, involves the production of antibodies against *Proteus* microbes following infections of the urinary tract particularly in women.

Further evidence into the suggestion that RA occurs as the result of the cross-reactivity reactions between external microbial factors and the auto-antigens, is the failure to detect microbial DNA products at the main pathological sites, the articular tissues, when analysed with gas chromatography-mass spectrometry and pan-bacterial polymerase chain reaction (Chen et al, 2003). However, the identification of *Proteus* microbes at a remote site in the urinary tract system of RA patients (Ebringer et al, 1993) would apparently support the involvement of the molecular mimicry mechanism in the development of RA.

The presence of homologous antigens in both *Proteus* and tissues of genetically susceptible individuals suggests that antibodies produced against haemolysins and urease enzymes of *Proteus* bacteria, would bind to cross-reactive self-antigens of HLA-DR4/1 molecules and collagen type XI respectively. These bacterially-induced cross-reactive antibodies probably comprise only a small proportion of the whole antibody repertoire, among which other as yet unidentified antibodies that have auto-pathogenic and auto-destructive potentials may exist. Binding of these cross-reactive antibodies, especially if they are present in sufficient amount, to the joint tissues particularly the synoviocytes and collagens of hyaline cartilages could trigger the activation of inflammatory cascades through the mechanism of type II immune-mediated reaction or complement-dependent antibody-mediated cytotoxicity (Wilson et al, 2003). These preliminary activations will lead to tissue-injurious immune reactions through the production of pro-inflammatory mediators, such as cytokines, proteolytic enzymes, chemotactic factors, vasoactive amines as well as the recruitment of other inflammatory cells, which might all contribute to the local destruction of the joint structures (Figure 2).

There are many other autoimmune diseases, which could be explained on the basis of molecular mimicry or cross-reactivity mechanisms, among these are rheumatic fever, multiple sclerosis and ankylosing spondylitis to name a few.

## *Molecular Mimicry in other Autoimmune Diseases*

### Rheumatic Fever

Rheumatic fever is considered as the prototype of the cross-reactivity or molecular mimicry pathological mechanism, which has been extensively studied. In this disease, antibodies against *Streptococcal* cell wall components were found to be reacting specifically with heart muscle tissues (Friemer and McCarty, 1965) and brain tissues (Husby et al, 1976) of patients with rheumatic carditis and Sydenham's chorea respectively.

INFECTION
by *Proteus mirabilis* in the upper urinary tract of middle aged and elderly women

↓

ANTIBODIES
against these microbes produced in the local lymph nodes, such as those draining the genitourinary tract

↓

INFLAMMATION
induced because anti-*Proteus* antibodies bind to HLA-DR4 positive cells as well as to collagen type XI in the peripheral joints, and through their activation of the complement cascade these antibodies will help in releasing inflammatory mediators and cytokines produced by other immune cells which have been recruited to the site of inflammation. As the result of these inflammatory reactions pathological damage to the joint tissues would follow

↓

*PROTEUS*-REACTIVE ARTHRITIS
formed due to the recurrent waves of *Proteus* urinary infections occurring especially in women, because of the existing differences in the anatomical features of the genitourinary system

↓

RHEUMATOID ARTHRITIS
would appear to be the end result of repeated episodes of *Proteus* reactive arthritis occurring in genetically predisposed individuals possessing HLA-DR4/1 molecules

Figure 2. Proposed aetiopathogenetic sequence from *Proteus* urinary infection to the development of RA.

## Multiple Sclerosis

Multiple sclerosis (MS) is a demyelinating neurological disease having severe and disabling consequences. It is considered as an autoimmune disease with suggested molecular mimicry hypothesis as the main pathogenetic mechanism implicated in the development of this condition.

The main targeted neuronal antigens, myelin basic protein (MBP) and myelin oligodendrocyte glycoprotein (MOG), were found to carry peptide amino acid sequences, which are cross-reactive with similar sequences present in 4-carboxy-munonolactone decarboxylase and 3-oxoadipate coA transferase enzymes respectively, found in *Acinetobacter* bacteria (Ebringer et al, 1997). Furthermore, antibodies against these amino acid peptides were found to be elevated among patients with MS when compared to patients with cerebro vascular accidents and healthy controls (Hughes et al, 2003). In an earlier study carried out on the same group of patients and controls, MS patients were found to have significantly elevated antibodies against six *Acinetobacter* species as well as to MBP and neurofilament neuronal antigens when compared to disease or healthy control groups (Hughes et al, 2001).

## Ankylosing Spondylitis

Ankylosing spondylitis (AS), another rheumatic disease with a similar pathogenetic mechanism, is considered as the prototype of seronegative spondyloarthropathies and is strongly linked to the presence of HLA-B27 genetic markers, where more than 90% of patients with AS were found to carry this gene, whereas its occurrence among healthy control populations is about 8% (Schlosstein et al, 1973). This remarkable observation could be linked to an association between AS and the presence of a bowel microbe, *Klebsiella pneumoniae* on the basis of molecular mimicry mechanism.

There is substantial evidence for the involvement of *Klebsiella* in AS. These entail the results of various independent groups which showed molecular, microbiological and immunological associations between *Klebsiella* microbes and AS (Ebringer, 1992). For example, antibodies against *K. pneumoniae* microbes or their products were detected in sera of 1330 patients with AS from fifteen different countries when compared to 1191 healthy controls (Ebringer et al, submitted). *Klebsiella* nitrogenase (Schwimmbeck et al., 1987) and pullulanase (Fielder et al, 1995b) enzymes possess molecular similarities to HLA-B27 molecules. Antibodies to the peptides within these molecules bind specifically to the synovial tissues of AS patients (Husby et al, 1989) and were shown to be cytotoxic in-vitro (Wilson et al, 2003). Furthermore, temporal relationships between the acquisition of *Klebsiella* in the faeces and the exacerbation of symptoms were observed in two longitudinal studies carried out in patients with AS (Ebringer et al, 1977; Eastmond et al, 1980).

### The *Proteus* Molecular Mimicry Hypothesis could Explain Many features of RA

Unlike other theories, which have been proposed in the aetiopathogenesis of RA, molecular mimicry between *Proteus* and self tissues provides an explanation for most of the prominent features found to occur in RA patients:

a) The predominance of RA in females (female:male ratio = 3:1) could be attributed to the higher incidence of *Proteus* UTIs in women.
b) RA occurs mainly in the age group of between 30 to 70 years because of the increased frequency of UTIs in these potentially vulnerable age groups.
c) Women with RA show characteristic onset of exacerbation after pregnancy, because of the higher incidence of UTIs among these groups of patients. The characteristic remission during pregnancy has been attributed to the increased production of gonadotrophic hormones by the placenta which display steroid-like functional activities.
d) Observation of the low concordance rate, that is the possibility of the second twin to develop the disease when the first one has developed the disease, among monozygotic twins with RA is considerably low (<15%) signifying the role of other non-genetic (environmental) factors in this condition.
e) The presence of both molecular and immunological cross-reactivity between the "IRRET" amino acid sequences of the *Proteus* urease enzyme and the "LRREI" amino acid sequences of the collagen XI self molecules, could explain the predominance of the peripheral small joint involvements in RA.
f) The observation of high frequency (>90%) of HLA-DR4/1 subtypes, especially those with "SE" moieties, in association with RA could mainly be explained on the basis of molecular mimicry theory.
g) Results of multiple studies suggest the presence of RF as a secondary effect of triggering infectious agents, giving an explanation to the high frequency of these autoantibodies among patients with RA.

## Proposed New Diagnostic Criteria

Although extensive studies have been carried out on RA patients to develop empirical and precise diagnostic criteria, debate is still active in trying to detect the disease in its relatively early stages.

Currently the requirement for a combination of clinical, laboratory and radiological observations is essential for the establishment of the diagnosis of classical RA. However, delay of considerably long periods exist between the disease onset and the appearance of some of these diagnostic parameters. For example, the distinguishing radiological signs of RA sometimes take up to two years or more to become manifest. Furthermore, some patients with RA remain sero-negative for RF, which is one of the ACR classification criteria, till late stages of the disease by which time irreversible pathological damages have already occurred.

The search for some new approaches to identify patients with possible RA in the very early stages of the disease is of vital importance. To achieve this goal, reliance on the following diagnostic tools could be useful (Figure 3):

1) *Clinical presentation*: Middle-aged female patients presenting with acute or insidious peripheral polyarthritis or monoarthritis and associated with morning stiffness (>60 minutes), preferably with signs of joint swelling and tenderness.
2) *Laboratory signs of inflammation*: Elevated levels of C-reactive protein (CRP) (>10 mg/L) and/or erythrocyte sedimentation rate (ESR) (>30 mm/hr).
3) *Tissue typing*: Identification of the "SE" within the RA-associated haplotypes, using polymerase chain reaction (PCR) and oligonucleotide sequencing.
4) *Immunological and/or microbiological evidence of Proteus infections*:
   - Increased serum antibodies (IgM and/or IgG) against *P. mirabilis* (>95% confidence limit above the mean of healthy controls).
   - Increased urinary isolation rate ($\geq 10^4$ colony forming units/ml) of *P. mirabilis*.

It is proposed that diagnosis of "RA" could be made, on the basis of the following two taxonomic groups:

A) Early "RA" (Pre-RA): occurs in an individual who
   - Has arthritis of the small joints of the hands and feet for at least three months.
   - Is HLA-DR1/DR4 positive.
   - Has an ESR $\geq$ 30 mm/hr or CRP > 10 mg/L.
   - Has high titre of antibodies to *Proteus* bacteria.
   - Has no sings of "erosions" on X-ray examination.

B) Advanced "RA" (Classical RA): occurs in an individual who
   - Has arthritis of the small joints of the hands and feet for at least three months.
   - Is HLA-DR1/DR4 positive.
   - Has an ESR $\geq$ 30 mm/hr or CRP > 10 mg/L.
   - Has high titre of antibodies to *Proteus* bacteria.
   - Has signs of "erosions" on X-ray examination.

The basic goal for using these diagnostic criteria is in trying to detect very early cases of RA, mainly for therapeutic purposes. Furthermore, these investigations could be accomplished through the outpatient services by the general practitioners, hence abolishing the time needed by the patients for their preliminary referral to specialist clinics.

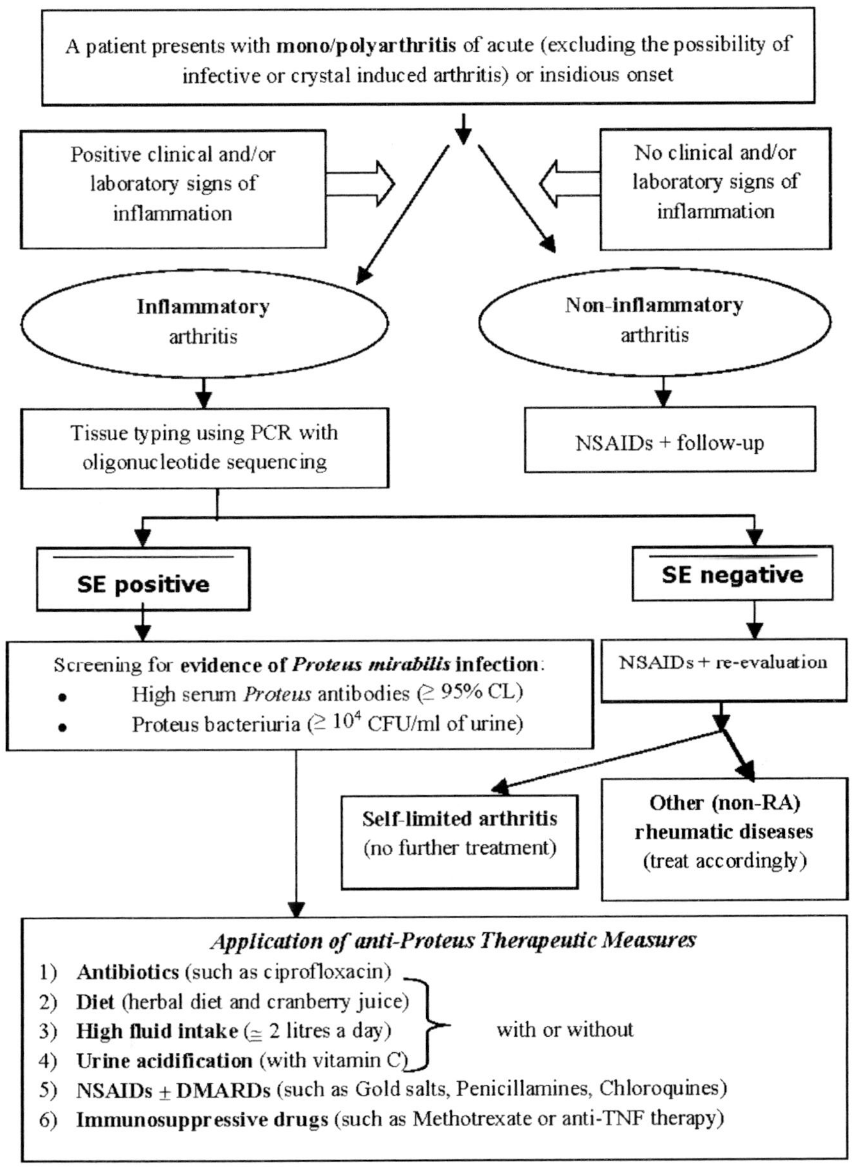


Figure 3. Proposed strategy in the identification and treatment of early cases with RA. Modified from Ebringer et al, 2003. With permission.

**PCR**: Polymerase Chain Reactionж **SE**: Shared Epitopeж **CL**: Confidence Limitж **NSAIDs**:Non-steroidal Anti-inflammatory Drugsж **TNF**: Tumour Necrosis Factorж **CFU**: Colony Forming Unit.

# Strategic Regimen for Early Treatment in RA

## Current Treatment Used in RA

So far no specific curative treatment has been found for RA. However, many immunologically targeted modalities have been used in this disease and currently they are still the only therapeutic regimens available. This group of drugs includes the following:

a) *Non-steroidal anti-inflammatory drugs (NSAIDs)*, such as ibuprofen and indomethacin. Nearly all of these pharmacological agents act by inhibiting the pro-inflammatory cyclo-oxygenase enzyme. More recently a group of related drugs called cyclo-oxygenase-2 (COX-2) inhibitors were introduced in the treatment of RA. This group of drugs has the beneficial characteristics of lacking the gastrointestinal side effects, which are considered as the main disadvantage associated with the use of other NSAIDs.
b) *Glucocorticoids or steroidal products*, such as prednisolone. These are mainly reserved for treatment of patients with very active disease or as maintenance therapy used in conjunction with other anti-rheumatic drugs.
c) *Second-line or disease modifying anti-rheumatic drugs (DMARDs)*, such as penicillamine, sodium aurothiomalate, hydroxychloroquine and methotrexate. Nearly all DMARDs, were found serendipitously, where their initial use in RA was based on chance observations with yet unanswered explanations for their effective therapeutic responses. However, most if not all are acting through modulating or reducing the cellular and humoral activities of the immune system.
d) *Biological agents*, such as anti-cytokine preparations. These include anti- tumour necrosis factor (TNF)-alpha blockers and the recombinant human interleukin-1 (IL-1) receptor antagonist (anakinra). Most of the newer treatments in the management of RA are currently based on the use of anti-TNF-alpha biological agents. These anti-cytokine measures include three types of preparations: the chimeric (infliximab) or humanized (adalimumab) monoclonal antibodies to TNF-alpha receptors and the TNF-alpha receptor-binding proteins (etanercept) (Braun and Sieper, 2003; Bresnihan and Cobby, 2003). Apart from these anti-cytokine measures other biologically acting therapeutic modalities such as those aimed against T cells (Mason et al, 2002), B cells (Cambridge et al, 2003), or against chemokines (Haringman et al, 2003) have shown some promising results.

Most of these therapeutic agents, which induce clinical remissions and potentially halt the disease progression, basically act by targeting the immune-activated cells and inflammatory products with consequent decrease or blockage of the inflammatory processes occurring in RA. Generally speaking, these anti-inflammatory and immunomodulatory agents are only temporarily effective and do not induce permanent remission. Some patients may even continue to suffer from progressive and disabling RA despite the continuation of these treatments. Moreover, most if not all of these drugs possess various side effects, such as gastrointestinal, mucocutaneous, haematological, renal, hepatic, neurological and immunological adverse reactions and toxicities (Wollheim, 1998). Some of these side effects may not be tolerated and are even potentially life-threatening. For example, patients with RA or other autoimmune diseases taking anti-TNF therapy were reported to have higher risk of developing serious systemic fungal (Lee et al, 2002) or bacterial (Kroesen et al, 2003) infections.

In a 5 year follow-up inception cohort study, carried out to assess the impact of RA on the functional outcomes in a group of 732 RA patients with less than 2 years duration and in spite of receiving traditional second-line drugs, only 13% of patients achieved complete remission, whilst the remaining 87% have ended up with various poor functional status (Young et al, 2000). This difficulty could be resolved through the introduction of a regimen by which one can implement certain therapeutic measures that could possibly eradicate the causative agent(s) in this disease. This rationalises the search for more specific and long lasting treatments with as little side effects as possible. In the meantime, the introduction of other disease modifying and anti-inflammatory therapeutic modalities could be supportive to the cause-eradication treatment.

In the past 20 years a change in therapeutic strategy has occurred from the ‘pyramid therapeutic approach’ toward an earlier introduction of DMARDs which were used singly and then later started to be introduced in various combinations (Lee and Kavanaugh, 2003). In pyramid therapy, treatment of RA patients were started with NSAIDs and other non-pharmacological measures and changed progressively to more aggressive therapy with DMARDs especially in those patients demonstrating severe and persistent disease status.

Although pharmacotherapy remains the cornerstone of treatment for established RA, other therapeutic modalities are also used in the management of RA patients. These may include, physiotherapy, occupational therapy, and surgery as well as educating the patient and counselling.

## A New Therapeutic Approach in Very Early Cases of RA

Treatment of RA in the early stages of the disease is of paramount importance, because the time lag between the onset of synovitis and the occurrence of joint damage and dysfunction is relatively short (McQueen et al, 2001). Results of several studies indicate that early introduction of immune modulating drugs such as DMARDs can slow the progression of joint damage and improve the long-term outcome (Geletka and St Clair, 2003). Furthermore, severe morbidity and structural damage of the joints requires early and effective treatment (Lee and Weinblatt, 2001). In one particular study, it was shown that the earlier (less than 4 months) treatment started the better the outcome in clinical state and radiological progressions in patients with initially active RA (Peltomaa et al, 2001).

One fundamental problem in the commencement of treatment at the very early stages of RA is the delay to diagnosis or the time lapse between the diagnosis and the referral to a rheumatologist for further evaluation and treatment. For example, Sokka and Pincus from USA have found that 60% of patients with early RA had at least 4 month delay before they were first seen by a specialist (Sokka and Pincus, 2002).

Decisions for the use of aggressive therapies with DMARDs in patients with RA, are mainly based on the presence of certain markers of disease severity and/or poor prognostic signs, such as the resistance to the use of NSAIDs, the presence of RFs and the radiological evidence of joint erosions. However, a NSAID agent may be tried for several weeks before a decision for its lack of effectiveness can be reached. Serological markers for disease severity, such as RF, are often absent in early cases with RA, and the radiological signs of joint damage usually appear in the late stages of the disease. Furthermore, most of these drugs must be taken for months before they show any positive effects.

The selection of the early cases with possible RA based on the previously described diagnostic criteria is, therefore, necessary for the establishment of a proper management of RA. The introduction of a new therapeutic strategy mainly involves the use of drugs that directly target the causes of the disease rather than attempting to alleviate symptoms or postpone joint destructions, and these might involve the use of anti-microbial therapies (Figure 3).

### *Treatment of RA through Eradications of* Proteus *Microbes from Urinary Tract*

#### Use of Antibiotics

So far several chemotherapeutic agents have been tried in RA patients with encouraging results. Among these are sulphasalazine, metronidazole, rifampicin and minocycline (Ebringer et al, 2003). The therapeutic effects of these antibiotics were suggested to be attributed to their immunomodulating effects rather than to their anti-microbial actions. However, this explanation has been partially disputed in studies involving the anti-inflammatory, 5-amino salicylic acid, and the anti-microbial, sulphapyridine, parts of the sulphasalazine separately, where it has been shown that the active moiety of sulphasalazine is mainly confined to its anti-microbial component (Pullar et al, 1985; Neumann et al, 1986).

Some problems exist concerning the commonly used antibiotics in patients with chronic or recurrent *Proteus* UTIs. Firstly, *P. mirabilis* bacteria readily develop resistance to some antibiotics (Stock, 2003). Secondly, *Proteus* infection affects mainly the kidneys and the upper urinary tract (Fairley et al, 1971) where the use of ordinary urinary sterilizing substances and antibiotics can be less effective. Thirdly, *P. mirabilis* possesses various virulence factors which enhance its urinary epithelial invasiveness and hence rendering this microbe relatively resistant to antibiotics due to the safe haven provided by the urinary epithelial cells (Mathoera et al, 2002). Fourthly, when an infected struvite stone is present in the kidney (Mobley and Hausinger, 1989), none of the antibiotic agents seem to be effective unless the stone is removed by surgery or shock-wave therapy. Finally, because of the late age onset and associated disability in patients with RA, proper personal maintenance for the urinary tract hygiene is impeded, therefore, increasing the chance of bacterial contamination.

In order to test the effects of antibiotics in patients with RA through prospective longitudinal studies, the search for an effective anti-*Proteus* chemotherapeutic agent is mandatory. *Proteus* microbes are apparently susceptible to many of the synthetic penicillin products such as ciprofloxacin as well as to cephalosporin and aminoglycoside derivatives (Farrell et al, 2003).

A single course of commonly used antibiotics could be initiated in suspected patients with very early RA before the results of urine culture are available, hence increasing the chance of proper eradication of *Proteus mirabilis* microbes from the urinary tract. The selection of an appropriate antibiotic is, therefore, of fundamental importance in the treatment of *Proteus* urinary infections and hence in the management of RA.

### Other Supplementary Urinary Sterilizing Measures

Apart from using chemotherapeutic agents other non-phamacological measures are also available to be used in the treatment and/or prevention of attacks of UTIs. Such urinary sterilizing strategies are generally safe and could be used with relative ease by the patient.

## Dietary Measures

### *Vegetarian Diet*

For the last two decades various diets have been tried in the management of RA patients with some encouraging results (Haugen et al, 1999). Kjeldsen-Kragh and colleagues used a vegetarian diet preceded by fasting in patients with RA and found significantly long lasting benefits on the clinical disease status (Kjeldsen-Kragh et al, 1991) as well as on the biological parameters of disease activity (Kjeldsen-Kragh et al, 1995a). Furthermore, in a controlled longitudinal study carried out on the same group of RA patients who were receiving a one-year fasting and vegetarian diets, significantly reduced *Proteus* but not *E. coli* antibody levels were observed at all the time points during the study when compared with base line values, whilst those patients on the omnivorous diet did not show significant changes in the anti-bacterial antibody profile (Kjeldsen-Kragh et al, 1995b). This latter result was also found to be correlated with the decrease in the disease activity status. It has been suggested that vegetarian diets could exert their anti-microbial effects both on the colonic (Peltonen et al, 1997) and urinary (Kjeldsen-Kragh et al, 1995c) pathogens, because of the lignans and phytoestrogen present in the plant products (Aldercreutz et al, 1986).

### *Cranberry Juice*

Although cranberry juice (CJ) products have not yet been used in the treatment of RA, their basic property as a urinary sterilizing substance in cystitis could be used in the management of RA. Extensive evidence exists which indicate that consumption of CJ beverages is effective at preventing UTIs (Lowe and Fagelman, 2001). This is attributed to fructose and other bacterial anti-adherence substances, which prevent pathogens from adhering to the urinary epithelium. Fructose, which is present in the CJ as well as in orange, pineapple and other fruit juices, inhibits type I (mannose-sensitive) fimbriae (Papas et al, 1966), whereas other factors present mainly in cranberry and blueberry juices, appear to inhibit P-fimbriae (mannose-resistant) adherence (Zafriri et al, 1989; Howell et al, 1998).

In a placebo-controlled randomised trial, elderly women who were given 300 ml of CJ (+1% fructose), showed significant reduction in the incidence of bacteriuria and pyuria, as well as a drop in the use of antibiotics when compared to the placebo group of women who were given 300 ml of water (+ saccharin) (Avorn et al, 1994). In a later randomised controlled longitudinal study, a group from Finland has shown that regular drinking of CJ but not lactobacillus drink among women could significantly reduce the incidence of recurrences of UTIs (Kontiokari et al, 2001). In a recent study from Canada, it has been shown that cranberry juice, whether in a juice or tablet form is a cost-effective preventive measure in women with recurrent UTIs (Stothers, 2002). Furthermore, based on its urine acidifying effect, cranberry juice could be useful in the treatment or prevention of struvite stones, which are usually associated with *Proteus* UTIs (Kessler et al, 2002).

Apart from CJ beverages, other fruit juices such as apricot and peach juices, which contain fructose, could also be used in the treatment of RA (Rashid et al, 2001).

## High Fluid Intake

Daily intake of ≥2 litres of fluids of any type (water, tea, coffee, lemonade or other soft drinks) with regular voiding at 2 or 3 hourly intervals by day may have a flushing effect on the kidneys. It has been reported that good hydration and urine flow is important in maintaining sterilization in the urinary tract (Cox and Hinman, 1961).

## Acidification of the Urine

Urinary acidification with vitamin C (ascorbic acid) or hexamine (methenamine) and restriction of alkalizing agents such as milk or sodium bicarbonate may help to lower the urinary pH (Fowler, 1989). *Proteus mirabilis* is a potent producer of urease enzyme, which has a urea-splitting property with production of ammonia and the resultant elevation of urinary pH. Chronic infection by this microbe could result in the induction of alkaline urine with increased chance of urinary stone formations through precipitation of struvite and apatite crystals. Acidification of the urine may therefore help in reducing the size and number of the infected urinary calculi and hence in decreasing the frequency of recurrent urinary tract infections caused by these microorganisms.

# General Conclusions

RA is most likely to be triggered and maintained by infection with *Proteus mirabilis* bacteria in the urinary tract. Recurrent bouts of *Proteus* UTIs are necessary for the production of considerably sufficient amount of cross-reactive antibodies in order to bind and attack the targeted antigens within the synovial tissues with consequent immunodestructive effects on joint structures and the eventual development of RA. Hence, early identification and treatment of susceptible individuals is of basic importance. To achieve this goal appropriate selections of patients with "SE" positive HLA type who possess high *Proteus* antibody levels are necessary for starting proper anti-microbial therapeutic measures in combination with other currently used anti-RA treatments.

If patients with RA respond to anti-microbial measures, prophylaxis of susceptible individuals could be implemented by immunizations against the causative microbe in the form of whole killed *Proteus* microbes not possessing the cross-reactive sequences. If such early therapy is undertaken the possibility arises that RA may be eradicated in the same way that rheumatic fever has been eliminated in the Western World by the early treatment of *Streptoccocal* tonsillitis with penicillin and other related antibiotics.

The discovery that RA is linked to *Proteus* UTIs leads to a new clinical approach, which requires early and aggressive anti-microbial therapy. *Proteus* upper UTI in a woman who is HLA-DR1/DR4 positive raises the strong possibility that such an individual has a high probability of becoming an RA patient. To prevent such a development it is suggested that anti-*Proteus* therapy is started before the appearance of arthritic symptoms. RA is a severe and common disease whose early treatment, together with other established measures, requires anti-*Proteus* therapies.

# References

Adlercreutz H, Fotsis T, Bannwart C, Wahala K, Makela T, Brunow G, Hase T Determination of urinary lignans and phytoestrogen metabolites, potential antiestrogens and anticarcinogens, in urine of women on various habitual diets. *J Steroid Biochem* 1986;25:791–7.

Arnett FC, Edworthy SM, Bloch DA, McShane DJ, Fries JF, Cooper NS, et al. The American Rheumatism Association 1987 revised criteria for the classification of rheumatoid arthritis. *Arthritis Rheum* 1988;31:315-24

Avorn J, Monane M, Gurwitz JH, Glynn RJ, Choodnovskiy I, Lipsitz LA. Reduction of bacteriuria and pyuria after ingestion of cranberry juice. *JAMA* 1994;271:751–4.

Braun J, Sieper J. Overview of the use of the anti-TNF agent infliximab in chronic inflammatory diseases. *Expert Opin Biol Ther* 2003;3:141-68.

Bresnihan B, Cobby M. Clinical and radiological effects of anakinra in patients with rheumatoid arthritis. *Rheumatology* (Oxford) 2003;42 (Suppl 2):ii22-8.

Calin A. Spondylarthropathies. In: Maddison PJ, Isenberg DA, Woo P, and Glass DN, eds. *Oxford Textbook of Rheumatology*. Oxford: Oxford University Press. 1998;1037-49.

Cambridge G, Leandro MJ, Edwards JC, Ehrenstein MR, Salden M, Bodman-Smith M, Webster AD. Serologic changes following B lymphocyte depletion therapy for rheumatoid arthritis. *Arthritis Rheum* 2003;48:2146-54.

Chen T, Rimpilainen M, Luukkainen R, Mottonen T, Yli-Jama T, Jalava J, Vainio O, Toivanen P. Bacterial components in the synovial tissue of patients with advanced rheumatoid arthritis or osteoarthritis: analysis with gas chromatography-mass spectrometry and pan-bacterial polymerase chain reaction. *Arthritis Rheum* 2003;49:328-34.

Cox CE, Hinman F. Experiments with induced bacteriuria, vesical emptying and bacterial growth on the mechanism of bladder defence to infection. *J Urol* 1961;86:739–48.

Dalakos TG, MacSween RNM, Whaley K, Dick WC, Boyle JA, Jasani MK, Wilson ME et al. Conjugal prevalence of rheumatoid arthritis, rheumatoid factor and other autoantibodies in rheumatoid arthritis. *Clin Exp Immunol* 1968;3:761-9.

Deighton CM, Roberts DF, Walker DJ. Effect of disease severity on rheumatoid arthritis concordance in same sexed sublings. *Ann Rheum Dis* 1992a;51:943-5.

Deighton CM, Gray SW, Biant AJ, Walker DJ. Specificity of the *Proteus* antibody response in rheumatoid arthritis. *Ann Rheum Dis* 1992b; 51:1206-7.

Doran MF, Pond GR, Crowson CS, O'Fallon WM, Gabriel SE. Trends in incidence and mortality in rheumatoid arthritis in Rochester, Minnesota, over a forty-year period. *Arthritis Rheum* 2002;46:625-31.

Eastmond CJ, Willshaw HE, Burgess SE, Shinebaum R, Cooke EM, Wright V. Frequency of faecal *Klebsiella aerogenes* in patients with ankylosing spondylitis and controls with respect to individual features of the disease. *Ann Rheum Dis* 1980;39:118-23.

Ebringer A. Ankylosing spondylitis is caused by *Klebsiella*. Evidence from immunogenetic, microbiologic and serologic studies. *Rheum Dis Clin North Am* 1992; 18: 105-21.

Ebringer R, Cooke D, Cawdell DR, Cowling P, Ebringer A. Ankylosing spondylitis: *Klebsiella* and HLA-B27. *Rheumatol Rehabil* 1977;16:190-6.

Ebringer A, Ptaszynska T, Corbett M, Wilson C, Mcafee Y, Avakian H, et al. Antibodies to *Proteus* in rheumatoid arthritis. *Lancet* 1985; ii:305-7.

Ebringer A, Cunningham P, Ahmadi K, Wrigglesworth J, Hosseini R, Wilson C. Sequence similarity between HLA-DR1 and DR4 subtypes associated with rheumatoid arthritis and *Proteus/Serratia* membrane haemolysins. *Ann Rheum Dis* 1992;51:1245–6.

Ebringer A, Wilson C, Ahmadi K, Corbett M, Rashid T, Shipley M, et al. Rheumatoid arthritis as a reactive arthritis to *Proteus* infection: Prospects for therapy. In: Machtey I, ed. "Sixth International Seminar on the Treatment of Rheumatic Diseases". *Prog Rheumatol* 1993;5:77–83.

Ebringer A, Pirt J, Wilson C, Cunningham P, Thorpe C, Ettelaie C. Bovine spongiform encephalopathy: Is it an autoimmune disease due to bacteria showing molecular mimicry with brain antigens? *Environ Health Perspect* 1997;105:1172-4.

Ebringer A, Rashid T, Wilson C. Rheumatoid arthritis: proposal for the use of anti-microbial therapy in early cases. *Scand J Rheumatol* 2003;32:2-11.

Ebringer A, Rashid T, Wilson C, Ptaszynska T, Fielder M. Ankylosing spondylitis as an immune-mediated disease linked to intestinal *Klebsiella* infection: proposal for a new therapeutic approach. *Curr Rheumatol Rev* (Submitted).

Fairley KF, Carson NE, Gutch RC, Leighton P, Grounds AD, Laird EC, et al. Site of infection in acute urinary tract infection in general practice. *Lancet* 1971;ii:615-8.

Farrell DJ, Morrissey I, De Rubies D, Robbins M, Felmingham D. A UK multicentre study of the antimicrobial susceptibility of bacterial pathogens causing urinary tract infection. *J Infect* 2003;46:94-100.

Ferraro AS, Newkirk MM. Correlative studies of rheumatoid factors and antiviral antibodies in patients with rheumatoid arthritis. *Clin Exp Immunol* 1993;92:425-31.

Fielder M, Tiwana H, Youinou P, Le Goff P, Deonarian R, Wilson C, and Ebringer A. The specificity of the anti-*Proteus* antibody response in tissue-typed rheumatoid arthritis (RA) patients from Brest. *Rheumatol Int* 1995a; 15:79-82.

Fielder M, Pirt SJ, Tarpey I, Wilson C, Cunningham P, Ettelaie C, et al. Molecular mimicry and ankylosing spondylitis: possible role of a novel sequence in pullulanase of *Klebsiella pneumoniae*. *FEBS* 1995b; 369:243-8.

Fowler JE. *Urinary Tract Infection and Inflammation*. Chicago: Year Book Medical Publishers. 1989.

Fox DA. Etiology and pathogenesis of rheumatoid arthritis. In: Koopman WJ, ed. *Arthritis and Allied Conditions*. Philadelphia: Lippincott Williams & Wilkins. 2001:1085-102.

Freimer EH, McCarty M. Rheumatic Fever. *Scientific American* 1965;213:67-74.

Geletka R, St Clair EW. Treatment of early rheumatoid arthritis. *Best Pract Res Clin Rheumatol* 2003;17:791-809.

Goldbach-Mansky R, Senior B, Susan S, Deville C, Hoxworth J, Newkirk M, et al. IgM and IgA antibodies to *Proteus mirabilis* are associated with early RF positive RA. *Arthritis Rheum* 2000; 43 Suppl:S190.

Gregersen PK, Silver J, Winchester RJ. The shared epitope hypothesis. An approach to understanding the molecular genetics of susceptibility to rheumatoid arthritis. *Arthritis Rheum* 1987;30:1205-13.

Hara Y, Kaneko T, Yoshimura A, Kato I. Serum rheumatoid factor induced by intraperitoneal administration of periodontopathic bacterial lipopolysaccharide in mice. *J Periodontal Res* 1996;31:502-7.

Haringman JJ, Kraan MC, Smeets TJM, Zwinderman KH, Tak PP. Chemokine blockade and chronic inflammatory disease: proof of concept in patients with rheumatoid arthritis. *Ann Rheum Dis* 2003;62:715-21.

Haugen M, Fraser D, Forre O. Diet therapy for the patients with rheumatoid arthritis? *Rheumatology* (Oxford) 1999;38:1039–44.

Hol C, Bloembergen P, van Dijk H. Bacterium-induced autoimmune reactivity. *Autoimmunity* 1993;15:49-54.

Howell AB, Vorsa N, Der Marderosian AD, Foo LY. Inhibition of the adherence of P-fimbriated *Escherichia coli* to uro-epithelial-cell surfaces by proanthocyanidin extracts from cranberries. *N Engl J Med* 1998;339:1085–6.

Hughes LE, Bonell S, Natt RS, Wilson C, Tiwana H, Ebringer A, et al. Antibody responses to *Acinetobacter* spp. and *Pseudomonas aeruginosa* in multiple sclerosis: prospects for diagnosis using the Myelin-*Acinetobacter*-Neurofilament antibody index. *Clin Diag Lab Immunol* 2001;8:1181-88.

Hughes LE, Smith PA, Bonell S, Natt RS, Wilson C, Rashid T, Amor S, Thompson EJ, Croker J, Ebringer A. Cross-reactivity between related sequences found in *Acinetobacter* sp., *Pseudomonas aeruginosa*, myelin basic protein and myelin oligodendrocyte glycoprotein in multiple sclerosis. *J Neuroimmunol* 2003;144:105-15.

Husby G, Rijn I van der, Zabriskie JB, Abdin ZH, Williams RC. Antibodies reacting with cytoplasm of subthalamic and caudate nuclei neurons in chorea and acute rheumatic fever. *J Exp Med* 1976;144:1094-110.

Husby G, Tsuchiya N, Schwimmbeck PL, Keat A, Pahle JA, Oldstone MB et al. Cross-reactive epitope with *Klebsiella pneumoniae* nitrogenase in articular tissue of HLA-B27+ patients with ankylosing spondylitis. *Arthritis Rheum* 1989;32:437-45.

Jacobsson LT, Hanson RL, Knowler WC, Pillemer S, Pettitt DJ, McCance DR, Bennett PH. Decreasing incidence and prevalence of rheumatoid arthritis in Pima Indians over a twenty-five-year period. *Arthritis Rheum* 1994;37:1158-65.

Kessler T, Jansen B, Hesse A. Effect of blackcurrant-, cranberry- and plum juice consumption on risk factors associated with kidney stone formation. *Eur J Clin Nutr* 2002;56:1020-3.

Khalafpour S, Ebringer A. Cross-reactivity between HLA-DR4 and *Proteus mirabilis*. *Period Biol* (Zagreb) 1987;89 Suppl.1:203.

Kjeldsen-Kragh J, Haugen M, Brochgrevink CF, Laerum E, Eek M, Mowinkel P, et al. Controlled trial of fasting and one-year vegetarian diet in rheumatoid arthritis. *Lancet* 1991;338:899–902.

Kjeldsen-Kragh J, Rashid T, Dybwad A, Sioud M, Haugen M, Forre O, et al. Decrease in anti-*Proteus mirabilis* but not anti-*Escherichia coli* antibody levels in rheumatoid arthritis patients treated with fasting and a one year vegetarian diet. *Ann Rheum Dis* 1995a;54:221–4.

Kjeldsen-Kragh J, Mellbye OJ, Haugen M, Mollnes TE, Hammer HB, Sioud M et al. Changes in laboratory variables in rheumatoid arthritis patients during a trial of fasting and one-year vegetarian diet. *Scand J Rheumatol* 1995b;24:85–93.

Kjeldsen-Kragh J, Kvaavik E, Bottolfs M, Lingaas E. Inhibition of growth of *Proteus mirabilis* and *Escherichia coli* in urine in response to fasting and vegetarian diet. *APMIS* 1995c;103:818–22.

Kontiokari T, Sundqvist K, Nuutinen M, Pokka T, Koskela M, Uhari M. Randomised trial of cranberry-lingonberry juice and Lactobacillus GG drink for the prevention of urinary tract infections in women. *Br Med J* 2001;322:1571-3.

Kroesen S, Widmer AF, Tyndall A, Hasler P. Serious bacterial infections in patients with rheumatoid arthritis under anti-TNF-alpha therapy. *Rheumatology* (Oxford) 2003;42:617-21.

Lee DM, Weinblatt ME. Rheumatoid arthritis. *Lancet* 2001;358:903-11.

Lee SJ, Kavanaugh A. Pharmacological treatment of established rheumatoid arthritis. *Best Pract Res Clin Rheumatol* 2003;17:811-29.

Lee JH, Slifman NR, Gershon SK, Edwards ET, Schwieterman WD, Siegel JN et al. Life-threatening histoplasmosis complicating immunotherapy with tumor necrosis factor alpha antagonists infliximab and etanercept. *Arthritis Rheum* 2002;46:2565-70.

Lowe FC, Fagelman E. Cranberry juice and urinary tract infections: what is the evidence? *Urology* 2001;57:407-13.

MacGregor AJ, Silman AJ. Rheumatoid arthritis, classification and epidemiology. In: Klippel JH, Dieppe PA, eds. *Rheumatology*. London: Mosby. 1998;5.2.1–5.2.6.

MacGregor AJ, Snieder H, Rigby AS, Koskenvuo M, Kaprio J, Aho K, Silman AJ. Characterizing the quantitative genetic contribution to rheumatoid arthritis using data from twins. *Arthritis Rheum* 2000;43:30-7.

Mason U, Aldrich J, Breedveld F, Davis CB, Elliott M, Jorgensen C, Keystone E et al. CD4 coating, but not CD4 depletion, is a predictor of efficacy with primatized monoclonal anti-CD4 treatment of active rheumatoid arthritis. *J Rheumatol* 2002;29:220-9.

Mathoera RB, Kok DJ, Verduin CM, Nijman RJ. Pathological and therapeutic significance of cellular invasion by *Proteus mirabilis* in an enterocystoplasty infection stone model. *Infect Immun* 2002;70:7022-32.

McQueen FM, Benton N, Crabbe J, Robinson E, Yeoman S, McLean L, Stewart N. What is the fate of erosions in early rheumatoid arthritis? Tracking individual lesions using X rays and magnetic resonance imaging over the first two years of disease. *Ann Rheum Dis* 2001;60:859-68.

Mobley HLT, Hausinger RP. Microbial ureases: Significance, regulation, and molecular characterization. *Microbiol Rev* 1989;53:85–108.

Mobley HLT, Chippendale GR, Swihart KG, Welch RA. Cytotoxicity of the HpmA haemolysin and urease of *Proteus mirabilis* and *Proteus valgaris* against cultural human renal proximal tubular epithelial cells. *Infect Immun* 1991;59:2036-42.

Nepom GT, Nepom B. Genetics of the MHC in rheumatoid arthritis. In: Klippel JH, Dieppe PA, eds. *Rheumatology*. London, Mosby. 1998;5.7.1-12.

Neumann VC, Taggart AJ, Le Gallez P, Astbury C, Hill J, Bird HA. A study to determine the active moiety of sulphasalazine in rheumatoid arthritis. *J Rheumatol* 1986;13:285-7.

Newkirk MM. Rheumatoid factors: host resistance or autoimmunity? *Clin Immunol* 2002;104:1-13.

Papas PN, Brusch CA, Ceresia GC. Cranberry juice in the treatment of urinary tract infections. *Southwest Med* 1966;47:17–20.

Peltomaa R, Paimela L, Helve T, Leirisalo-Repo M. Effect of treatment on the outcome of very early rheumatoid arthritis. *Scand J Rheumatol* 2001;30:143-8.

Peltonen R, Nenonen M, Helve T, Hanninen O, Toivanen P, Eerola E. Faecal microbial flora and disease activity in rheumatoid arthritis during a vegan diet. *Br J Rheumatol* 1997;36:64–8.

Pincus T, Callahan LF. What is the natural history of rheumatoid arthritis? *Rheum Dis Clin North Am* 1993;19:125-51.

Pullar T, Hunter JA, Cappell HA. Which component of sulphasalazine is active in rheumatoid arthritis? *Br Med J* 1985;290:1535-8.

Rashid T, Tiwana H, Wilson C, Ebringer A. Rheumatoid arthritis as an autoimmune disease caused by *Proteus* urinary tract infections: a proposal for a therapeutic protocol. *IMAJ* 2001;3:675-80.

Rashid T, Leirisalo-Repo M, Tani Y, Hukuda S, Kobayashi S, Wilson C, Bansal S, Ebringer A. Anti-bacterial and anti-peptide antibodies in Japanese and Finnish patients with early and advanced RA. *Clin Rheumatol* 2004;23:134-41.

Rozalski A, Sidorczyk Z, Kotelko K. Potential virulence factors of *Proteus* bacilli. *Microbiol Mol Biol Rev* 1997;61:65–89.

Schiff B, Mizrachi Y, Organd S, Yaron M, Gasit E. Association of Aw31 and HLA-DR1 with adult rheumatoid arthritis. *Ann Rheum Dis* 1982;41:403-4.

Schlosstein L, Terasaki PI, Bluestone E, Pearson CM. High association of an HLA antigen, W27, with ankylosing spondylitis. *N Engl J Med* 1973;288:704-6.

Schwimmbeck PL, Yu DTY, Oldstone MBA. Autoantibodies to HLA-B27 in the sera of HLA-B27 patients with ankylosing spondylitis and Reiter's syndrome: Molecular mimicry with *Klebsiella pneumoniae* as potential mechanism of autoimmune disease. *J Exp Med* 1987;166:173-81.

Senior BW, Anderson GA, Morley KD, Kerr MA. Evidence that patients with rheumatoid arthritis have asymptomatic 'non-significant' *Proteus mirabilis* bacteriuria more frequently than healthy controls. *J Infect* 1999;38:99–106.

Silman AJ, MacGregor AJ, Thomson W, Holligan S, Carthy D, Farhan A, et al. Twin concordance rates for rheumatoid arthritis: results from a nation-wide study. *Br J Rheumatol* 1993;32:903-7.

Silman AJ, Harrison B, Barrett E, Symmons D. The existence of geographic clusters of cases of inflammatory polyarthritis in a primary care based register. *Ann Rheum Dis* 2000;59:152-4

Silman AJ. The changing face of rheumatoid arthritis: why the decline in incidence? *Arthritis Rheum* 2002;46:579-81.

Sokka T, Pincus T. First visit to a rheumatologist of U.S. patients with early rheumatoid arthritis occurs after a median of 5 months of symptoms. *Arthritis Rheum* 2002;46:S543.

Spector TD. Epidemiology of rheumatic diseases: rheumatoid arthritis. *Rheum Dis Clin North Am* 1990;16:513-37.

Stastny P. Mixed lymphocyte cultures in rheumatoid arthritis. *J Clin Invest* 1976;57:1148-57.

Stastny P. Association of the B-cell alloantigen DRw4 with rheumatoid arthritis. *N Engl J Med* 1978;298:869-71.

Stock I. Natural antibiotic susceptibility of *Proteus* spp., with special reference to *P. mirabilis* and *P. penneri* strains. *J Chemother* 2003;15:12-26.

Stothers L. A randomised trial to evaluate effectiveness and cost effectiveness of naturopathic cranberry products as prophylaxis against urinary tract infection in women. *Can J Urol* 2002;9:1558-62.

Subair H, Tiwana H, Feilder M, Binder A, Cunningham K, Ebringer A, Wilson C, and Hudson MJ. Elevation in anti-*Proteus* antibodies in patients with rheumatoid arthritis from Bermuda and England. *J Rheumatol* 1995; 22:1825-8.

Sussman M. Microbiology and defences of the urinary tract. In: Davidson AM, Cameron JS, Grunfeld JP, Kerr DN, Ritz E, Winearls CG, eds. *Oxford Textbook of Nephrology*. Oxford, Oxford Medical Publications, 1998:1213-30.

Svendsen AJ, Holm NV, Kyvik K, Petersen PH, Junker P. Relative importance of genetic effects in rheumatoid arthritis: historical cohort study of Danish nationwide twin population. *Br Med J* 2002;324:264-6.

Tishler M, Caspi D, Aimog Y, Segal R, Yaron M. Increased incidence of urinary tract infection in patients with rheumatoid arthritis and secondary Sjogren's syndrome. *Ann Rheum Dis* 1992;51:601–6.

Tiwana H, Wilson C, Cunningham P, Binder A and Ebringer A. Antibodies to four Gram-negative bacteria in rheumatoid arthritis which share sequences with the rheumatoid arthritis susceptibility motif. *Br J Rheumatol* 1996; 35:592-4.

Tiwana H, Wilson C, Alvarez A, Abuknesha R, Bansal S, Ebringer A. Cross-reactivity between the rheumatoid arthritis-associated motif EQKRAA and structurally related sequences found in *Proteus mirabilis*. *Infect Immun* 1999;67:2769–75.

Turesson C, O'Fallon WM, Crowson CS, Gabriel SE, Matteson EL. Extra-articular disease manifestations in rheumatoid arthritis: incidence trends and risk factors over 46 years. *Ann Rheum Dis* 2003;62:722-7.

Valenzuela A, Gonzalez-Escribano MF, Rodriguez R, Moreno I, Garcia A, Nunez-Roldan A. Association of HLA shared epitope with joint damage progression in rheumatoid arthritis. *Hum Immunol* 1999;60:250-4.

Vandenbroucke JP, Kaaks R, Valkenburg HA, Boersma JW, Cats A, Festen JJ, et al. Frequency of infections among rheumatoid arthritis patients, before and after disease onset. *Arthritis Rheum* 1987;30:810-3.

Vencovsky J, Machacek S, Sedova L, Kafkova J, Gatterova J, Pesakova V, Ruzickova S. Autoantibodies can be prognostic markers of an erosive disease in early rheumatoid arthritis. *Ann Rheum Dis* 2003;62:427-30.

Williams RC, Kunkel HG. Rheumatoid factor, complement and conglutinin aberrations in patients with subacute bacterial endocarditis. *J Clin Invest* 1962;41:666-75.

Wilson C, Ebringer A, Ahmadi K, Wrigglesworth J, Tiwana H, Fielder M, et al. Shared amino acid sequences between major histocompatibility complex class II glycoproteins, type XI collagen and *Proteus mirabilis* in rheumatoid arthritis. *Ann Rheum Dis* 1995;54:216–20.

Wilson C, Thakore D, Isenberg D, Ebringer A. Correlation between anti-*Proteus* antibodies and isolation rates of *P. mirabilis* in rheumatoid arthritis. *Rheumatol Int* 1997;16:187–9.

Wilson C, Rashid T, Tiwana H, Beyan H, Hughes L, Bansal S, Ebringer A, Binder A. Cytotoxicity responses to peptide antigens in rheumatoid arthritis and ankylosing spondylitis. *J Rheumatol* 2003;30:972-8.

Wollheim FA. Rheumatoid arthritis—clinical picture. *In*: Maddison PJ, Isenberg DA, Woo P, Glass DN, eds. *Oxford Textbook of Rheumatology*. Oxford, Oxford University Press. 1998: 1004-31.

Woodrow JC, Nichol FE, Zaphiropoulos G. DR antigens in rheumatoid arthritis: a study of two populations. *Br Med J* 1981;283:1287-8.

Young A, Dixey J, Cox N, Davies P, Devlin J, Emery P, Gallivan S et al. How does functional disability in early rheumatoid arthritis (RA) affect patients and their lives? Results of 5 years of follow-up in 732 patients from the Early RA Study (ERAS). *Rheumatology* (Oxford) 2000;39:603-11.

Zafriri D, Ofek I, Adar R, Pocino M, Sharon N. Inhibitory activity of cranberry juice on adherence of type I and type P fimbriated *Escherichia coli* to eucaryotic cells. *Antimicrob Agents Chemother* 1989;33:92–8.

In: Arthritis Research: Treatment and Management
Editor: F. Columbus, pp. 27-57
ISBN 1-59033-984-3


*Chapter II*

# New Diagnostic and Treatment Approaches for Spondyloarthritis

***Suzanne Sanders**, Kenneth J. Hardy and Robert W. McMurray***
Rheumatology Section, G.V. (Sonny) Montgomery VA Hospital and
the Division of Rheumatology and Molecular Immunology, Department of Medicine,
University of Mississippi Medical Center, Jackson, MS 39216

## Abstract

### Objective

The spondyloarthropathies can be difficult to diagnose and resistant to treatment. Diagnosis has primarily been based upon clinical characteristics and plain radiographic changes; however, radiographic changes are slow to progress. Similarly, treatment has been largely empiric with minimal impact on disease progression and disability. Herein, we review the diagnosis and treatment of spondyloarthropathies with special emphasis on more recent advances.

### Methods

Case reports, investigations, and reviews were identified using Medline searches of various key words including, but not limited to, the following: spondyloarthropathy, ankylosing spondylitis, psoriatic arthritis, reactive arthritis, Reiter's syndrome, inflammatory bowel disease, psoriasis, arthritis, therapy, treatment, sulfasalazine, methotrexate, cyclosporine, anti-tumor necrosis factor alpha, etanercept, infliximab, leflunomide, thalidomide, pamidronate, bromocriptine, magnetic reasonance imaging,

* Address correspondence to: Suzanne Sanders, MD, Medical Service – 111, G.V. (Sonny) Montgomery VA Hospital, 1500 East Woodrow Wilson, Jackson, MS 39216, Fax: 601 984 5535, Telephone: 601 364-1251, E-mail: SSandersl@medicine.umsmed.edu

computed tomography, and radiographs. Additional references were identified by thorough review of identified manuscripts as well as review of recent journal issues and scientific meeting abstracts.

### Results

The spondyloarthropathies are frequently associated with recalcitrant disease activity and cause significant disability. While clinical features and plain radiographs are occasionally useful, magnetic resonance imaging is moving to the forefront in the detection and localization of inflammation in the sacroiliac joints and spine in early spondyloarthropathy. MRI also predicts later sacroiliac changes on plain radiographs and can be useful in monitoring for response to therapy. Although much of the evidence is anecdotal or from uncontrolled trials, sulfasalazine and methotrexate have been traditionally used as initial treatment for NSAID-resistant spondyloarthropathies. Although alternative therapies such as thalidomide and pamidronate are also being investigated, controlled trials have recently demonstrated the dramatic efficacy of anti-TNF-α therapy in the treatment of spondyloarthropathies.

### Conclusions

Recent advances in imaging techniques in the spondyloarthropathies have the potential to expedite the diagnosis in early disease and may prove beneficial in earlier initiation and monitoring the response to therapy. Recent advances, especially in the utilization of TNF-α inhibitors, are very promising, particularly for the control of axial skeleton inflammation. Along with continued research in these areas, more rigorous trials of less expensive drugs such as methotrexate or leflunomide would be beneficial in delineating treatment paradigms in the spondyloarthropathies.

## Introduction

The spondyloarthropathies - ankylosing spondylitis (AS), psoriatic arthritis (PsA), reactive arthritis or Reiter's syndrome (ReA), enteropathic spondylarthropathy, and undifferentiated spondyloarthropathy (UspA) are an interrelated group of arthritides classically characterized by an inflammatory arthritis of the axial skeleton ( spine and sacroiliac joints), hips, and shoulders. Some patients have a component of peripheral arthritis and, indeed, this presentation may predominate. Additional or alternative presentations may include enthesitis, inflammatory eye disease (uveitis or conjunctivitis), oral ulceration, skin rashes, and gastrointestinal inflammation.

The epidemiology of the different spondyloarthropathies varies. AS is commonly seen in young adults, is three times more common in males, and is highly associated with the HLA-B27 haplotype. Psoriatic arthritis is seen in young to middle age adults, is equally distributed in males and females, and is less often associated with the HLA-B27 haplotype [1,2]. The prevalence of the spondyloarthropathies varies depending on the population studied and the diagnostic criteria used [3,4]. The prevalence of AS in most population studies ranges from 0 to 1.8 % [3]. Whereas, the prevalence of psoriatic arthritis in community-based studies ranges from 0.2 to 1.01 per 1000 [4].

Despite an indolent course in many patients, the spondyloarthropathies can have aggressive and treatment-resistant disease that leads to significant disability and social financial burden. Review of a German rheumatological database revealed that, for comparable ages, disability in female AS patients was similar to disability in female patients with rheumatoid arthritis (RA), while men with AS were rated as more disabled than men with RA [5]. In a cross-sectional study of Dutch patients with AS, work disability was 16.9% and 15.7% higher than expected for the general population of female and male patients respectively. Employed AS patient's used 10.1 additional days of sick leave per patient compared to a national average of 12.3 unspecified days of sick leave [6] Significant disability also complicates psoriatic arthropathy. In one study, 19% of 180 patients with psoriatic arthritis were found to have marked physical limitations [7].

## Diagnosis and Monitoring of the Spondyloarthropathies

Because spondyloarthropathies can initially present with an indolent or incomplete course, diagnosis of these disorders can sometimes be difficult and delayed. Two sets of diagnostic criteria have proven useful in this regard. The European Spondyloarthropathy Study Group proposed a set of diagnostic criteria for spondyloarthropathies [8]. Those criteria require the patient to have inflammatory spinal pain or synovitis which is asymmetric or predominantly in the lower extremities, along with at least one of the following: a positive family history, psoriasis, inflammatory bowel disease, urethritis or acute diarrhea, alternating buttock pain, enthesopathy, or sacroiliitis on radiographs of the pelvic region. These criteria have a diagnostic sensitivity and specificity for a spondyloarthropathy of 87% [8]. For the specific diagnosis of ankylosing spondylitis, the Modified New York Criteria are frequently utilized and include both clinical and radiological components [9]. The clinical criteria include the following: low back pain and stiffness for greater than 3 months (which improves with exercise and is not relieved by rest), limitation of motion of the lumbar spine in both the sagittal and frontal planes, and limitation of chest expansion relative to normal values corrected for age and sex. Radiological criterion include documented sacroiliitis (grade $\geq 2$ bilaterally or sacroiliitis grade 3-4 unilaterally). Patients are considered to have definite ankylosing spondylitis if the radiologic criterion and at least one clinical criterion are present. Probable ankylosing spondylitis is determined to be present if there are three clinical criteria present or if the radiological criterion is present without any clinical criteria [9].

In spite of the fact that radiographic changes may be a vital part of some criteria for diagnosis of spondyloarthropathies, and even more so for the diagnosis of AS, the utility of plain radiographs in the diagnosis and monitoring of the spondyloarthropathies is considerably limited. For instance, in AS sacroiliitis, obvious radiological change may not appear for months or years after the initial symptoms. Moreover, early changes of sacroiliitis can be difficult to recognize, especially to the untrained eye [10] Several radiological scoring methods have been partially validated for investigative evaluation and monitoring of AS - the Bath Ankylosing Spondylitis Radiology Index (BASRI), the BASRI-s (a newer BASRI score with a composite score of the lumbar spine, cervical spine, and SI joints), and the Stoke Ankylosing Spondylitis Spine Score (SASSS) [11]. Their primary usefulness is in determining disease progression and not assisting in diagnosis. The SASSS and BASRI-s showed good to excellent interobserver reliability, while the BASRI showed moderate interobserver reliability. After extensive training, it became possible to attain good to moderate intraobserver reliability with all of these methods. However, a one year follow up period was noted to be too short to quantitatively demonstrate sensitivity to axial skeletal radiographic change with any of these scoring methods [11]. In another study of 470 patients with AS, the sensitivity to change using the BASRI-s method did become apparent at 2 years of followup [12]. Therefore, earlier clinical use of plain radiographs in evaluating and monitoring spondyloarthropathies appears to be severely limited both by the ability of observers to detect and classify radiographic changes, as well as, by the naturally slow progression of significant changes on plain radiographs. Further, it is also unclear as to what extent radiographic changes actually correlate with patient outcome, or to what extent, if any, plain radiographic changes can be reversed by treatment [10].

Computed tomography (CT) has been shown to be more sensitive and equally specific in the recognition of sacroiliitis [13]. CT offers improved delineation of the SI joints and thus reveals abnormalities earlier and more accurately. While this latter method of evaluation does uncover sacroiliitis at various grades and in patients with early AS (≤3 years duration) [13,14], more recent investigations of imaging in spondyloarthropathies have focused on magnetic resonance imaging (MRI). Especially when used with special enhancement programs, early sacroiilitis can be demonstrated by dynamic MRI in patients who otherwise have no changes evident on plain radiographs [15]. Furthermore, abnormalities in both subchondral bone and periarticular bone marrow can also be seen quite early in patients with symptoms compatable with sacroiliitis [16]. MRI also differentiates which structures are involved in the sacroiliac joints in early versus late disease [17], and predicts later changes on plain radiographs [18]. In one small study the positive predictive value of ≥ grade 2 sacroiliitis on MRI for the development of ≥ grade 2 sacroiliitis on plain radiographs after 3 years was 60% with a sensitivity of 85% and specificity of 47% [18]. MRI has been recently used to localize the site of inflammation to distinct regions of the spine in AS and other spondyloarthropathies [19], and to evaluate the response of spondyloarthritis patients to anti-tumor necrosis factor α (anti-TNF α) therapy as discussed later in this chapter [20-26]. Although the expense of an MRI may preclude its widespread use, preliminary studies would argue that MRI may be helpful, if not essential, in the diagnosis of patients with early disease, as well as, for evaluation of patient response to therapy.

## Treatment of the Spondyloarthropathies

### Traditional Therapy

Historically, treatment of the spondyloarthropathies consisted primarily of education, exercise, and nonsteroidal anti-inflammatory drugs (NSAIDS). However, a large percentage of patients fail conservative therapy, necessitating the use of disease modifying drugs. For many years the choice of disease modifying agents has been largely based on an emperic choice or anecdotal evidence. Sulfasalazine and methotrexate are commonly used for persistent spondyloarthropathic pain and inflammation. Likewise, cyclosporine is used frequently in psoriatic arthritis. However, despite their widespread use, objective evidence of the efficacy of these medications in the spondyloarthropathies is somewhat limited.

### *Sulfasalazine*

Several placebo-controlled trials have shown limited clinical success of sulfasalazine in patients with ankylosing spondylitis, psoriatic arthritis, and reactive arthritis (Reiter's Syndrome) [27-36]. Most studies showed significant clinical improvement in measures of pain, physician or patient global assessment, and inflammatory markers [27-33,36]. Sulfasalazine also reduced extrarticular manifestations of disease activity, such as the frequency of anterior uveitis [27,37,38] or severity of psoriatic skin lesions [29]. Patients with peripheral arthritis, especially those with psoriatic arthritis, have also been noted to respond to sulfasalazine [27,35,39] Conversely, several studies suggest that there is essentially no improvement of spinal disease with sulfasalazine [27,28,35,39]; however, most of these patients had had spinal disease for many years. In two small trials, radiological progression in AS or psoriatic arthritis patients treated with sulfasalazine was examined. AS patients followed for 12 months showed no evidence that sulfasalazine retarded radiological progression [36]. Similarly, psoriatic arthritis patients treated with sulfasalazine had no statistically significant mean change in axial skeleton radiographic scores over a 24 month period [40]. To our knowledge, sulfasalazine, while standard treatment for inflammatory bowel disease (IBD) [41] has not been thoroughly evaluated in patients with enteropathic-associated spondyloarthropathy. However, as the activity of peripheral arthritis in IBD has been associated with intestinal disease activity, sulfasalazine has been recommended as maintenance therapy in patients with inflammatory bowel disease and peripheral arthritis [42]. Several anecdotal reports also suggest that sulfasalazine is useful in HIV- associated reactive arthritis (e.g. Reiter's syndrome) in association with increased CD4+ lymphocyte counts [43-45].

### *Methotrexate*

Although methotrexate is commonly used in resistant spondyloarthropathies, the majority of the literature regarding it's use consists of case reports or uncontrolled trials. One small randomized, double-blind, placebo controlled trial has evaluated the efficacy of methotrexate in psoriatic arthritis [46]. In this 12 week trial, sixteen patients received oral pulse methotrexate therapy (7.5-15mg weekly) and twenty-one patients received placebo therapy. Although there was some improvement reported in grip strength, morning stiffness, and patient assessment, statistically significant improvement only occurred in physician assessment of disease severity [46]. Surface area involvement of psoriatic lesions improved significantly in 14 methotrexate patients, although the lesions themselves showed no significant changes in scaling, induration, or erythema [46]. In a separate prospective evaluation, patients were treated with methotrexate for 24 months and the radiologic outcome was assessed [47]. Worsening of the damage score was observed in 63% of the 19 methotrexate treated patients. There was no significant difference in radiographic damage progression compared to matched controls [47].

Despite these seemingly poor results, Cuellar et al in their 1997 review of the use of methotrexate in psoriasis and psoriatic arthritis suggested that methotrexate may be the most effective agent in the systemic treatment of psoriasis and psoriatic arthritis, noting that most patients experienced significant clinical responses of skin, nail, and joint involvement. Although minor adverse events were relatively common, serious reactions, including liver cirrhosis, were uncommon [48]. Nevertheless, liver biopsy was recommended at baseline in psoriatic patients with a history of excessive alcohol intake, persistently abnormal baseline AST or ALT, or chronic hepatitis B or C infection, or during treatment if patients develop persistently elevated liver function tests or hypoalbuminemia [48].

The efficacy of methotrexate in the treatment of ankylosing spondylitis is also not well documented. Anecdotal reports have shown favorable responses [49,50]; however, small open-label trials and two controlled trials have shown conflicting results. For example, Ostendorf et al. found no significant response to methotrexate in patients with ankylosing spondylitis compared to psoriatic arthritis or RA [51,52]. In contrast, Sampaio-Barros et al. found favorable results in 53% of patients, but most responders had peripheral arthritis [53]. Creemers et al. reported efficacy of methotrexate in 5 of 9 patients and observed no difference in the clinical response of axial versus peripheral disease [54]. In a small 3 year open-label study, methotrexate induced response in axial disease was reported and verified by radiographic evidence, but essentially no response in peripheral arthritis was found [55]. It is important to note that patients in this study [55] had a mean duration of spondyloarthropathic disease of 4.8 years, which is much lower than many of the other studies cited. Low doses of methotrexate were also used in this study (mean dose of 7.3 mg/wk at 3 years) [55]. Surprisingly, neither of the referenced studies [54,55] showed a significant effect of methotrexate on flares of AS-associated iridocyclitis.

More recently, Alton et al. published a randomized trial of 51 AS patients treated with naproxen 1000 mg/day or naproxen 1000 mg/day and methotrexate 7.5 mg weekly for 12 months. Patients in the methotrexate plus naproxen group showed a significant improvement in physician global evaluation compared to naproxen alone. However, no other parameter was found to be significantly different between the two groups [56]. A small double-blinded placebo-controlled trial has examined the use of methotrexate in AS [57]. A total of 30 patients received methotrexate 10mg weekly or placebo for 24 weeks. Of the 28 patients who completed the study, there were no significant changes in the disease activity or metrology score in patients receiving methotrexate compared to placebo. Many of the patients in this study had disease duration of greater than 10 years [57]. Contradictory results from these trials raise many questions. Does early axial disease respond to methotrexate while longstanding axial disease does not? Would the arthritis or iridocyclitis respond to higher doses of methotrexate? Clearly larger, controlled trials are needed to further evaluate these issues.

The use of methotrexate in Reiter's syndrome is supported primarily by anecdotal reports. Lally et al, in a review of the medical literature from 1965 to 1985, reported 21 patients with Reiter's syndrome treated with methotrexate. Eighteen of the patients noted dramatic improvement in skin lesions within 2 weeks. Fifteen of the 21 patients had significant improvement in arthritis, but response was slower than that of the skin manifestations [58].

A paucity of data exists regarding the use of methotrexate in enteropathic spondyloarthropathy. Two recent reviews of methotrexate use for inflammatory bowel disease (IBD) came to similar conclusions. Both groups concluded that methotrexate was safe and effective in treatment of Crohn's disease, but not ulcerative colitis [59,60]. It is still unclear to what extent methotrexate might be useful in patients with arthritis associated with IBD.

The use of methotrexate and other immunosuppressive agents in HIV- related spondyloarthropathies is relatively contraindicated due to concerns for worsening HIV disease, leukopenia, opportunistic infections and Kaposi's sarcoma [61-63]. However, methotrexate in severe HIV-related psoriatic arthritis and Reiter's syndrome patients has been utilized [64-66] with the caveat that it only be considered when all other treatments have been exhausted and appropriate retroviral and prophylactic antimicrobial agents are administered [64-66].

### *Cyclosporine*

Cyclosporine has been primarily evaluated in psoriatic arthritis patients. Reviewed in a 1997 publciation [67], the majority of available clinical trials demonstrated significant improvement from baseline in psoriasis and psoriatic arthritis at cyclosporine doses of 3-6 mg/kg/day. Important side effects included moderate nephrotoxicity (approximately 6% of patients), uncontrolled hypertension, or gastrointestinal discomfort [67]. None of the trials were randomized or placebo controlled. Several small open-labeled prospective studies have shown cyclosporine induces significant improvement in psoriatic arthritis joint tenderness, swelling, patient and physician activity rating, morning stiffness, and pain score [67].

While not compared to placebo, cyclosporine has been compared to other DMARDS in controlled studies. In a prospective, randomized, open, controlled study, ninety-nine psoriatic arthritis patients treated for 24 weeks with cyclosporine (3mg/kg/day) plus standard therapy (NSAIDS, analgesics, and/or prednisone 5mg/day or less), were compared to similar patients treated with sulfasalazine (2000mg/day) plus standard therapy, or standard therapy alone [68]. Compared to both sulfasalazine and standard therapy, there were statistically significant differences in favor of cyclosprine in pain score, swollen joint count, tender joint count, joint/pain tenderness score, patient and physician global assessment, total arthritis impact measurement scale score, and spondylitis functional index, and Psoriatic Area and Severity Index (PASI) [68]. Statistically significant differences were also seen in the ACR 50% and ACR 70% response rates between cyclosporine and standard therapy [68]. Only the spondylitis functional index and eyrthrocyte sedimentation rate (ESR) were significantly different when comparing the sulfasalazine and standard therapy groups [68].

In a prospective, controlled randomized trial (n=35 patients), cyclosporine (at 3-5mg/kg/day) was compared to methotrexate (at 7.5 to 15mg weekly) in the treatment of psoriatic arthritis, similar clinical responses were seen in both treatment cohorts [69]. At 6 and 12 months significant improvement were found in the number of painful joints, number of swollen joints, the Ritchie index, the duration of morning stiffness, grip strength, C-reactive protein (CRP), the patient's and physician's assessment of PsA activity, and the

PASI in both the cyclosprine and methotrexate groups compared to baseline. ESR improved significantly only in the methotrexate group [69]. Unfortunately, after one year, cyclosporine and methotrexate were discontinued in 41.2% and 27.8 % of psoriatic patients respectively (not a statistically significant difference). Withdrawals in the cyclosporine group (n=7) were from hypertension, abnormal renal function, or gastrointestinal discomfort, or unsatisfactory response. Withdrawals in the methotrexate group (n=4) were from gastrointestinal symptoms, elevation of liver enzymes, or intercurrent infections [69]. In a prospective study comparing cyclosporine to other potential disease modifying drugs in psoriatic arthritis, Spadaro et al. concluded that patients taking cyclosporine are less likely than patients taking methotrexate to continue long-term treatment, although the inefficacy rates of these drugs was not significantly different [70].

Cyclosporine has been used successfully in combination with methotrexate in patients with severe psoriasis or psoriatic arthritis resistant to single agent therapy [71,72]. Patients that had previously failed cyclosporine or methotrexate as single agents showed good response to these medications in combination [71]. Preliminary reports of a randomized, double-blind, placebo controlled trial of combination therapy with methotrexate and cyclosporine versus methotrexate alone in psoriatic arthritis suggests that combination therapy may be more effective, particularly in severe disease [73].

Responsiveness of severe recurrent Reiter's syndrome to cyclosporine has been documented in one case report [74]. Cyclosporine has also been used in refractory cases of IBD with arthritis, but relapse was frequent upon stopping therapy [41,75]. Successful cyclosporine treatment of HIV- associated psoriatic arthritis has also been reported, without worsening of HIV disease or opportunistic infections [76]. Traditional and possible alternative therapies (discussed below) for spondyloarthropathies are listed in Table 1.

### *Leflunomide*

Leflunomide is a pyrimidine synthesis inhibitor that has been shown to be effective in RA [77]. Despite the relative lack of information on the use of leflunomide in the spondyloarthropathies, it may be a useful alternative especially in psoriatic patients who have failed methotrexate (personal observation). Scarpa et al [78] reported preliminary results of an open pilot study of leflunomide in psoriatic arthritis. Six patients were treated for 3 months. Marked improvement was noted in tender joint count, swollen joint count, and pain on visual analogue scale; however, no significant improvement was seen in the extent of the skin disease or sedimentation rate [78]. Others have reported that psoriasis and psoriatic arthritis may improve [79,80]. In preliminary data (n=9 patients) in patients with recalcitrant, polyarticular, symmetrical, rheumatoid type pattern of psoriatic arthritis eight had an improvement in arthritis and six had an improvement in psoriasis from baseline with leflunomide ttherapy [80] [80]. Cuchacovich and Soto [81] reported clinical remission of psoriatic arthritis involving the peripheral joints and sacroiliac joint with leflunomide in a patient who had failed sulfasalazine and failed to tolerate methotrexate. Radiographs of the feet showed partial filling of a subchondral cyst with bony sclerosis, progressive bone absortion of the erosion in the right fifth interphalangeal joint, and no new erosions after one year [81].

**Table 1. Traditional and Alternative Therapies for Spondylarthritis**

| ***Traditional*** |
|---|
| Methotrexate |
| Sulfasalazine |
| Cyclosporine |
| ***Alternative*** |
| Leflunomide |
| ***Azathioprine*** |
| Gold |
| Etretinate |
| Mycophenolate mofetil |
| Antimalarials |
| Penicillamine |
| Cyclophosphamide |
| Antibiotics |
| Bromocriptine |
| Pamidronate |
| Thalidomide |

## Alternative Therapy

Most recently, preliminary data from a double-blind, randomized, placebo-controlled trial (n=190 psoriatic arthritis and psoriasis patients) over 24 weeks showed significant differences in favor of leflunomide in the Psoriatic Arthritis Response Ccriteria (PsARC), modified ACR 20% and PASI at endpoint [82]. Improvements in skin and joint counts occurred as early as 3 months and were sustained throughout the study. Leflunomide induced significant reductions in tender and swollen joint counts and three psoriasis severity assessments [82]. Data regarding the use of leflunomide in psoriatic arthritis with significant spinal involvement and in other spondyloarthropathies, to our knowledge, is otherwise not available.

### *Azathioprine*

Azathioprine use in spondyloarthropathies originated from its application in the treatment of inflammatory bowel disease (IBD) [41,42]. Therapeutic response can be expected in the peripheral arthritis of IBD (as peripheral arthritis activity usually correlates with bowel disease activity) [42]. Case reports further suggest that ankylosing spondylitis, psoriatic arthritis, and Reiter's syndrome may also respond to azathioprine [83-86]. One small trial comparing azathioprine to sulfasalazine in ankylosing spondylitis showed positive responses to both drugs in 66% of patients; however, azathioprine was less well tolerated [87].

### *Gold*

Administration of gold has been most thoroughly examined in psoriatic arthritis patients. Therapeutic trials of both intramuscular gold thiomalate or auranofin have been reported. Palit et al. showed that IM gold was effective and safe for the treatment of psoriatic arthritis compared to auranofin (which showed no significant benefit) [88]. Other authors have shown clinical efficacy for either agent [89,90]. Scarpa et al. concluded that auranofin was more effective in patients with polyarthritis than spondylitis [89]. Bruckle et al. noted a higher percentage of psoriatic patients responded to auranofin; however, patients responding to IM gold had a more rapid and more impressive response [90]. Mucocutaneous side effects were more common with IM gold, while gastrointestinal side effects were more common with auranofin [88,90]. Occasionally exacerbations of psoriasis have been noted in a small percentage of patients treated with either agent [90]. A small study showed no prevention of radiographic progression of peripheral joint disease with IM gold therapy [91]. Efficacy and toxicity of IM gold versus methotrexate in psoriatic arthritis were compared and showed that patients with earlier disease were more likely to respond to either medication [92]. Methotrexate, however, was shown to be superior to gold in the likelihood of achieving a clinical response, in allowing reduction of prednisone, in correcting anemia, and in the likelihood of discontinuing therapy [92]. Auranofin has been reported as successful and safe treatment of psoriatic arthritis in one patient with HIV (in association with an increase in CD4 lymphocyte count) [93]. In a single report, gold therapy was useful in the treatment of Reiter's syndrome [94].

### *Etretinate*

Etretinate is effective in the treatment of psoriasis [95], in improving psoriatic arthritis, and in reducing psoriatic nail dystrophy [95,96]. In a 24 week pilot study involving 40 patients, significant improvements in tender joints, morning stiffness, patient and physician global assessment, pain by visual analogue scale (VAS), PASI, and ESR were seen [97]. Thirty-nine of 40 patients had moderate mucocutaneous side effects, but side effects were only severe enough to result in treatment termination in 9 patients. Elevation of AST was noted in 8 patients and elevation of triglycerides were noted in 15 patients [97]; therefore, liver tests and lipid panels should be monitored in patients on retinoids. In a two-year follow up study of 20 patients with psoriatic arthropathy, beneficial effects were maintained with low, well tolerated maintenance doses of etretinate [98]. Similarly responsiveness of HIV-associated psoriasis has been reported with etretinate [63], and it has been successfully used in Reiter's Syndrome in both immunocompetent and HIV patients [99-103]. It is noted that etretinate is metabolized to an active metabolite, acetretin (currently marketed as Psoriatane) and etretinate is no longer available (personal communication). Studies of psoriatic arthritis responses to acetretin are not currently available.

### *Mycophenolate Mofetil*

Mycophenolate mofetil (MMF) has been widely used in organ transplantation and has more recently been expanded into other autoimmune disorders and inflammatory skin disorders [104,105]. Mycophenolic acid, a precursor of mycophenolate mofetil, has a remote history of being used successfully to treat psoriasis [106]. In 1998, Tong and Walder reported a case of recalcitrant plaque psoriasis and psoriatic arthritis treated with MMF. The patient's psoriasis showed good response; however, the patient subjectively noted better control of arthritis during treatment with cyclosporine or methotrexate [107]. More recently, Grundmann-Kollmann et al described 6 patients with refractory psoriatic arthritis treated with MMF for 10 weeks; half of the patients showed significant improvement in pain, with a reduction in the mean visual analog scale from 7.1 to 4.7. Significant improvement in range of motion of their hip joints, knee joints, and spine flexion, and in quality of life was also observed. MMF was well tolerated in these patients [105]. In a similar study, relative improvement in pain, mobility and degree of psoriatic skin effluorescences in 4 of 6 patients and improvement in life quality in 3 patients was seen with MMF treatment [108].

### *Antimalarials*

Antimalarial use in spondyloarthritis has primarily been limited to psoriatic arthritis. Chloroquine administration to patients over a period of at least 6 months produced a >30% reduction in the inflamed joint count (in 18/32 patients); however, this was not significantly different from the control group. Worsening of psoriasis in the treatment group was not different from that of controls [109]. In another trial, aspirin and hydroxychloroquine (n=32 patients) were compared to hydroxychloroquine alone (n=18 patients) [110]. Twenty – three patients and 11 patients respectively had remission, improvement, or stabilization of disease. Hydroxychloroquine did not palliate or aggravate existing psoriasis [110]. A high discontinuation rate secondary to inefficacy in psoriatic arthritis patients treated with hydroxychloroquine has been suggested [70]. While antimalarials have been implicated in the worsening of psoriasis [111,112], recent publications suggest that this adverse reaction is infrequent, minor, and not a contraindication for antimalarial use [70,113] although antimalarial efficacy in spondyloarthritis, at best, is questionable [114,115].

### *Penicillamine*

Anecdotal reports of the successful treatment of AS with penicillamine [116-119] are contradicted by a placebo controlled trial of penicillamine in AS which showed no significant improvement [120]. Reports of penicillamine use in the other spondyloarthropathies could not be identified.

## Cyclophosphamide

Cyclophosphamide, in an uncontrolled trial, was administered to 12 ankylosing spondylitis patients with high disease activity and involvement of peripheral joints [121]. An aggressive regimen of 200mg cyclophosphamide intravenously every second day for 3 weeks followed by 100mg orally once weekly for 3 months produced significant reductions in spinal and peripheral joint pain, number of swollen peripheral joints, and the mean ESR; however, no difference in the mobility of the spine could be established [121].

### *Antibiotics*

The role of antibiotic therapy in reactive arthritis has been investigated and remains controversial. Antibiotics (tetracycline primarily) may be most beneficial if used early during the pathogenesis of reactive arthritis [122]. However, long-term antibiotic therapy for the spondyloarthropathies is probably not indicated [122,123].

### *Bromocriptine*

Bromocriptine, a dopamine agonist, has been used successfully in the treatment of psoriasis and psoriatic arthritis [124,125]. Weber et al reported a significant improvement in 77% of 35 patients with resistant psoriatic arthritis treated with bromocriptine [124]. Additionally, acute remissions of Reiter's syndrome related to infectious gastroenteritis have been described following treatment with bromocriptine [126]. er, others have reported failed treatment of reactive arthritis with bromocriptine [127]. er controlled studies might be warranted to evaluate the efficacy of bromocriptine in spondyloarthropathies.

### *Pamidronate*

Administration of pamidronate in refractory AS (n=16 patients) suggested that it may possess anti-inflammatory activity, particularly with prolonged administration [128]. her study involving nine patients showed significant improvement in clinical and laboratory parameters in refractory peripheral spondyloarthritis treated with intravenous pamidronate, as well as, significant reduction in the maximal rate of synovial augmentation assessed by MRI [129]. Data from a randomized double-blinded dose response comparison of IV pamidronate in AS showed significantly greater reduction in Bath Ankylosing Spondylitis Disease Activity Index (BASDAI) and Bath Ankylosing Spondylitis Functional Index (BASFI) in patients treated with pamidronate 60mg IV once monthly for 6 months than those treated with 10mg IV once monthly for 6 months [130]. In a separate observational study (n=12 patients), Haibel et al. reported somewhat less impressive results [131]. Patients were given IV pamidronate 60mg at days 0, 2, 14, 28, and 56 and were observed for 6 months. One patient dropped out secondary to disease flare. In the remainder, there was a significant change in the mean BASDAI after 3 months which was not maintained at 6 months. Patient's global assessment was improved significantly after 1 and 2 months and physician's global assessment improved after 1, 2, and 3 months. However, no significant changes were noted in BASFI, BASMI (Bath Ankylosing Spondylitis Metrology Index ), pain, NSAID usage, CRP or ESR at any time [131].

### *Thalidomide*

The use of thalidomide, a selective inhibitor of tumor necrosis factor, in refractory spondyloarthropathy has also been investigated in the spondyloarthropathies [132-134]. Initial anecdotal reports showed a positive response to thalidomide in 2 patients [132]. Thereafter, eight additional patients were included with the 2 patients in an open study. The patient population included 7 with AS, 1 with psoriatic arthritis, and 3 with undifferentiated spondyloarthropathy. Preliminary results of this study confirm the initial impression regarding the efficacy of thalidomide in refractory spondyloarthropathy, showing improvement in clinical and biological parameters in 50% of patients [133]. More recently, a 12 month open study of the use of thalidomide (200mg/day) in 30 patients with refractory AS has been reported [134]. Twenty-six of thirty patients completed the study. Seven indices including BASDAI, BASFI, total body pain, total spinal pain, patient global assessment, physician global assessment, and duration of morning stiffness were measured as primary outcome measures. Of these measures, >20% improvement in 4 of 7 indices was observed in the majority of patients. Nine of the patients became pain free. Secondary outcome measures, ESR and CRP, were both significantly decreased. Of particular interest, tumor necrosis factor α transcripts in peripheral blood mononuclear cells were significantly decreased [134]. Despite these encouraging results, the availability of thalidomide remains a practical problem (personal communication).

## Anti-tumor Necrosis Factor Therapies

### *Infliximab*

Several important trials utilizing infliximab in the treatment of spondyloarthropathies are summarized in Table 2. Infliximab was initially shown to be efficacious and safe in the treatment of patients with Crohn's disease [135] and Van den Bosch et al reported significant improvement in 4 patients with Crohn's related spondyloarthropathy [136]. Small, open-label studies have shown relatively significant improvements in arthritic manifestations of AS, psoriatic arthritis, and undifferentiated spondyloarthritis [20-23,137-141]. One year follow up studies of spondyloarthropathic patients have shown a sustained response upon continuation of infliximab therapy 22,23,142,143]. As documented by studies shown in Table 2, infliximab not only improves psoriatic arthritis but also significantly improves skin disease [22,137,139-141]. Magnetic resonance imaging (MRI) has shown improvement of inflammation of the ileosacral joints, spine, and peripheral joints in ankylosing spondylitis [20,21,23-25]. In a randomized, placebo-controlled trial (n=20 patients), clinical improvement correlated with significant regression of spinal inflammation using MRI activity scores [24]. Antoni et al showed a reduction of gadolinium uptake by MRI of 82% in affected joints in psoriatic arthritis after infliximab treatment [22]. An additional infliximab benefit of improvement in ocular symptoms of AS patients with anterior uveitis has also been observed [20]. Preliminary reports of a prospective trial of infliximab therapy in patients with refractory non-infectious uveitis (n=12) show subjective and objective improvement in a majority of patients treated with infliximab for a minimum of 12 weeks [144].

Controlled studies in spondyloarthropathies (primarily psoriasis and AS) have shown significant improvement in arthritis disease activity following infliximab administration [145-147]. A recent placebo- controlled study of 40 spondyloarthropathy patients receiving infliximab showed significant improvements were noted in patient global assessment, patient pain assessment, and physician global assessment at 12 weeks [145]. Morning stiffness, erythrocyte sedimentation rate, and C-reactive protein values also improved significantly with infliximab therapy. Spinal pain, as assessed by visual analogue scale (VAS), improved from a median of 30 to a median of 16 in treated patients. The BASDAI and BASFI improved from a median of 58.9 to 26.6 and from a median of 46.5 to 27.4 respectively. All of these measures where statistically significant for infliximab compared to placebo [145].

## Table 2. Use of Infliximab in the Spondyloarthropathies

| First Author | Year | Design | Patients | Disease | Follow Up | Inflammatory Markers | VAS | BASDAI | BASFI | PASI | MRI | Other |
|---|---|---|---|---|---|---|---|---|---|---|---|---|
| Stone [20] | 2000 | Open | 21 | AS | 14wks | Improved | | Improved >60% | Improved>60% | | Improved | |
| Brandt [21] | 2000 | Open | 11 | AS | 12 wks | Improved | Improved | Improved | Improved | N/A | Improved 2 of 3 | |
| Brandt [142] | 2001 | Follow Up | 10 of 11 | AS | 1 year | | | Lesser Magnitude | | | | |
| Van den Bosch [137] | 2000 | Open | 21 | 10 AS 9 PsA 2 USpA | 12 wks | Improved | | Improved | Improved | Improved | | |
| Kruithof [143] | 2001 | Follow Up | 19 of 21 | | 1 year | Sustained | | Sustained | Sustained | Unknown | | |
| Maksymo-wych [23] | 2001 | Open | 17 | AS | 14wks | Improved | | Improved 6.2 to 2.8 | Improved | | Improved | Remission 5/11 peripheral joints |
| Cauza [141] | 2002 | Open | 9 | PsA | 22wks | | | | | Improved | | ACR20/50/70 89% 56% 22% |
| Antoni [22] | 2002 | Open | 10 | PsA | 10 wks | Improved | 67.7 to 11.8 | | | Improved 71% | Improved By 82 % | ACR50 in 10, ACR70 in 8/10. |
| Antoni [22] | 2002 | Follow Up | 10 | PsA | 54 wks | Continued response | 67.7 to 20.2 | | | | | ACR50 in 10, ACR70 in 6/10 |
| Braun [24] | 2003 | Open | 20 | AS | 3mo. | Improved | | Improved by 47.2% | Improved by 36.8% | | Improved by 40% and 60% | MRI correlated with clinical improvement |
| Proven-zano [140] | 2003 | Open | 12 | PsA | 6mo. | CRP-Improved | | | | Improved | | ACR20 10/12 ACR50 6/12 |
| Salvarani [139] | 2003 | Open | 14/16 completed | PsA | 30wks | Improved | Improved | | | Improved by 86% | | ACR 20/50/70 64% 57% 57% |

**Table 2. Use of Infliximab in the Spondyloarthropathies (Continued)**

| First Author | Year | Design | Patients | Disease | Follow Up | Inflammatory Markers | VAS | BASDAI | BASFI | PASI | MRI | Other |
|---|---|---|---|---|---|---|---|---|---|---|---|---|
| Van den Bosch [145] | 2002 | Control | 40 | SpA | 12 wks | Improved | Improved-Median 30 to 16 | Improved – Median 58.9 to 26.6 | Improved-Median 46.5 to 27.4 | | | Most Measures of Activity Improved |
| Braun [146] | 2002 | Control | 70 | AS | 12 wks | Improved | | 50% improvement in 53% | Improved | | | |
| Brandt [148] | 2003 | Follow Up | 54 of 70; 49 completed | AS | 2 year | | | 50% improvement in 43.5% | | | | |
| Antoni [147] | 2003 | Control | 102 | PsA | 1 year | | | | | Improved See text | | ACR 20/50/70 See text |

AS = Ankylosing Spondylitis.
PsA = Psoriatic Arthritis.
UspA = Undifferentiated Spondyloarthropathy.
VAS =Visual Analogue Scale –Pain.
BASDAI=Bath Ankylosing Spondylitis Activity Index.
BASFI = Bath Ankylosing Spondylitis Functional Index.
PASI = Psoriatic Area Severity Index.

In a separate 12 week randomized placebo controlled trial (n= 70 patients), AS patients were treated with infliximab (5mg/kg) at 0, 2, and 6 weeks [146]. The primary endpoint for this study was the improvement of disease activity (measured by BASDAI) by 50% between baseline and week 12. Results reveal that 53% of patients treated with infliximab achieved a 50% improvement in BASDAI at week 12 compared to 9% of control patients. Improvement was rapid in the infliximab group with 41% of these patients achieving a 50% improvement by week 2. It is also important to note that both peripheral pain and spinal pain improved significantly in infliximab treated patients. The mean activity index for spinal pain improved from 7.9 to 3.7 between baseline and week 12. While mean activity index for peripheral joint pain improved from 5.2 to 2.4 between baseline and week 12. Significant improvements were also noted in multiple secondary outcomes including BASFI, BASMI, quality of life, concentration of C-reactive protein, and erythrocyte sedimentation rate [146]. One – year follow-up data on these patients suggested that infliximab remains effective over time if given at 6-week intervals [146]. Preliminary data from 2 years of follow up of these patients was recently reported. Forty-nine patients (70%) completed 2 years of therapy. Although twenty-one patients dropped out (14 secondary to adverse events), the magnitude of improvement of disease activity in remaining patients was sustained in every outcome measure assessed [148].

Results of a multinational randomized double blind placebo controlled trial of infliximab in psoriatic arthritis are also available [147]. One-hundred and two patients were randomized to infliximab (5mg/kg) verus placebo for 16 weeks followed by open-label treatment through week 50. The infliximab group had an ACR 20% response of 69% at week 16 and 72% at week 50 compared to an ACR 20% response of 8% at week 16 in the placebo group and an ACR 20% response of 77% at week 50 after switching to infliximab. The ACR 50% and ACR 70% were 49% and 29% respectively for infliximab at 16 weeks and 54% and 35% respectively for infliximab at 50 weeks. The ACR 50% and ACR 70% increased from 0% at week 16 in the placebo group to 49% and 30% respectively after switching to infliximab. In patients with a baseline PASI $\geq$ 2.5 treated with infliximab, their mean PASI improved from 8.4 to 1.6 at week 16 and 1.8 at week 50. Placebo patients intitially worsened from a PASI of 8.4 to a mean of 9.3 at 16 weeks, but then improved to a mean PASI of 2.3 after switching to infliximab [147].

One case of reactive arthritis improving dramatically with infliximab has been reported previously [149]. The successful use of infliximab in an HIV positive patient with Reiter's has also been reported [150].

### *Etanercept*

As shown in Table 3, etanercept, as anti-TNFα therapy, has been widely utilized in psoriasis and psoriatic arthritis. Individual case reports as well as open-label and controlled studies support the role of etanercept as significantly effective for treatment of both skin and joint spondyloarthropathic disease as well as associated inflammatory markers [151-157]. In a 12 week randomized, double-blind, placebo-controlled trial (n=60 patients), an ACR 20% response was noted in 73% of etanercept treated psoriatic patients compared to 13% of placebo patients. ACR 50% and ACR 70% responses were documented in 50% and 13 % of treated patients respectively [155]. A 24 week open label extension of this trial showed similar sustained improvement in psoriatic arthritis disease activity [156]. A phase III clinical trial involving 205 patients verified etanercept's efficacy in psoriatic joint and skin disease (see table 2) [157]. Patients were randomized to twice weekly etanercept or placebo for 24 weeks. ACR 20% response at 12 weeks, the primary endpoint, was achieved by 59% of the etanercept group compared to 15% of the placebo group. At 24 weeks the ACR 20% response was 50% compared to 13 % in the placebo group. Significant responses by PsARC criteria and in psoriasis activity were also noted [157]. Extension results of this study are now available and improvements in psoriatic arthritis and psoriasis were maintained. With etanercept therapy, 66% achieved an ACR 20%, 47% achieved an ACR 50%, and 16% achieved an ACR 70% [158]. These impressive results have lead to the Food and Drug Administration (FDA) approval of etanercept for the treatment of psoriatic arthritis.

Case reports, open-label studies, and controlled trials of etanercept use in ankylosing spondylitis, Crohn's related spondyloarthropathy, and undifferentiated spondyloarthropathy are establishing its efficacy in these spondyloarthropathies as well [26,159-162]. In an open study, ten patients with various spondyloarthropathies treated with etanercept for a period of six months had statistically significant improvements in all clinical and functional parameters, including VAS spinal pain score during the day and night, BASFI, BASDAI, and quality of life. Eighty-six percent of MRI detected enthesial lesions involving the sacroiliac joints, cervical or lumbar spine, and peripheral joints in this study were noted to improve or regress completely with etanercept treatment [26].

Recent results of a controlled trial of etanercept with an open-label extension in ankylosing spondylitis appear to confirm the efficacy of etanercept in AS [160]. In this trial, 40 patients were randomized to receive etanercept 25mg SQ twice weekly or placebo for four months. Thirty-seven patients completed the study and were followed in an open-label extension study for another 6 months [160]. Results of the controlled trial revealed response rates at 4 months of 80% with etanercept and 30% with placebo. Statistically significant improvement was noted in morning stiffness, spinal pain, patient's global assessment of disease activity, BASFI, physician's global assessment of disease activity, chest expansion, enthesitis, ESR and C-reactive protein [160]. No statistically significant difference was noted in the modified Schober's index, mean occiput-to-wall measurement, score for peripheral-joint tenderness, mean swollen-joint score, or fatigue severity index [160]. The lack of improvement in peripheral joint scores was somewhat surprising considering the response of peripheral joints in psoriatic arthritis to etanercept. The most common adverse events included reactions at the injection site and minor infections (primarily respiratory); no serious adverse events were reported [160]. During the open-label extension period a similar rapid response was seen in those patients previously in the placebo group. During this period the dose was decreased or the medication discontinued in 66% of patients receiving corticosteroids, 63% of patients receiving methotrexate, 63% of patients receiving sulfasalazine, and 73 percent of patients receiving NSAIDs [160].

**Table 3. Use of Etanercept in the Spondyloarthropathies**

| First Author | Year | Design | Patients | Disease | Follow Up | Inflammatory Markers | VAS | BASDAI | BASFI | PASI | MRI | Other |
|---|---|---|---|---|---|---|---|---|---|---|---|---|
| Yazici [153] | 2000 | Open | 10 | PsA | 1 year | | | | | | | 8 of 10 good response, good skin response. |
| Cuellar [154] | 2000 | Open | 12 | PsA | 5-14mo | Improved 10 of 12 | | | | Improved 10 of 12 | | Joint disease Resolved 10 of 12. |
| Marza-Ortega [26] | 2001 | Open | 10 | 7AS, 2 Crohns 1USpA | 6mo | Improved | Improved | Improved | Improved | | 38 of 44 lesions resolved/improved | |
| Mease [155] | 2000 | Control | 60 | PsA | 12 wks | Improved | | | | Improved Median 46.2% | | PsARC 77-87%, ACR20 73% ACR50 50% ACR70 13% |
| Mease [156] | 2000 | Open Exten- sion | 58 of 60 | PsA | 24wks 9mo total | Improved | | | | Improved Median 62% | | PsARC 82% ACR20 74% ACR50 56% ACR70 30% |
| Mease [157] | 2001 | Control | 205 | PsA | 24 wks | | | | | Improved Median 47% | | PsARC 70% ACR20 50% ACR50 37% ACR70 9% |
| Mease [158] | 2003 | Open Exten-sion | 145 of 205 | PsA | 48 wks | | | | | Improved 50% in 67% | | ACR20 66% ACR50 47% ACR 70 16% |
| Gorman [160] | 2002 | Control | 40 | AS | 4 mo | Improved | | | Improved | | | Extension study – text. |

AS=Ankylosing Spondylitis, PsA= Psoriatic Arthritis, UspA= undifferentiated spondyloarthropathy, VAS=Visual Analogue Scale –Pain, BASDAI=Bath Ankylosing Spondylitis Disease Activity Index, BASFI=Bath Ankylosing Spondylitis Functional Index, PASI=Psoriatic Area and Severity Index, PsARC=Psoriatic Arthritis Response Criteria.

A separate placebo-controlled, randomized trial (n= 30 patients) in AS showed that etanercept treatment resulted in at least a 50% regression of disease activity in 57% of patients at week 6 compared to only 6% of the placebo group. When placebo patients switched to etanercept, 56% improved. Similarly, pain, function, mobility and quality of life improved with etanercept at week 6 and mean CRP levels decreased significantly with etanercept. There was ongoing improvement throughout the etanercept treatment period [161]. When etanercept was stopped, 87% of patients relapsed, with relapses occurring 6.2 ± 3.0 (mean ± SD) weeks after stopping etanercept [161,162]. Patients who relapsed entered into an open extension of the trial and re-administration of etanercept resulted in a rapid and sustained improvement in a significant portion of patients [162]. Etanercept has recently been approved by the Food and Drug Administration for the treatment of ankylosing spondylitis.

With respect to the other spondyloarthropathies, Aboulafia et al. reported one case of HIV-associated PsA treated with etanercept, showing improvement of both joint and skin disease. However, etanercept was discontinued after four months because of frequent polymicrobial infections [163].

## Summary

The spondyloarthropathies are a heterogeneous group of arthritidies that are difficult to diagnose and treat effectively. The utility of magnetic resonance imaging in the early diagnosis of the spondyloarthropathies, as well as, in monitoring responses to potential disease modifying therapies is becoming evident. However, it is unclear how cost-effective MRI will be in clinical practice and further studies are needed.

The treatment of the spondyloarthropathies has been largely empirical in the past. A review of the literature reveals that many of our traditionally utilized drugs may be effective in treating peripheral arthritis and skin manifestations in the spondylarthropathies. The only medications that are clearly effective in the treatment of spinal inflammation in the spondyloarthropathies appear to be the anti-TNFα therapies. Controlled trials have shown improvement of spinal pain and MRI findings with these therapies. These therapies have also been proven to be effective in peripheral joint disease, psoriasis, and uveitis. The FDA approval of etanercept for the treatment of psoriatic arthritis and, more recently, ankylosing spondylitis heralds a new era in the treatment of these recalcitrant diseases.

Based on the above review, some might argue that all patients with spondyloarthropathies, particularly those with axial skeletal disease, should be treated with anti-TNF α therapies, given the high risk of disability. However, this would currently appear impractical considering the current cost of these medications. Also, the risks might outweigh the benefits in patients with mild disease or in patients with relative or absolute contraindications to anti-TNF α therapies. It would seem reasonable that patients with mild to moderate peripheral disease could be tried initially on less expensive and potentially less toxic agents such as sulfasalazine, methotrexate, or leflunomide. Also, considering that many of the patients who failed methotrexate therapy already had advanced spine disease, it might be useful to pursue earlier diagnosis of axial skeletal disease with MRI to direct therapy. Another important consideration is that caution must be used in the treatment of patients with HIV-associated spondyloarthropathies because they may not tolerate further immunosuppression. Despite the above considerations, it is clear that patients with aggressive spondylarthropathic spinal disease and no contraindications should be considered for aggressive intervention with anti-TNF α therapy early on in their disease process.

## References

[1] Khan MA. Ankylosing Spondylitis: Clinical Features. In: Klippel JH, Dieppe PA, eds. *Rheumatology. 2nd ed.* London, UK: Mosby, Harcourt Publishers Limited; 2000: 6, 16.8.

[2] Arnett FC, Khan MA, Wilkens RF: A new look at ankylosing spondylitis. *Patient Care.* 1989; 23: 82-101.

[3] Gran JT, Husby G: The Epidemiology of Ankylosing Spondylitis. *Seminars in Arthritis and Rheumatism.* 1993; 22: 319-34.

[4] Taylor, WJ: Epidemiology of psoriatic arthritis. *Current Opinion in Rheumatology.* 2002; 14: 98-103.

[5] Zink A, Braun J, Listing J, Wollenhaupt J: Disability and Handicap in Rheumatoid Arthritis and Ankylosing Spondylitis – Results from the German Rheumatological Database. *J of Rheumatol.* 2000; 27:613-22.

[6] Boonen A, Chorus A, Miedema H, van der Heijde D, van der Tempel H, van der Linden S: Employment, work disability, and work days lost in patients with ankylosing spondylitis: a cross sectional study of Dutch patients. *Annals of Rheumatic Diseases.* 2001; 60: 353-58.

[7] Torre Alonso JC, Rodrigues Perez A, Arribas Castrillo JM, Ballina Garcia J, Riestra Noriega JL, Lopez Larrea C: Psoriatic arthritis: a clinical, immunologic and radiological study. *British Journal of Rheumatology.* 1991; 30: 245-50.

[8] Dougados M, van der Linden S, Juhlin R, Huitfeldt B, Amor B, Calin A, et al: The European Spondylarthropathy Study Group Preliminary Criteria For The Classification of Spondylarthropathy. *Arthritis and Rheum.* 1991; 34: 1218-27.

[9] van der Linden S, Valkenburg HA, Cats A: Evaluation of Diagnostic Criteria for Ankylosing Spondylitis. *Arthritis and Rheum.* 1984; 27: 361-68.

[10] Calin A: Radiology and spondyloarthritis. *Bailliere's Clinical Rheumatology.* 1996; 10: 455-76.

[11] Spoorenberg A, de Vlam K, van der Heijde D, de Klerk E, Dougados M, Mielants H, et al. Radiologic Scoring Methods in Ankylosing Spondylitis: Reliability and Sensitivity to Change Over One Year. *J Rheumatol.* 1999; 26: 997-1002.

[12] Mackay K, Mack C, Brophy S, Calin A: The Bath Ankylosing Spondylitis Radiology Index (BASRI). *Arthritis and Rheum*. 1998; 41: 2263-70.

[13] Kozin F, Carrera GF, Ryan LM, Foley D, Lawson T: Computed Tomography in the Diagnosis of Sacroiliitis. *Arthritis and Rheum*. 1981; 24: 1479-85.

[14] Fam AG, Rubenstein JD, Chin-Sang H, Leung FYK: Computed Tomography in the Diagnosis of Early Ankylosing Spondylitis. *Arthritis and Rheum*. 1985; 28: 930-37.

[15] Braun J, Bollow M, Eggens U, Kőnig H, Distler A, Sieper J: Use of Dynamic Magnetic Resonance Imaging with Fast Imaging in the Detection of Early and Advanced Sacroiliitis in Spondylarthropathy Patients. *Arthritis and Rheum*. 1994; 37: 1039-45.

[16] Ahlstrőm H, Feltelius N, Nyman R, Hallgren R: Magnetic Resonance Imaging of Sacroiliac Joint Inflammation. *Arthritis and Rheum*. 1990; 33: 1763-69.

[17] Muche B, Bollow M, Francois RJ, Sieper J, Hamm B, Braun J: Anatomic Structures Involved in Early- and Late-Stage Sacroiliitis in Spondylarthritis. *Arthritis and Rheum*. 2003; 48: 1374-84.

[18] Oostveen J, Prevo R, den Boer J, van de Laar M: Early Detection of Sacroiliitis on Magnetic Resonance Imaging and Subsequent Development of Sacroiliitis on Plain Radiography. A Prospective, Longitudinal Study. *J Rheumatol*. 1999; 26: 1953-58.

[19] Bollow M, Enzweiler C, Taupitz M, Golder W, Hamm B, Sieper J, et al: Use of contrast enhanced magnetic resonance imaging to detect spinal inflammation in patients with spondyloarthritides. *Clin Exp Rheumatol*. 2002; 20 (Suppl. 28): S167-S174.

[20] Stone M, Salonen D, Lax M, Payne U, Lapp V, Inman R: Clinical and Imaging Correlates of Response to Treatment with Infliximab in Patients with Ankylosing Spondylitis. *J of Rheumatol*. 2001; 28: 1605-14.

[21] Brandt J, Haibel H, Cornely D, Golder W, Gonzalez J, Reddig J, Thriene W, Sieper J, Braun J: Successful Treatment of Active Ankylosing Spondylitis with the Anti-Tumor Necrosis Factor _ Monoclonal Antibody Infliximab. *Arthritis and Rheum*. 2000; 43: 1346-52.

[22] Antoni C, Dechant C, Lorenz PDH, Wendler J, Ogilvie A, Lueftl M, et al: Open-Label Study of Infliximab Treatment for Psoriatic Arthritis: Clinical and Magnetic Resonance Imaging Measurements of Reduction of Inflammation. *Arthritis and Rheum*. 2002; 47: 506-12.

[23] Maksymowych WP, Jhangri GS, Lambert RG, Mallon C, Buenviaje H, Pedrycz E, et al: Infliximab in Anklylosing Spondylitis: A Prospective Observational Inception Cohort Analysis of Efficacy and Safety. *J Rheumatol*. 2002; 29: 959-65.

[24] Braun J, Baraliakos X, Golder W, Brandt J, Rudwaleit M, Listing J, et al: Magnetic Resonance Imaging Examinations of the Spine in Patients With Ankylosing Spondylitis, Before and After Successful Therapy With Infliximab. *Arthritis and Rheum*. 2003; 48: 1126-36.

[25] Boeger CA, Wittwer H, Schattenkirchner M, Kellner H, Kellner W: Treatment of ankylosing spondylitis with infliximab. *Annals of Rheumatic Diseases*. 2001; 60: 115 – 60.

[26] Marza-Ortega H, McGonagle D, O'Connor P, Emery P: Efficacy of Etanercept in the Treatment of the Entheseal pathology in Resistant Spondylarthropathy: A Clinical and Magnetic Resonance Imaging Study. *Arthritis and Rheum*. 2001;44: 2112-17.

[27] Dougados M, van der Linden S, Leirisalo-Repo M, Huitfeldt B, Juhlin R, Veys E, et al: Sulfasalazine in the Treatment of Spondylarthropathy: a Randomized, Multicenter, Double-Blind, Placebo-Controlled Study. *Arthritis Rheum*. 1995; 38: 618-27.

[28] Clegg DO, Reda DJ, Weisman M, Blackburn WD, Cush JJ, Cannon GW, et al: Comparison of Sulfasalazine and Placebo in the Treatment of Ankylosing Spondylitis: A Department of Veterans Affairs Cooperative Study. *Arthritis Rheum*. 1996; 39:2004 – 2012.

[29] Gupta AK, Grober JS, Hamilton TA, Ellis CN, Siegel MT, Voorhees JJ, et al: Sulfasalazine Therapy for Psoriatic Arthritis: A Double Blind, Placebo Controlled Trial. *J of Rheumatol*. 1995; 22: 894-98.

[30] Clegg DO, Reda DJ, Mejias E, Cannon GW, Weisman MH, Taylor T, et al: Comparison of Sulfasalazine and Placebo in the Treatment of Psoriatic Arthritis: a Department of Veterans Affairs Cooperative Study. *Arthritis and Rheum*. 1996; 39: 2013-20.

[31] Combe B, Goupille P, Kuntz JL, Tebib J, Liotes F, Bregeon C: Sulphasalazine in Psoriatic Arthritis: A Randomized, Multicentre, Placebo-Controlled Study. *British Journal of Rheumatology*. 1996; 35: 664-68.

[32] Clegg DO, Reda DJ, Weisman MH, Cush JJ, Vasey FB, Schumacher, Jr. HR, et al: Comparison of Sulfasalazine and Placebo in the Treatment of Reactive Arthritis ( Reiter's Syndrome): A Department of Veterans Affairs Cooperative Study. *Arthritis and Rheum*. 1996; 39: 2021-27.

[33] Egsmose C, Hansen TM, Andersen LS, Beier JM, Christensen L, Ejstrup L, et al: Limited effect of sulphasalazine treatment in reactive arthritis. A randomised double blind placebo controlled trial. *Annals of Rheumatic Diseases*. 1997; 56: 32-36.

[34] Fraser SM, Hopkins R, Hunter JA, Neumann V, Capell HA, Bird HA: Sulphasalazine in the Management of Psoriatic Arthritis. *British Journal of Rheumatology*. 1993; 32: 923-25.

[35] Kirwan J, Edwards A, Huitfeldt B, Thompson P, Currey H: The Course of Established Ankylosing Spondylitis and the Effects of Sulphasalazine Over 3 Years. *British Journal of Rheumatology*. 1993; 32: 729-33.

[36] Taylor HG, Beswick EJ, Dawes PT: Sulphasalazine in Ankylosing Spondylitis. A Radiological, Clinical and Laboratory Assessment. *Clinical Rheumatology*. 1991; 10: 43-48.

[37] Dougados M, Berenbaum F, Maetzel A, Amor B: The use of sulfasalazine for the prevention of attacks of acute anterior uveitis associated with spondylarthropathy. *Rev Rhum Engl Ed.* 1993; 60: 80-82.

[38] Munoz-Fernandez S, Hildalgo V, Fernandez-Melon J, Schlincker A, Bonilla G, Ruiz-Sancho D, et al: Sulfasalazine Reduces the Number of Flares of Acute Anterior uveitis Over a One-Year Period. *J Rheumatol.* 2003; 30: 1277-79.

[39] Clegg, DO, Reda DJ, Abdellatif M: Comparison of Sulfasalazine and Placebo for the Treatment of Axial and Peripheral Articular Manifestations of the Seronegative Spondylarthropathies: A Department of Veterans Affairs Cooperative Study. *Arthritis and Rheum.* 1999; 42: 2325-29.

[40] Rahman P, Gladman DD, Cook RJ, Zhou Y, Young G: The Use of Sulfasalazine in Psoriatic Arthritis: A Clinical Experience. *J of Rheumatol.* 1998; 25: 1957-61.

[41] De Keyser F, Van Damme N, De Vos M, Mielants H, Veys EM: Opportunities for immune modulation in the spondyloarthropathies with special reference to gut inflammation. *Inflammation Research.* 2000; 49: 47-54.

[42] De Vos M, De Keyser F, Mielants H, Cuvelier C, Veys E: Review article: bone and joint diseases in inflammatory bowel disease. *Aliment Pharmacol Ther.* 1998; 12: 397-404.

[43] Youssef PP, Bertouch JV, Jones PD: Successful treatment of human immunodeficiency virus – associated Reiter's syndrome with sulfasalazine. *Arthritis and Rheum.* 1992; 35: 723-24.

[44] Adebajo AO: Sulfasalazine and human immunodeficiency virus – associated reactive arthritis: comment on the article by Cleg et al. *Arthritis and Rheum.* 1997;40: 1911.

[45] Disla E, Rhim HR, Reddy A, Taranta A: Improvement in CD4 lymphocyte count in HIV-Reiter's syndrome after treatment with sulfasalazine. *J of Rheumatol.* 1994; 21: 662-64.

[46] Willkens RF, Williams HJ, Ward JR, Egger MJ, Reading JC, Clements PJ, et al: Randomized, double-blind, placebo controlled trial of low-dose methotrexate in psoriatic arthritis. *Arthritis and Rheum.* 1984; 27: 376-81.

[47] Abu-Shakra M, Gladman DD, Thorne JC, Long J, Gough J, Farewell VT: Longterm methotrexate therapy in psoriatic arthritis: clinical and radiological outcome. *J Rheumatol.* 1995; 22: 241-45.

[48] Cuellar ML, Espinoza LR: Methotrexate use in Psoriasis and Psoriatic Arthritis. *Rheumatic Disease Clinics of North America.* 1997; 23: 797-809.

[49] Handler RP: Favorable results using methotrexate in the treatment of patients with ankylosing spondylitis. *Arthritis and Rheum.* 1989; 32: 234.

[50] Ferraz MB, Da Silva HC, Atra E: Low Dose Methotrexate With Leucovorin Rescue in AS. *J of Rheumatol.* 1991; 18: 146-47.

[51] Ostendorf B, Specker C, Schneider M: Ankylosing Spondylitis: Clinical and Serological Response to Methotrexate Therapy Compared with Rheumatoid Arthritis [abstract]. *Arthritis and Rheum.* 1995; 38 Suppl.: S203.

[52] Ostendorf B, Specker C, Schneider M: Methotrexate lacks efficacy in the treatment of severe ankylosing spondylitis compared with rheumatoid arthritis and psoriatic arthritis. *Journal of Clinical Rheumatology*. 1998; 4: 129-36.

[53] Sampaio-Barros PD, Costallat LTL, Bertolo MB, Neto JFM, Samara AM: Methotrexate in the treatment of ankylosing spondylitis. *Scandinavian Journal of Rheumatology*. 2000; 29:160-62.

[54] Creemers MCW, Franssen MJAM, van de Putte LBA, Gribnau FWJ, van Riel PLCM: Methotrexate in Severe Ankylosing Spondylitis: An Open Study. *J Rheumatol*. 1995; 22: 1104-1107.

[55] Biasi D, Carletto A, Caramaschi P, Pacor ML, Maleknia T, Bambara LM: Efficacy of Methotrexate in the Treatment of Ankylosing Spondylitis: A Three -Year Open Study. *Clinical Rheumatology*. 2000; 19: 114-17.

[56] Altan L, Bingol U, Karakoc Y, Aydiner S, Yurtkuran Mu, Yurtkuran Me: Clinical investigation of methotrexate in the treatment of anylosing spondylitis. *Scand J Rheumatol*. 2001; 30: 255-59.

[57] Roychowdhury B, Bintley-Bagot S, Bulgen DY, Thompson RN, Tunn EJ, Moots RJ: Is methotrexate effective in ankylosing spondylitis? *Rheumatology*. 2002; 41: 1330-32.

[58] Lally EV, Ho,Jr. G: A Review of Methotrexate Therapy in Reiter Syndrome. Seminars *in Arthritis and Rheumatism*. 1985; 15: 139-145.

[59] Vandell AG, DiPiro JT: Low-Dosage Methotrexate for Treatment and Maintenance of Remission in Patients with Inflammatory Bowel Disease. *Pharmacotherapy*. 2002; 22: 613-20.

[60] Schroder O, Stein J: Low Dose Methotrexate in Inflammatory Bowel Disease: Current Status and Future Directions. *The American Journal of Gastroenterology*. 2003; 98: 530-37.

[61] Keat A: HIV and overlap with Reiter's syndrome. Bailliere's Clinical *Rheumatology*.1994; 8: 363-77.

[62] Winchester R, Bernstein DH, Fischer HD, Enlow R, Solomon G: The Co -occurrence of Reiter's Syndrome and Acquired Immunodeficiency. *Annals of Internal Medicine*. 1987; 106: 19-26.

[63] Duvic M, Johnson TM, Rapini RP, Freese T, Brewton G, Rios A: Acquired Immunodeficiency Syndrome – Associated Psoriasis and Reiter's Syndrome. *Archives of Dermatology*. 1987; 123: 1622-32.

[64] Maurer TA, Zackheim HS, Tuffanelli L, Berger TG: The use of methotrexate for treatment of psoriasis in patients with HIV infection. *J Am Acad Dermatol*. 1994; 31: 372-75.

[65] Mason C, Chennebault JM, Leclech C: Is Hiv Infection Contraindication to the Use of Methotrexate in Psoriatic Arthritis? *J of Rheumatol*. 1995; 22:2191.

[66] Berenbaum F, Duvivier C, Prier A, Kaplan G: Successful Treatment of Reiter's Syndrome in a Patient with AIDS with Methotrexate and Corticosteroids. *British Journal of Rheumatology*. 1996; 35: 295-301.

[67] Olivieri I, Salvarani C, Cantini F, Macchioni L, Padula A, Niccoli L, Boiardi L, Portioli I: Therapy with Cyclosporine in Psoriatic Arthritis. *Seminars in Arthritis and Rheumatism*. 1997; 27: 36-43.

[68] Salvarani C, Macchioni P, Olivieri I, Marchesoni A, Cutolo M, Ferraccioli G, et al: A Comparison of Cyclosporine, Sulfasalazine, and Symptomatic Therapy in the Treatment of Psoriatic Arthritis. *J Rheumatol*. 2001; 28: 2274-82.

[69] Spadaro A, Riccieri V, Sili-Scavalli A, Sensi F, Taccari E, Zoppini A: Comparison of cyclosporin A and methotrexate in the treatment of psoriatic arthritis: a one-year prospective study. *Clinical and Experimental Rheumatology*. 1995; 13: 589-93.

[70] Spadaro A, Taccari E, Mohtadi B, Riccieri V, Sensi F, Zoppini A: Life-table analysis of cyclosporin A treatment in psoriatic arthritis: Comparison with other disease – modifying antirheumatic drugs. *Clinical and Experimental Rheumatology*. 1997; 15: 609-14.

[71] Mazzanti G, Coloni L, De Sabbata G, Paladini G: Methotrexate and Cyclosporin Combined Therapy in Severe Psoriatic Arthritis. A pilot study. *Acta Derm Venereol; Suppl*. 1994; 186: 116-17.

[72] Clark CM, Kirby B, Morris AD, Davison S, Zaki I, Emerson R, Saihan EM, Chalmers RJG, Barker JNWN, Allen BR, Griffiths CEM: Combination treatment with methotrexate and cyclosporin for severe recalcitrant psoriasis. *British Journal of Dermatology*. 1999; 141: 279-82.

[73] Fraser AD, van Kuryk A, Westhovens R, Karim Z, Gerards A, Landewe RBM, et al. A Randomised, Double-Blind, Placebo Controlled Multi-Centre Trial of Combination Therapy with Methotrexate Plus Cyclosporin Vs Methotrexate Plus Placebo in Patients with Active Psoriatic Arthritis (PsA) [abstract]. *Arthritis and Rheum*. 2003; 48 Suppl.: S170.

[74] Kiyohara A, Takamori K, Niizuma N, Ogawa H: Successful treatment of severe recurrent Reiter's syndrome with cyclosporine. *J Am Acad Dermatol*. 1997; 36:482-83.

[75] Allison MC, Pounder RE. Cyclosporin for Crohn's disease. *Alimentary Pharmacology and Therapeutics*. 1987; 1:39-43.

[76] Tourne L, Durez P, Vooren JV, Farber CM, Liesnard C, Heenen M, Parent D: Alleviation of HIV-associated psoriasis and psoriatic arthritis with cyclosporine. *J Am Acad Dermatol*. 1997; 37: 501-502.

[77] Sanders S, Harisdangkul V: Leflunomide for the Treatment of Rheumatoid Arthritis and Autoimmunity. *The American Journal Of The Medical Sciences*. 2002; 323: 190-93.

[78] Scarpa R, Manguso F, Oriente A, Peluso R, Oriente P: Leflunomide in Psoriatic Polyarthritis: an Italian Pilot Study [abstract]. *Arthritis and Rheum*. 2001;44 Suppl.: S92.

[79] Reich K: Treatment of severe psoriasis and psoriatic arthritis with leflunomide. *British Journal of Dermatology*. 2002;146: 335-6.

[80] Liang GC, Barr WG: Long Term Follow-Up of the Use of Leflunomide (LF) in Recalcitrant Psoriatic Arthritis (PA) and Psoriasis (PS)[abstract]. *Arthritis and Rheum.* 2001; 44 Suppl. S121.

[81] Cuchacovich M, Soto L: Leflunomide decreases joint erosions and induces reparative changes in a patient with psoriatic arthritis [Letters]. *Annals of Rheum Dis.* 2002; 61: 942-43.

[82] Mease P, Nash P, Gladman D, Rosen C, Behrens F, Kaltwasser P, On behalf of the TOPAS Study Group: Leflunomide in the Treatment of Psoriatic Arthritis and Psoriasis: Joint and Skin Effficacy and Safety in the TOPAS Study [abstract]. *Arthritis and Rheum.* 2003; 48 Suppl.: S169.

[83] Durez P, Horsmans Y: Dramatic response after an intravenous loading dose of azathioprine in one case of severe and refractory ankylosing spondylitits. *British Society for Rheumatology.* 2000; 39: 182-84.

[84] Le Quintrec JL, Menkes CJ, Amor B: Severe psoriatic rheumatism: treatment with azathioprine: report of 11 cases. *Rev Rheum Mal Osteoartic.* 1990; 57: 815- 19.

[85] Hacker SM, Ramos-Caro FA, Ford MJ, Flowers FP: Azathioprine: A Forgotten Alternative For Treatment Of Severe Psoriasis. *International Journal of Dermatology.* 1992; 31: 873-74.

[86] Calin A: A placebo controlled, crossover study of azathioprine in Reiter's syndrome. *Annals of Rheumatic Diseases.* 1986; 45: 653-55.

[87] Brandt J, Buss B, Sieper J, Braun J: Treatment with Sulfasalazine vs. Azathioprine of Ankylosing Spondylitis Patients with a Disease Duration < 10 Years [abstract]. *Arthritis and Rheum.* 2000; 43 Suppl.: S103.

[88] Palit J, Hill J, Capell HA, Carey J, Daunt SO'N, Cawley MID, Bird HA, Nuki G: A Multicentre Double- Blind Comparison of Auranofin, Intramuscular Gold Thiomalate and Placebo in Patients with Psoriatic Arthritis. *British Journal of Rheumatology.* 1990; 29: 280-83.

[89] Scarpa R, Pucino A, Iocco M, Sollazzo M, Oreinte CB, Oriente P: The Management of 138 Psoriatic Arthritic Patients. *Acta Derm Venereol; Suppl.* 1989; 146: 199-200.

[90] Bruckle W, Dexel T, Grasedyck K, Schattenkirchner M: Treatment of Psoriatic Arthritis with Auranofin and Gold Sodium Thiomalate. *Clinical Rheumatology.* 1994; 13: 209-16.

[91] Mader R, Gladman DD, Long J, Gough J, Farewell VT: Does injectable gold retard radiographic evidence of joint damage in psoriatic arthritis?. *Clinical and Investigative Medicine.* 1995; 18: 139-43.

[92] Lacaille D, Stein HB, Raboud J, Klinkhoff AV: Longterm Therapy of Psoriatic Arthritis: Intramuscular Gold or Methotrexate? *J of Rheumatol.* 2000; 27: 1922- 27.

[93] Shapiro DL, Masci J: Treatment of HIV Associated Psoriatic Arthritis with Oral Gold. *J of Rheumatol.* 1996; 23: 1818-20.

[94] Kovalev IN, Il'in II: The crysotherapy of patients with Reiter's disease. *Terapevticheskii Arkhiv.* 1991; 63: 123-25.

[95] Orfanos CE, Ehlert R, Gollnick H: The retinoids. A review of their clinical pharmacology and therapeutic use. *Drugs*. 1987; 34: 459-503.
[96] Rabinovitz HS, Scher RK, Shupack JL: Response of Psoriatic Nails to the Aromatic Retinoid Etretinate. *Arch Dermatol*. 1983, 119: 627-28.
[97] Klinkhoff AV, Gertner E, Chalmers A, Gladman DD, Stewart WD, Schachter GD, Schachter RK. Pilot Study of Etretinate in Psoriatic Arthritis. *J of Rheumatol*. 1989; 16: 789-91.
[98] Chieragato GC, Leoni A: Treatment of Psoriatic Arthropathy with Etretinate: A Two-year Follow-up. *Acta Derm Venereol (Stockh)*. 1986; 66: 321-24.
[99] Benoldi D, Alinovi A, Bianchi G, Buticchi G: Reiter's Disease: Successful Treatment of the Skin Manifestations with Oral Etretinate. *Acta Derm Venereol (Stockh)*. 1984; 64: 352-54.
[100] Richman TB, Kerdel FA: Reiter's Syndrome. *Arch Dermatol*. 1988; 124: 1007- 9.
[101] Williams HC, Du Vivier AWP: Etretinate and AIDS-related Reiter's disease. *British Journal of Dermatology*. 1991; 124: 389-92.
[102] Belz J, Breneman DL, Nordlund JJ, Solinger A: Successful treatment of a patient with Reiter's syndrome and acquired immunodeficiency syndrome using etretinate. *J Am Acad Dermatol*. 1989; 20: 898-903.
[103] Louthrenoo W: Successful Treatment of Severe Reiter's Syndrome Associated with Human Immunodeficiency Virus Infection with Etretinate. Report of 2 Cases. *J of Rheumatol*. 1993; 20: 1243-46.
[104] McMurray RW, Harisdangkul V: Mycophenolate Mofetil: Selective T Cell Inhibition. *The American Journal of The Medical Sciences*. 2002; 323: 194-96.
[105] Grundmann-Kollmann M, Mooser G, Schraeder P, Zollner T, Kaskel P, Oschsendorf F, et al: Treatment of chronic plaque-stage psoriasis and psoriatic arthritis with mycophenolate mofetil. *J Am Acad Dermatol*. 2000; 42: 835-37.
[106] Epinette WW, Parker CM, Jones EL, Greist MC: Mycophenolic acid for psoriasis. A review of pharmacology, long-term efficacy, and safety. *J. Am. Acad. Dermatol*. 1987; 17: 962-71.
[107] Tong DW, Walder BK: Widespread plaque psoriasis responsive to mycophenolate mofetil. *Australasian J of Dermatol*. 1998; 40: 135-37.
[108] Schrader P, Mooser G, Peter RU, Puhl W:[Preliminary results in the therapy of psoriatic arthritis with mycophenolate mofetil]. [German] *Zeitschrift fur Rheumatologie*. 2002; 61: 545-50.
[109] Gladman DD, Blake R, Brubacher B, Farewell VT: Chloroquine Therapy in Psoriatic Arthritis. *J of Rheumatol*. 1992; 19: 1724-26.
[110] Kammer GM, Soter NA, Gibson DJ, Schur PH: Psoriatic Arthritis: A Clinical, Immunologic and HLA Study of 100 Patients. *Seminars in Arthritis and Rheumatism*. 1979; 9: 75-97.
[111] Luzar MJ: Hydroxychloroquine in psoriatic arthropathy: Exacerbations of psoriatic skin lesions. *J of Rheumatol*. 1982; 9: 462-64.

[112] Trnavsky K, Zbojanova M, Vlcek F: Antimalarials in Psoriatic Arthritis. *J of Rheumatol.* 1983; 10: 833.

[113] Sayers ME, Mazanec DJ: Use of Antimalarial Drugs for the Treatment of Psoriatic Arthritis. *The American Journal of Medicine.* 1992; 93: 474-75.

[114] Laurent R: Are there any antirheumatic drugs that modify the course of ankylosing spondylitis? *Bailliere's Clinical Rheumatology.* 1991; 4: 387- 400.

[115] Dougados M, Revel M, Khan MA: Spondylarthropathy treatment: progress in medical treatment, physical therapy and rehabilitation. *Bailliere's Clinical Rheumatology.* 1998; 12: 717-36.

[116] Golding DN: D-penicillamine in ankylosing spondylitis and polymyositis. *Postgraduate Medical Journal.* 1974; 50: 62-64.

[117] Scharf Y, Nahir M: Penicillamine in Ankylosing Spondylitis. *Arthritis Rheum.* 1976; 19:122.

[118] Bird HA, Dixon ASJ: Failure of D-penicilamine to affect peripheral joint involvement in ankylosing spondylitis or HLA B27-associated arthropathy. *Annals of Rheumatic Diseases.* 1977; 36: 289.

[119] Jaffe IA: Penicillamine in seronegative polyarthritis. *Annals of Rheumatic Diseases.* 1977; 63: 593.

[120] Steven MM, Morrison M, Sturrock RD: Penicillamine in Ankylosing Spondylitis: A Double Blind Placebo Controlled Trial. *J of Rheumatol.* 1985; 12: 735-37.

[121] Sadowska-Wroblewska M, Garwolinska H, Maczynska-Rusiniak B: A Trial of Cyclophosphamide in Ankylosing Spondylitis with Involvement of Peripheral Joints and High Disease Activity. *Scandinavian Journal of Rheumatology.* 1986; 15: 259-64.

[122] Toivanen A: Bacteria-Triggered Reactive Arthritis: Implications for Antibacterial Treatment. Drugs. 2001; 61: 343-51.

[123] Sieper J, Braun J: Treatment of Reactive Arthritis with Antibiotics. *British Journal of Rheumatology.* 1998; 37: 717-20.

[124] Weber G, Frey H: Treatment of psoriatic arthritis with bromocriptine. *J Am Acad Dermatol.* 1987; 16: 388-89.

[125] Buskilla D, Sukenik S, Holcberg G, Horowitz J: Improvement of Psoriatic Arthritis in a Patient Treated with Bromocriptine for Hyperprolactinemia. *J Rheumatol.* 1991; 18: 611-2.

[126] Bravo G, Zazueta B, Lavalle C: An Acute Remission of Reiter's Syndrome in Male Patients Treated with Bromocriptine. *J of Rheumatol.* 1992; 19: 747-50.

[127] Eulry F, Mayaudon H, Bauduceau B, Lechevalier D, Crozes P, Magnin J, et al: [Blood prolactin under the effect of protirelin in spondylarthropathies. Treatment trial of 4 cases of reactive arthritis and 2 cases of psoriatic arthritis with bromocriptine]. [French]. *Annales de Medecine Interne.* 1996; 147: 15-9.

[128] Maksymowych WP, Jhangri GS, LeClercq S, Skeith K, Yan A, Russell AS: An Open Study of Pamidronate in the Treatment of Refractory Ankylosing Spondylitis. *J of Rheumatol.* 1998; 25: 714-17.

[129] Maksymowych WP, Lambert R, Jhangri GS, LeClercq S, Chiu P, Wong B, et al: Clinical and Radiologic Ameriolation of Refractory Peripheral Spondyloarthritis by Pulse Intravenous Pamidronate Therapy. *J Rheumatol.* 2001; 28: 144-55.

[130] Maksymowych WP, Jhangri GS, Fitzgerald AA, LeClercq S, Chiu P, Yan A, et al: A Six-Month Randomized, Controlled, Double-Blind, Dose-Response Comparison of Intravenous Pamidronate (60mg Versus 10 mg) in the Treatment of Nonsteroidal Antiinflammatory Drug- Refractory Ankylosing Spondylitis. *Arthritis and Rheum.* 2002;46: 766-73.

[131] Haibel H, Brandt J, Rudwaleit M, Soerensen H, Sieper J, Braun J: Treatment of active ankylosing spondylitis with pamidronate. *Rheumatology (Oxford).* 2003; 42: 1018-20.

[132] Breban M, Gombert B, Amor B, Dougados M: Efficacy of thalidomide in the treatment of refractory ankylosing spondylitis. *Arthritis and Rheum.* 42: 580- 581, 1999.

[133] El Hassani S, Dougados M, Gombert B, Amor B, Breban M: Treatment of Severe Refractory Spondylarthropathy (SPA) with Thalidomide: Results of an Open Study [abstract]. *Arthritis and Rheum.* 42 Suppl.: S373, 1999.

[134] Huang F, Gu J, Zhao W, Zhu J, Zhang J, Tak Yan Yu D: One-Year Open-Label Trial of Thalidomide in Ankylosing Spondylitis. *Arthritis and Rheum.* 2002; 47: 249-54.

[135] Bondeson J, Maini RN: Tumour Necrosis Factor as a Therapeutic Target in Rheumatoid Arthritis and Other Chronic Inflammatory Diseases: The Clinical Experience with Infliximab (Remicade). *International Journal of Clinical Practice.* 2001; 55:211-16.

[136] Van den Bosch F, Kruithof E, De Vos M, De Keyser F, Mielants H: Crohn's disease associated with spondyloarthropathy: effect of TNF α blockade with infliximab on articular symptoms. *Lancet.* 2000; 356:1821-22.

[137] Van den Bosch F, Kruithof E, Baeten D, De Keyser F, Mielants H, Veys EM: Effects of a loading dose regimen of three infusions of chimeric monoclonal antibody to tumour necrosis factor α (infliximab) in spondyloarthropathy: an open pilot study. *Annals of Rheumatic Disease.* 2000; 59: 428-33.

[138] Brandt J, Haibel H, Reddig J, Sieper J, Braun J: Successful Short Term Treatment of Severe Undifferentiated Spondyloarthropathy with the Anti-Tumor Necrosis Factor α Monoclonal Antibody Infiliximab. *J of Rheumatol.* 2002; 29:118-22.

[139] Salvarani C, Cantini F, Olivieri I, Macchioni P, Padula A, Niccoi L: Efficacy of Infliximab in Resistant Psoriatic Arthritis. *Arthritis and Rheum.* 2003; 49: 541- 545.

[140] Provenzano G, Termini A, Le Moli C, Rinaldi F: Efficacy of infliximab in psoriatic arthritis resistant to treatment with disease modifying antirheumatic drugs: an open pilot study. *Ann Rheum Dis.* 2003; 62: 680-81.

[141] Cauza E, Spak M, Cauza K, Hanusch-Enserer U, Dunky A, Wagner E: Treatment of psoriatic arthritis and psoriasis vulgaris with the tumor necrosis factor inhibitor infliximab. *Rheumatology International.* 2002; 22: 227-32.

[142] Brandt J, Haibel H, Sieper J, Reddig J, Braun J: Infliximab treatment of severe ankylosing spondylitis: one-year followup. *Arthritis and Rheum.* 2001; 44: 2936-45.

[143] Kruithof E, Van den Bosch F, Baeten D, De Keyser F, Mielants H, Veys EM: Repeated infusions of infliximab, a chimeric anti-TNFα monoclonal antibody, in patients with active spondyloarthropathy: one year follow up. *Annals of Rheumatic Diseases*. 2002; 61: 207-12.

[144] Suhler EB, Smith JR, Kurz DE, Lauer AK, Pickard TD, Rosenbaum JT: A Prospective Trial of Infliximab Therapy for Patients with Refractory Uveitis: Preliminary Results [abstract]. *Arthritis and Rheum*. 2003; 48 Suppl.: S442.

[145] Van den Bosch F, Kruithof E, Baeten D, Herssens A, De Keyser F, Mielants H, et al: Randomized Double-Blind Comparison of Chimeric Monoclonal Antibody to Tumor Necrosis Factor α ( Infliximab) Versus Placebo in Active Spondyloarthropathy. *Arthritis and Rheum*. 2002; 46: 755-65.

[146] Braun J, Brandt J, Listing J, Zink A, Alten R, Golder W, et al: Treatment of active ankylosing spondylitis with infliximab; a randomized controlled multicentre trial. *The Lancet*. 2002; 359: 1187-93.

[147] Antoni C, Kavanaugh A, Kirkham B, Burmester G, Manger B, Schneider U, et al: The One Year Results of the Infliximab Multinational Psoriatic Arthritis Controlled Trial (IMPACT) [abstract]. *Arthritis and Rheum*. 2003; 48 Suppl.: S265.

[148] Brandt J, Listing J, Alten R, Bumester G, Gromnica-Ihle E, Kellner H, et al: Two Year Follow Up Results of a Controlled Trial of the Anti-TNF Alpha Antibody Infliximab in Active Ankylosing Spondylitis [abstract]. *Arthritis and Rheum*. 2003; 48 Suppl.: S172.

[149] Braun J, De Keyser F, Brandt J, Mielants H, Sieper J, Veys E: New treatment options in spondyloarthropathies: increasing evidence for significant efficacy of anti-tumor necrosis factor therapy. *Current Opinion in Rheumatology*. 2001; 13: 245-49.

[150] Gaylis N: Infliximab in the Treatment of an HIV Positive patient with Reiter's Syndrome. *J Rheumatol*. 2003; 30: 407-11.

[151] Elkayam O, Yaron M, Caspi D: From wheels to feet: a dramatic response of severe chronic psoriatec arthritis to etanercept. *Annals of Rheumatic Diseases*. 2000; 59: 839.

[152] Kurschat P, Rubbert A, Poswig A, Scharffetter-Kochanek K, Krieg T, Hunzelmann N: Treatment of psoriatic arthritis with etanercept. *J Am Acad Dermatol*. 2001; 44: 1052.

[153] Yazici Y, Erkan D, Lockshin MD: A preliminary study of etanercept in the treatment of severe, resistant psoriatic arthritis. *Clinical and Experimental Rheumatology*. 2000; 18: 732-34.

[154] Cuellar ML, Mendez EA, Collins RD, Burford S, Espinoza LR: Efficacy of Etanercept in Refractory Psoriatic Arthritis [abstract]. *Arthritis and Rheum*. 2000; 43 Suppl.: S106.

[155] Mease PJ, Goffe BS, Metz J, VanderStoep A, Finck B, Burge DJ: Etanercept in the treatment of psoriatic arthritis and psoriasis: a randomised trial. *Lancet*. 2000; 356: 385-90.

[156] Mease PJ, Goffe BS, Metz J, VanderStoep A, Burge DJ: Enbrel (Etanercept) in Patients with Psoriatic Arthritis and Psoriasis [abstract]. *Arthritis and Rheum*. 2000; 43 Suppl.: S403.

[157] Mease P, Kivitz A, Burch F, Siegal E, Cohen S, Burge D: Improvement in Disease Activity in Patients with Psoriatic Arthritis Receiving Etanercept (Enbrel): Results of a 3 Multicenter Clinical Trial [abstract]. *Arthritis and Rheum.* 2001;44 Suppl.: S90.

[158] Mease PJ, Ruderman EM, Kivitz AJ, Burch FX, Siegel EL, Cohen SB, et al: Continued Efficacy and Safety of Etanercept (Enbrel ®) in Patients With Psoriatic Arthritis and Psoriasis [abstract]. *Arthritis and Rheum.* 2003; 48 Suppl.: S169.

[159] Barthel HR: Rapid remission of treatment-resistant ankylosing spondylitis with etanercept – a drug for refractory ankylosing spondylitis? *Arthritis Care and Research.* 2001; 45: 404.

[160] Gorman JD, Sack KE, Davis JC: Treatment of Ankylosing Spondylitis By Inhibition of Tumor Necrosis Factor α. *N Engl J Med.* 2002; 346: 1349-56.

[161] Brandt J, Khariouzov A, Listing J, Haibel H, Sorensen H, Grassnickel L, et al: Six-Month Results of a Double-Blind, Placebo-Controlled Trial of Etanercept Treatment in Patients With Active Ankylosing Spondylitis. *Arthritis and Rheum.* 2003; 48: 1667-75.

[162] Brandt J, Khariouzov A, Listing J, Haibel H, Sorensen H, Rudwaleit M, et al: One Year Follow Up Results of a Controlled Trial of a German Double-Blind Placebo Controlled Trial of Etanercept in Active Ankylosing Spondylitis [abstract]. *Arthritis and Rheum.* 2003; 48 Suppl.: S173.

[163] Aboulafia DM, Bundow D, Wilske K, Ochs UI: Etanercept for the Treatment of Human Immunodeficiency Virus – Associated Psoriatic Arthritis. *Mayo Clinic Proc.* 2000; 75: 1093-98.

In: Arthritis Research: Treatment and Management
Editor: F. Columbus, pp. 59-80
ISBN 1-59033-984-3


*Chapter III*

# Current Aspects of Colchicine Therapy: Classical Indications and New Therapeutic Uses

***Uwe Lange***
Kerckhoff Clinic and Foundation, Department of Rheumatology,
Bad Nauheim, Germany

## Abstract

Medical researchers are reporting new applications for an old medicine. Over the centuries colchicine has been used preponderantly to treat and prevent gout, but an astonishing array of therapeutic properties is now being ascribed to this age-old substance. Besides its stabilizing effect on the cytoskeleton and cell membranes, colchicine has anti-inflammatory and antifibrotic properties. The potential for applications beyond gout therapy has not gone unnoticed by researchers seeking to confirm the supposition that treatment with low-dose colchicine, even long-time use, could very probably be extended to a wide variety of other life-impairing conditions for which existing therapies sometimes fall short of expectations. Responses have been especially favorable in fibrotic and inflammatory systemic diseases. The outlook for further therapeutic possibilities is promising and due to the virtual absence of side effects when properly applied, a significant new phase in low-dose colchicine therapy can be predicted if controlled studies succeed in demonstrating its multiplicity and its benefits.

# Introduction

Colchicine is an alkaloid obtained from the seeds of meadow saffron, *Colchicum autumnale.* It has a long medical history as a substance for treating gout, an ailment known even in ancient times. Unrivalled by any other generally accepted gout medication, it is widely prescribed for acute attacks or for use as a prophylactic. The current licence authorizes only these applications. However, colchicine is known to have manifold pharmacological properties and over the past twenty years significant studies have yielded increasing evidence that it can serve as an effective medication for a large variety of illnesses: amyloidosis [27, 35], Behcet's syndrome [118], Dupuytren's contracture [31], familial Mediterranean fever [44], pulmonary fibrosis [32], recurrent pericarditis [3, 4], psoriatic arthritis [36, 99], Sweet's syndrome [103], vasculitis [53], alcohol-induced cirrhosis [59, 60], primary biliary cirrhosis [57], chondrocalcinosis or "pseudogout" [41], methotrexate-induced nodulosis [1, 116], seronegative spondylarthropathies [35] and calcinosis [41]. In many cases, colchicine therapy seems to be a successful alternative if a standard form of treatment fails. The complex actions of colchicine, which are mainly attributable to its stabilizing effect on the cytoskeleton and cell membranes, and its special pattern of distribution form the basis of the results presented in this chapter. As side effects are rare, some authors believe that low-dose colchicine should be considered as an alternative to traditional therapies, if not the first choice. Its application can be recommended particularly for fibrotic and inflammatory systemic diseases and those in which leucocytic chemotaxis is a feature.

Colchicine research has confirmed the possibility of considering entirely new therapeutic applications of the "gout medicine," and controlled studies could present proof of the effectiveness of this substance in treating diseases which have hitherto involved considerable life impairment. It seems imperative to critically evaluate current findings relating to this fascinating substance which ranks among the oldest known medicines.

# Pharmacology – Mechanism of Action

Colchicine can also be regarded as the oldest known cytostatic and has traditionally been referred to as "spindle poison." It is assumed that it blocks the polymerisation of tubulin dimers of the microtubuli, which affects the function of the mitotic spindle. The ability of two of the three rings of the colchicine molecule (Figure 1) to bind to microtubuli in the interphase stage is regarded as significant since this inhibits the movement of intercellular granules and thus the secretion of a variety of substances. This effect has been documented in detail [13]. Apart from high colchicine concentrations in leucocytes, the inhibitory actions on various leucocyte functions such as adhesivity, amoeboid motility, mobilization and lysosome degranulation have been observed as the most significant effects on *leucocyte chemotaxis* [26]. Only the latter activity is found at the lowest concentrations ($1 \times 10^{-8}$ mol/L). Although this effect is said to be the most significant for the *anti-inflammatory action* of colchicine, other effects on leucocytes have also been discovered. For instance, the expression of adhesion molecules of the neutrophil membrane is reduced so that migration and interaction with endothelial cells are inhibited, and cytokine production by polymorphonuclear cells is modulated. It is also important to note the *leucocyte membrane-stabilizing action* of this substance [86]. Basically, it can be said that the action of colchicine stems from its concentration in leucocytes and their role in inflammatory reactions. To date no explanation has been found for the special affinity of colchicine for leucocytes [13].

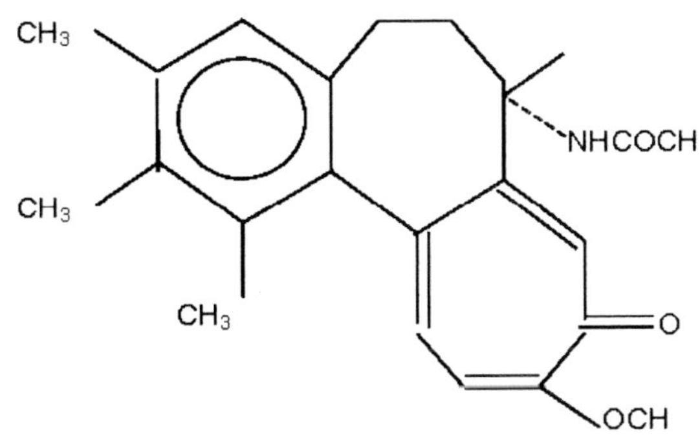


Figure 1. Colchicine molecule.

# Pharmacokinetics

The essential pharmacokinetic data for colchicine are listed in Table 1. Within 1 to 2 hours after oral administration, peak plasma levels are reached, regardless of whether the patients are given tablets or solutions. Although the plasma colchicine concentration decreases rapidly, excretion continues for several days after ingestion. Hence, it may be concluded that it remains bound in body tissues for a long time. The apparent volume of distribution of oral colchicine is 4.25 + 2.90 L/kg, indicating intensive tissue binding. Protein binding is 50%. There is evidence of colchicine passage into the placenta and foetus, as well as into breast milk. Approximately 20% of a colchicine dose is excreted via the kidneys and after a single subtherapeutic dose traces can still be found in urine after 7 to 10 days. There are also indications that colchicine undergoes intensive hepatic metabolism, especially involving demethylation by the cytochrome P-450 system (Isoform CYP 3A4). It is not clear how colchicine metabolites contribute to biological activity. An enterohepatic circulation has been proposed as an explanation. In patients with normal liver and kidney function the terminal elimination half-life of colchicine is about 9 hours after oral administration and 19 minutes after intravenous administration. The findings in cases with impaired liver and/or kidney damage have been dissimilar, but it can be said that functional impairment of these organs appears to markedly affect the clearance of colchicine. The elimination half-life is increased two- to threefold if there is severe kidney failure and as much as tenfold should there be additional cirrhosis of the liver. Hence the recommendation that such patients be closely monitored even if they are being given low doses of colchicine [13]. The pharmacology of colchicine has been extensively discussed in the articles by Achtert et al. [2], Sabouraud et al. [91, Rochdi et al. [88] and Ferron et al. [39].

**Table 1. Pharmacokinetics of Colchicine**

| Parameter / Presentation | Oral | Intravenous |
|---|---|---|
| Bioavailability | 25 – 50 % | 100 % |
| Plasma protein binding | 50 % | 50 % |
| Max. plasma level after 1 mg | No information | 0,32 + 1,17 μg/100 ml |
| Time to max plasma level (Tmax) | 1 – 3 h* | No information |
| Volume of distribution | 4,25 + 2,90 L/Kg | No information |
| Renal excretion (2 h / 24 h) | No information | 20 / 30 % |
| T1/2 | 9 ± 4 h | 19 Min. |
| T1/2 with impaired renal function | Prolonged 3-fold | No information |
| T1/2 with impaired renal and liver function | Prolonged 10-fold | No information |
| Dialysability | No† | No information |
| Passage into foetus / breast milk | Yes / Yes | Yes / Yes |

* 2nd peak after about 6 h.

† Bennet (15).

# Interactions

Interactions are summarized in Table 2. As mentioned above, colchicine undergoes intensive hepatic metabolism (CYP 3A4) [106]. Therefore, substances that are also metabolized via this isozyme of the cytochrome P-450 system inhibit the entire cytochrome system or are inhibitors of CYP 3A4.

**Table 2. Substances Possibly Interacting with Colchicine**

| Utilising CYP 3A4 | | Inhibitors of CYP 3A4 |
|---|---|---|
| Oestrogen | Midazolam | Diltiazem |
| Steroids | Quinidine | Gestodene |
| Dapsone | Terfenadine | Grapefruit juice |
| Diltiazem | Testosterone | Ketoconazole |
| Erythromycin | Nifedipine | Toleandomycin |
| Lidocaine | Verapamil | Erythromycin |
| Lovastatin | | |

Descriptions also exist for interaction with cyclosporin A [47]). P-gp, the product of the MDR-1 gene (Multi-Drug Resistance) is a cellular efflux pump for a variety of chemotherapeutic agents and is inhibited by cyclosporin A. This and other MDR modulators can also inhibit the metabolism of cytotoxins such as colchicine [100, 101].

# Toxicology

A dosage summary is given in the Appendix which shows that in all cases, with the exception of acute gout, doses of up to a maximum of 2mg/day were used. These low doses were seen to cause few adverse effects and for the most part no side effects at all. Nor were significant interactions reported. A higher daily dose, particularly for the treatment of acute gout, may cause gastrointestinal side effects, specifically diarrhoea, before the therapeutic effect occurs. If all guidelines are followed, colchicine therapy can be considered safe [84, 109]. The fatal dose is quite variable, ranging from 7 mg over a period of 4 days to 60 mg as a single dose [73]. Colchicine-specific monoclonal antibodies (Fab fragments) have been used for detoxification in cases of severe Colchicine overdoses [9]. Elevated toxicity is associated with the intravenous use, but it has been pointed out that this can very likely be attributed to incorrect i.v. administration [28] and recent studies of the risk factors stress the importance of adhering strictly to the existing guidelines [84, 109].

## Colchicine and Impaired Renal Function

The rapid distribution of colchicine in the tissues and the slow excretion process have been referred to above. The therapeutic dose should be reduced to half in patients with impaired renal function with glomerular filtration rates below 50ml/min. [16] and there should be an interval of 12 to 18 hours between the individual doses if the filtration rate is less than 10ml/min.; in cases of impaired liver function a larger proportion of the colchicine is renally excreted [65].

## Colchicine and Male Fertility

The life-long use of colchicine by patients with familial Mediterranean fever (FMF) often begins in their youth. This presents not only the problem of tolerability but also that of fertility. The sperm pathology is inconsistent and it is not likely that there is a monocausal link to colchicine. Frequent epididymitis and testicular vasculitis may predispose the oligospermia and azoospermia which often arise in Behcet's syndrome [96]. In FMF patients amyloidosis has occasionally been seen in the testes as well; however, it is not known why there is such a difference in the incidence of oligospermia and azoospermia to be found in FMF and Behcet's syndrome or gout [14].

### Colchicine and Female Fertility, Pregnancy and Nursing

As colchicine inhibits cell division, in theory female fertility should also be affected. In practice, however, there has been no indication that this assumption holds true [13]. It might also be assumed that colchicine has a teratogenic capability, but case-control studies conducted on as many as 36 pregnant women revealed an absolutely normal course of pregnancy. There were no effects observed on fertility, the incidence of miscarriage, birth weight or duration of pregnancy. Where FMF patients are concerned, it has been suggested that the use of colchicine during pregnancy may actually be quite beneficial because the expectant mothers suffer no FMF attacks. Indeed, it has been recommended that colchicine therapy be continued for FMF patients and that amniocentesis be practiced in the 4th to 5th month. In large studies with 500 and 1124 live births chromosome disruption rates were found to be somewhat higher, but to date the role that FMF itself plays here has not been determined. Studies involving nursing mothers found that colchicine concentrations in the serum and breast milk corresponded to about 1/10th of the weight-related dose in the mother. As yet no adverse effects on the infants have been discovered and, although their conclusion conflicts with official opinion, the researchers believe it is safe for nursing mothers to take colchicine [11, 13, 68]. It may well be possible to apply the findings of these FMF studies to other diseases for which long-term colchicine therapy is required.

## Treatment of Children

FMF can also be contracted by children under one year of age. Without treatment, they suffer FMF attacks and their physical development is impaired. Colchicine prevents the attacks, stimulates the appetite, and aids growth. Colchicine is recommended for the treatment of children irrespective of their age upon diagnosis. A study of long-term colchicine treatment involving 350 older children (under the age of 16) which included follow-up observation for a period of 13 years [122] showed no evidence of the development of amyloidosis, no ensuing growth or development disturbances, and no fertility problems later in life.

All studies, in particular those of FMF, have shown that in all respects colchicine, when administered in low doses below 1.5 to 2.0 mg/day is a safer medication than theoretical considerations tend to indicate, a remarkable finding since colchicine is generally taken for lengthy periods if not lifelong.

## Colchicine Therapy of Gout (Arthritis Urica)

Gout is an acute or chronic crystal-induced form of arthritis resulting from hyperuricaemia [28]. Epidemilogical studies have revealed that in Europe and the USA 20% of the population have hyperuricaemia and 2.8% of the men and 0.4% of the women between the ages of 30 and 59 have gout. The prevalence of this "disease of affluence" can be seen as a direct result of the standard of living. Women have gout about 10 times less frequently than men and rarely in their fertile period of life, but cases increase after menopause. There is a definite correlation between serum uric acid levels and the incidence of gout. When serum uric acid values are below 6.5 mg/dl, gout is an uncommon occurrence, but the condition can be found in about 90% of subjects with values over 9.0 mg/dl [46]. In the first stage of the disease, which can be brought on by elevated purine intake, medication (e.g. diuretics, penicillamine, uricosurics, allopurinol), trauma, infection, surgery, irradiation, unaccustomed physical strain, fasting or alcohol abuse, the metatarso-phalangeal joint of the large toe is affected. As the disease progresses it spreads to more joints along with the bursae, tendon sheaths and the soft tissues of the terminal phalanges. Patients who do not receive proper treatment, suffer recurring attacks with the intervals in between becoming shorter until eventually the condition becomes chronic. A much feared complication is uric acid nephropathy with its known consequences (renal hypertension, progressive loss of renal function, secondary pyelonephritis and uric acid nephrolithiasis). Of prime diagnostic relevance are the case history, the detection of urate deposits, the response to colchicine during attacks and the detection of hyperuricaemia [46]. The foremost objectives in the treatment of gout are the prevention of acute attacks with colchicine, still the medicine of first choice [46, 97], and the reduction of uric acid levels (to 5.0 - 5.5mg/dl) by means of dietary measures and drug therapy with uricostatics and/or uricosurics [46]. Hyperuricaemia on its own is not an indication for treatment with medication that lowers uric acid levels [51]; only when levels are over 8.5 mg/dl is treatment advised.

Optimal treatment of acute gout is obtained with the early oral administration of colchicine, beginning with a maximal 6-8 mg/day dose, then rapidly reducing it on the second day and as the curative effect becomes noticeable. The intravenous administration of colchicine brings about improvement within 6 to 12 hours [45]; nevertheless, due to the risk of toxicity, which was discussed above, corticosteroids or analgesics are to be preferred [51]. The main problems associated with oral administration, as already mentioned, are improper use and gastrointestinal disturbances.

The Appendix gives the recommended dosage for colchicine therapy of gout.

Recent reviews have discussed the clinical and therapeutic aspects of colchicine [38, 46, 51, 80, 117], the advantages and disadvantages of the various treatments [28], and the risks and benefits associated with this medication [87]. As is often the case with traditional medicines, insufficient information exists regarding placebo-controlled studies. Only one placebo-controlled study has been reported for colchicine [7].

## Colchicine Therapy In Chondrocalcinosis

In the first stage of chondrocalcinosis, a crystal arthropathy, there is storage of calcium pyrophosphate crystals in fibrous cartilage (menisci), surface layers of the hyaline cartilage and, more rarely, other tissues [41]. The condition is not as prevalent as gout, and age is not a factor. Its incidence is slightly higher in men than in women. No treatment of chondrocalcinosis should be undertaken unless clinical symptoms are present. Aetiological distinction is made between primary chondrocalcinosis (suspected enzyme deficiency in pyrophosphate metabolism) and a secondary form that may occur in patients with gout, haemochromatosis, hyperparathyroidism, hypothyroidism, rheumatoid arthritis, Wilson's disease and Paget's disease. The clinical picture varies: Apart from the asymptomatic form (usually a random radiographic finding), there is acute single-joint arthritis (rarely oligarthritis) that resembles a "pseudogout attack," as well as attacks of arthralgia (which sometimes last only a few hours), arthrotic complaints (with a clinical and radiomorphological picture of arthritis), occasionally with inflammatory flare-ups and severe destructive arthropathy (with the picture of a "neuropathic joint"). Chondrocalcinosis, unlike gout, does not entail visceral manifestations. Radiomorphologically evident chondrocalcinosis and/or the microscopic detection of crystals are the criteria for diagnosis. Treatment should be undertaken only in the presence of clinical symptoms.

The colchicine dose recommended for "pseudogout" is the same as that for gout and NSAR. The presence of destructive arthropathy may call for surgical intervention under some circumstances.

The Appendix gives the recommended colchicine dosage for chondrocalcinosis therapy.

## Colchicine Therapy in Familial Mediterranean Fever (FMF)

Familial Mediterranean fever (FMF) is an autosomal, recessive, hereditary disease that affects particularly Jews, Armenians, Arabs and Turks. Germany has a Turkish population of approximately 2.1 million, and there are thought to be around 2,000 FMF patients living here. However, the number may be as high as 10,000 according to the maximum figure calculated from the diagnostic register. Consequently, it is necessary for doctors in Germany to take FMF into diagnostic consideration.

FMF research has provided the best studies of the efficacy and safety of colchicine use beyond its application as a gout medicine [12,13], especially with regard to fertility, teratogenicity, the course of pregnancy and foetal development as well as the development of the breast-fed infant [13].In 50% of the cases the first manifestations occur before the age of 10, in only 5% after the age of 30. The publications of Samuels et al. [94], Ben-Chetrit & Levi [12], Ozen et al. [78], and Better & Zemer [18] include the epidemiology and the clinical presentation. Symptoms are periodic bouts of fever (beginning in the first decade of life), pleuritis, arthritis and myalgia; spenolmegaly is a feature in about 50% of the cases [12]. Typical of the attacks are sudden fever with acute sterile inflammation of the peritoneum, synovia or pleura, and pain. The attacks end spontaneously after 12 to 48 hours. Strenuous physical activity, stress, menstruation and fatty food may bring on an attack [12].

FMF may be associated with reactive, hereditary amyloidosis, whereby the amyloid is stored mainly in the kidneys (glomeruli), in the spleen and around the vessels. If the condition is not treated, most often the amyloidosis stage will be reached before the age of 40, ultimately ending in terminal kidney failure. FMF represents a clinical exclusion diagnosis [18]. A review by Livneh et al. [68] contains newly recognised symtoms of FMF and the changes in symptoms in the course of time. As yet no specific laboratory tests exist, but it is likely that a gene test will be developed presently to enable a positive diagnosis of FMF [104].

The first effective use of colchicine to prevent FMF attacks and to arrest its progression began with 5 case reports by Goldfinger [44]. He and his team went on to conduct a double-blind trial [30]. Low-dose colchicine is the standard medication for preventing and treating FMF today. Indeed, the attacks and their intensity can be almost completely suppressed, but when treatment is curtailed an attack almost inevitably occurs [11, 13, 68]. Amyloidosis has not occurred during this therapy in patients who had no proteinuria at the outset of the treatment which has been ongoing for almost two decades now, and in some cases pre-existing proteinuria has been completely eliminated [121]. Of course, the question of the risks involved in consistent colchicine treatment for FMF patients always arises when they wish to have children. Early diagnosis and consistent use of colchicine have dramatically boosted the possibility to have children and have led to a positive prognosis for the course of pregnancy. In cases with clinical manifestation in the first years of life early diagnosis and consistent colchicine use have altered the long-term prognosis; for the most part a premature death can be prevented and patients can enjoy a long life with enhanced quality.

The Appendix gives the recommended colchicine dose for familial Mediterranean fever therapy.

## Colchicine Therapy in Amyloidosis

Colchicine appears to be less effective in *primary amyloidosis [*70]. As is true with FMF, however, the situation is clearly better with *secondary amyloidosis*, and Gertz & Kyle [42], Escalante et al. [35], Zemer & Langevitz [123] and Fak et al. [37] have reported notable success in treating both small and large groups of amyloidosis patients with colchicine.

The Appendix gives the colchicine dose for Amyloidosis therapy.

Due to the achievement of a greater life expectancy, secondary amyloidosis has taken on increasing significance in patients with *mucoviscidosis*, for which there is a need for further research [63].

# Colchicine Therapy of Dupuytren's Contracture (DC)

Dupuytren's contracture (DC) is a spontaneous connective tissue disease affecting the palmar aponeurosis. It occurs predominantly in white males over the age of 40 [90, 113]. In Germany the number of people affected is possibly 1 million (1.25) [98]; in Sweden the reported number is 6% of the population over 55; and in Haugesund/Norway the figure is 9.4% of the men and 2.8% of the women over 16 years of age [90]. A genetic predisposition is considered to be confirmed [22].

The course the disease takes is not always progressive; reports include cases of arrest as well as regression [55], which makes it difficult to assess the success of conservative therapy such as the use of vitamin E, hyaluronic acid, hydrocortisone, collagenase, ultrasound, mechanical detachment or radiotherapy. Here again, placebo-controlled studies have not been undertaken to provide comparison. Studies with allopurinol have not been followed up [54].

Findings regarding Dupuytren's contracture have come from various sources: Borchardt & Lanz established that relapses after radical fasciectomy cannot be excluded [21]. Hazen and Krane (1971) showed in cell cultures that colchicine can increase collagenase activity 2 to 10 times. Deducing from this that colchicine could influence collagen formation in patients with fibromatosis, Dominguez-Malagon et al. [31] for the first time treated 3 different types of fibromatosis with colchicine: in a case of DC, in one of musculoaponeurotic desmoid fibromatosis and in a case of induratio penis plastica (Peyronie's disease). Optimal results were achieved with colchicine in the case of DC; there was extensive regression after 3 months and an absence of symptoms after 2 years. A case with rapid and extensive regression was reported by Pitts [81]. The doses administered were similar to those used in the treatment of FMF. There are no findings to date regarding the long-term use of colchicine in Dupuytren's contracture. It could turn out to be a cost-effective alternative to surgical therapy, which often is not ultimately convincing. Controlled studies must be performed to provide evidence of the efficacy of cholchicine before it can be recommended for general application in Dupuytren's contracture.

The Appendix gives the recommended colchicine dosage for treating Dupuytren's contracture.

# Colchicine Therapy of Behcet's Syndrome

Behcet's syndrome (after the Turkish dermatologist Hulusi Behcet) [10], is a chronic, multisystem disease of still unknown aetiology. An autoimmune background has been proposed as a possibility, but the question is still open [118]. The main characteristic is recurrent aphthae; the symptoms include both oral and genital ulcerations and inflammation of the skin and eyes. A publication by Kaklamani et al. [56] provides a review of the condition. The symptomatic therapy is based mainly on corticosteroids and immunosuppressives [43].

Behcet's syndrome is concentrated in specific geographic locations, namely in the Mediterranean regions and the Far East, where the number of people afflicted is from 80 to 370 per 100,000 adults [118]. The figure in Japan is around 8 cases per 100,000 adults. These instances can be compared with the Yorkshire number which is a mere 0.6 [112].

The disease appears in the 2nd to 4th decades of life. A diagnosis of Behcet's syndrome in a patient over 50 is most often incorrect [112]; there are, however, reports of an ever increasing number of children being diagnosed with the disease [62, 118].

The first reports on the use of colchicine in Behcet's syndrome came from Japanese authors in the 1970s [69, 74] followed by presentations of evidence of the efficacy of colchicine with regard to the ocular symptoms [74], with 66% improvement in 157 patients. Within the next decade there were more reports of the successful use [33, 95]. By the late 1990's several studies showed positive results with a daily colchicine dose of up to 1.8 mg [23, 43, 112]. Its benefits were also reported for the treatment of children [62].

As far as toxicological apects are concerned, patients with Behcet's syndrome generally show frequent oligo-/azoospermia subsequent to colchicine treatment [13], but this might be a result of the disease itself (vasculitis, epididymitis) [50]. Some authors believe that colchicine is preferable to steroids or immunosuppressives, especially regarding the aspect of long-term tolerability.

The Appendix gives the recommended colchicine dosage for the treatment of Behcet's syndrome.

## Colchicine Therapy of Vasculitis

Leucocytoclastic vasculitis is an inflammatory reaction in postcapillary venules that is characterized by lysis of infiltrated leucocytes. No clear treatment recommendations exist at the present time, and therapy with corticosteroids, immunosuppressives, antihistamines or prednisone has not proved satisfactory on the whole. Colchicine use in vasculitis is based mainly on its inhibition of the chemotaxis of polymorphonuclear leucocytes and stabilization of the leucocyte membrane (as discussed in the PHARMACOLOGY section). There have been a number of reports of the success of colchicine therapy in various forms of vasculitis [8, 20, 53, 75, 83, 114, 15]. Callen [24] reported treating 13 patients with leucocytoclastic vasculitis; 9 responded positively to the initial dose of 1.2 mg/day, whereas 3 patients showed only minor improvement. The only randomized study was carried out on 41 patients with cutaneous leucocytoclastic vasculitis but showed no superiority of colchicine over agents currently in use [93].

The Appendix contains the recommended colchicine dosage for treating vasculitis.

## Colchicine Therapy of Alcohol-Induced Cirrhosis, Primary Biliary Cirrhosis and Viral Hepatitis (B)

When *cirrhosis of the liver* is the result of chronic alcohol abuse or occurs within the context of virus hepatitis (B), there is progressive conversion of the liver parenchyma into scar-connective tissue in addition to progressive impairment of function and a variety of complications. The outcome can be fatal even before complete loss of liver function occurs. In the early 1970s the first studies were conducted to determine the therapeutic potential of colchicine in cirrhosis of the liver. Subsequent to these, a placebo-controlled study was begun by Kersenobich et al. [59] that eventually included 100 patients followed over a period of 14 years. The survival time with colchicine use was much longer (11 years) than for the placebo (3.5 years). In contrast to the placebo, no histological progression of fibrosis occurred with colchicine, and there were surprisingly normal findings in 2 cases. *Primary biliary cirrhosis* (*PBC*) is the cirrhotic late stage of a chronic non-purulent, destructive cholangitis. The cause is not known, although autoimmune processes are thought to be pathogenetically significant. Contrary to the results obtained in pilot studies [19, 11], those of Kaplan et al. [57] in their placebo-controlled trial yielded evidence of improved values for serum albumin, bilirubin, alkaline phosphatase, cholesterol and aminotransferases after 2 years of therapy. However, no change was noted in the symptoms, physical findings or biopsy findings. At the beginning of the third year colchicine treatment of all patients was begun. At the end of the fourth year the cumulative mortality rate was 47% for the patients receiving the placebo ($p<0.05$) and only 21% for those on colchicine. The medication was found to be therapeutically effective and safer for PBC patients even though it did not influence inflammation and fibrosis. Recently combinations of colchicine with ursodesoxycholic acid or steroids have been tested for use in PBC. Lindor et al. [67] treated 12 subjects with colchicine and low-dose prednisone for 2 years and were able to observe only a slight advantage over untreated patients. A placebo-controlled study of colchicine and ursodesoxycholic acid (UDCA) carried out by Vuoristo et al. [108] achieved beneficial results for both active treatments after 2 years, whereby the therapuetic effects of UDCA were more obvious on several parameters than those of colchicine. It must be said that the overall effect on survival rates was but minor with both active treatments. Most notably, colchicine led to a clear reduction of interleukin-2 and tumor necrosis factor-*a* levels, a feature of colchicine activity that requires further characterization. After a 2-year placebo-controlled study conducted by Miettinen et al. [71] there was evidence that treatment with UDCA or colchicine had a significant beneficial effect on some parameters of PBC and thus on the progression. These authors consider the treatment to be suitable for delaying liver transplantation for several years. Peterson et al. [79] investigated the effects of various cytokines on fibroproliferation and found that colchicine reduced PDGF (platelet-derived growth factor)-stimulated fibroproliferation by about 75%, which is comparable to the value obtained with other medication. The analysis of the authors points out, however, that the dose required for this effect is not achieved under normal circumstances, liver patients being a possible exception. In a randomized controlled trial of colchicine in patients with *chronic hepatitis B*, it was found that the substance shortened the acute phase considerably [66, 110]. Floreani et al. [40] conducted an open pilot study and reported antiviral effects against DNA viruses in 9 patients with chronic hepatitis B who had been treated with colchicine for 6 months. They found seronegativity in some patients for up to 12 months.

These studies, though minor in number, are of major importance as they provide evidence that colchicine appears to be very effective in the treatment of certain liver conditions. Certainly, the unsatisfactory situation in the therapy of these diseases makes it imperative that further controlled studies be carried out to clarify the potential of colchicine.

With regard to the recommended colchicine dosage refer to the Appendix.

# Colchicine Therapy of Idiopathic Pulmonary Fibrosis

## Pulmonary Fibrosis

Idiopathic pulmonary fibrosis (IPF) is a collagenosis, i.e. an inflammatory systemic disease of the connective tissue, a disease with poor prognosis, reduced survival time and high lethality. IPS is of unknown aetiology; the nature of the pathogenesis is for the most part (auto)immune [120]. It is characterized by inflammation, fibrosis and connective tissue alterations in the lung parenchyma. Its diagnosis must be preceded by the exclusion of other diseases such as neoplasms, other vascular conditions, environmental factors or granulomatous diseases such as sarcoidosis [77]. The various pathogenetic mechanisms involved in the (auto)immune processes essentially determine the medicinal-therapeutic options: corticosteroids, cyclosporin A, and pentoxifylline. Lately there have been reviews of the use of colchicine in IPF therapy [76, 77,120]. Even though the data base is still relatively small and based essentially on the work of the Mayo Clinic [29, 32], the existing theoretical basis for the use of colchicine [13, 34] is good enough to justify further study or, as some authors believe, good enough to recommend its use if other medicines prove ineffective or are poorly tolerated. Entzian et al. [34] studied closely its site of action in the pathogenetic cascade of idiopathic pulmonary fibrosis, achieving a breakthrough in a rationally grounded combination therapy that includes colchicine. There has also been a search for immunomodulators in *asthma therapy* since inflammatory elements seem to play a role in this condition. Kelly et al. [58] investigated colchicine with regard to its anti-inflammatory effects in early and late allergen-induced, IgE-mediated reactions of the respiratory tracts and found that partial inhibition of the IgE-mediated reaction resulted with clinically normal doses of colchicine.

The Appendix gives the recommended colchicine dosage for the treatment of idiopathic pulmonary fibrosis.

## Colchicine Therapy of Recurrent Pericarditis

Acute inflammation of the pericardium is usually of an idiopathic nature but may also be secondary, resulting from systemic infections, acute myocardial infarction, cardiac contusion or autimmune diseases. Relapses are seen in 15 to 32 percent of the cases [4]. Currently no optimal therapy or prophylaxis exists. Treatment options include nonsteroidal antirheumatics (NSAIDs), corticosteroids, immunosuppressives, and pericardectomy. Relapses are possible after dosage reduction or withdrawal of medication. The tested systemic anti-inflammatory efficacy of colchicine in FMF led to the use of this substance in recurrent pericarditis [89]. Further studies provided clear evidence of a negligible number of treatment failures with colchicine, and in most cases no relapses. However, in some instances relapses were only moderately inhibited [3, 48, 49, 72, 119]. At first colchicine was most often used in combination with other medicines, later alone. Some doubt has been expressed concerning the role of colchicine in preventing pericarditis relapses as no randomized, controlled studies have been undertaken [6], but because treatment failures have mainly occurred in patients previously treated with corticosteroids [4], colchicine is also recommended here as the preferable medication.

One of the most promising of the potential uses of colchicine may be as an alternative medication for the prevention of idiopathic recurrent pericarditis. In two cases of pericardial effusion in which treatment with NSAIDs, glucocorticoids and pericardiocentesis had been unsuccessful colchicine was said to have had a dramatic effect [5].

The Appendix gives the recommended colchicine dosage for treating pericarditis.

## Colchicine Therapy of Sweet's Syndrome

Four main features characterize Sweet's syndrome: fever, leucocytosis, inflammatory erythematous plaques and skin biopsy dominated by papillous dermal infiltrates with mature neutrophils [103]. Typically, steroids potassium iodide, dapsone or indometacin are chosen for treatment. Plantin et al. [82] reported the rapid, relapse-free improvement of a patient treated with colchicine in one case of Sweet's syndrome as well as a complete remission of symptoms within one one week in another case.

## Others

As postulated some time ago by Sterry [102], colchicine might be able to establish a place for itself among systemic therapies for various dermatoses. The treatment of *scleroderma* was reviewed in the early 1990s by Torres & Furst [107], who found no publications reporting improvement during colchicine administration. In a current review of the effects of colchicine in various skin diseases, Sullivan et al. [105] reported positive findings, whereby the results seemed to have depended on early and prolonged use and on the cumulative dose.

In the treatment of patients with FMF and Behcet's syndrome Sadjadi & Moshir [92] reported a very beneficial side effect on *acne vulgaris*, and there have been sporadic observations of this positive action in the therapy of panniculitis as well. [25].

A synergistic action on concomitant *psoriasis efflorescences* was discovered by Vuoristo et al. [108] in their study of the treatment of PBC with colchicine.

There are also case reports of an effect of colchicine on *methotrexate-induced nodulosis* in patients with rheumatoid arthritis [1, 116].

# Appendix

**Colchicine Dosage and Therapeutic Regimens**

| | Colchicine dose | Other therapeutic notes |
|---|---|---|
| Acute gout (Arthritis urica) and prophylaxis against attacks | up to 4 mg / 24 hours, max. 8 mg / attack | Then at least a 3-day colchicine-free interval |
| Chondrocalcinosis (Pseudogout) | | |
| FMF | 1 mg / day; weight-related in | 2 mg / day if insufficient |
| Amyloidosis | children | therapeutic response |
| Dupuytren's contracture | 0.5 – 1.5 mg / day | Initial 3 mg, maintenance 0.5 mg |
| Behçet's syndrome | 1 – 1.5 mg / day | |
| Vasculitis | 0.5 mg / day | |
| Primary biliary cirrhosis | 1 mg / day | |
| Alcoholic cirrhosis | 1 mg / day | On 5 days per week |
| Pulmonary fibrosis | 1 mg / day | |
| Pericarditis | 1 mg / day | Possibly initial dose of 3 mg / day |
| Sweet's syndrome | 0.5 – 1 mg / day | |
| Psoriasis vulgaris | 1 – 3 mg / day | Diarrhoea at higher doses |
| Acne vulgaris | 1 mg / day | |

# References


[1] Abraham Z, Rozenbaum M, Rosner I (1999) Colchicine therapy for low-dose-methotrexate-induced accelerated nodulosis in a rheumatoid arthritis patient. J Dermatol 26(10):691-4.

[2] Achtert G, Scherrmann JM, Christen MO (1989) Pharmacokinetics / bioavailability of Colchicinee in healthy male volunteers. Eur J Drug Metab Pharamcokinetics 14:317-22.

[3] Adler Y, Zandman-Godard G, Ravid M, et al. (1994) Usefulness of Colchicinee in preventing recurrences of pericarditis. Am J Cardiol 783:916-7.
[4] Adler Y, Finkelstein Y, Guindo J, et al. (1998) Colchicine treatment for recurrent pericarditis. A decade of experience. Circulation 97:2183-5.
[5] Adler Y, Guindo J, Finkelstein Y, et al. (1998) Colchicine for large pericardial effusions. Clin Cardiol 21:143-4.
[6] Adolph RJ (1990) Old drugs with new uses: Colchicine for treatment of recurrent pericarditis. Circulation 82:1505-6.
[7] Ahern MJ, Reid C, Gordon TP (1987) Does Colchicine work? Results of the first controlled study in gout. Aust N Z J Med 17:301-4.
[8] Asherson RA, Buchanan N, Kenwright S, et al. (1991) The normocomplemtemic urticarial vasculitis syndrome – report of a case and response to Colchicine. Clin Exp Dermatol 16:424-7.
[9] Baud FJ, Sabouraud A, Vicaut E, et al. (1995) Brief report: Treatment of severe Colchicine overdose with Colchicine-specific Fab fragments. N Engl J Med 332:642-5.
[10] Behcet H (1937) Über rezidivierende, aphthöse, durch einen Virus verursachte Geschwüre am Mund, am Auge und an den Genitalien. Dermatol Wschr 105:1152-7.
[11] Ben-Chetrit E, Levy M (1991) Colchicine prophylaxis in familial mediterranean fever: reappraisal after 15 years. Sem Arthritis Rheum 20:241-6.
[12] Ben-Chetrit E, Levy M (1998) Familial mediterranean fever. Lancet 351:659-64.
[13] Ben-Chetrit E, Levy M (1998) Colchicine: 1998 update. Semin Arthritis Rheum 28:48-59.
[14] Ben-Chetrit E, Backenroth R, Haimov-Kochman R, Pizov G (1998) Azoospermia in familial Mediterranean fever patients: role of Colchicine and amyloidosis. Ann Rheum Dis 57:259-60 (letter).
[15] Bennet WM (1988) Guide to drug dosage in renal failure. Clin Pharmacokinetics 15:326-54.
[16] Bennett WM, Aronoff GR, Morrison G, et al. (1983) Drug prescribing in renal failure: dosing guidelines for adults. Am J Kidney Dis III:155-171.
[17] Bergenudd H, Lindgärde F, Nilsson BE (1993) Prevalence of Dupuytren's contracture and its correlation with degenerative changes of the hands and feet and with criteria of general health. J Hand Surg Br 18:254-7.
[18] Better OS, Zemer D (1991) Familiäres Mittelmeerfieber. Dt Med Wschr 116:548-52.
[19] Bodenheimer H Jr, Schaffner F, Pezzullo J (1985) A randomised, double-blind controlled trial of Colchicine in primary biliary cirrhosis. Hepatology 5:968 (abstract).
[20] Bose SK (1996) Treatment of pustular vasculitis in rheumatoid arthritis with Colchicine. Natl Med J India 9:297-8.
[21] Borchardt B, Lanz U (1995) Dupuytren'sche Kontraktur – aktueller Stand in Forschung und Klinik. Therap Umschau 52:52-7.
[22] Burge P (1999) Genetics of Dupuytren's disease. Hand Clin 15:63-71.

[23] Çalgüneri M, Ertenli I, Kiraz S, et al. (1996) Effect of prophylactic benzathine penicillin on mucocutanous symptoms of Behçet's disease. Dermatology 192:125-8.
[24] Callen JP (1985) Colchicine is effective in controlling chronic cutaneous leucocytoclastic vasculitis. J Am Acad Dermatol 13:193-200.
[25] Callen JP (1998) Pannikulitis. In: Rheumatology; Second Edition, Klippel JH, Dieppe PA (eds.), pp 7/29.1-29.4, Mosby, London, Philadelphia, St. Louis, Sydney, Tokio.
[26] Caner JEZ (1965) Colchicine inhibition of chemotaxis. Arthritis Rheum 8:757-60.
[27] Cohen AS, Rubinow A, Anderson JJ, et al.(1987) Survival of patients with primary (AL) amyloidosis: Colchicine treated cases from 1971-1983 compared with cases seen in previous years, 1961-1973. Am J Med 82:1182-90.
[28] Conaghan PG, Day RO (1994) Risks and benefits of drugs used in the management and prevention of gout. Drug Safety 11:252-8.
[29] DeRemee RA (1994) New approaches to the treatment of pulmonary fibrosis (editorial). Eur Respir J 7:431-6.
[30] Dinarello CA, Wolff SM, Goldfinger SE, et al. (1974) Colchicine therapy for familial mediterranean fever. A double-blind trial. N Engl J Med 291:934-7.
[31] Dominguez-Malagon HR, Alfeiran-Ruiz, Chavarria-Xicotencatl P, Duran-Hernandez MS (1992) Clinical and cellular effects of Colchicine in fibromatosis. Cancer 69:2478-83.
[32] Douglas WW, Ryu JH, Bjoraker JA, et al. (1997) Colchicine versus prednisone as treatment of usual interstitial pneumonia. Mayo Clin Proc 72:201-9.
[33] Dührsen U, Kirch W (1985) Therapie des Behçet-Syndroms. Dtsch Med Wschr 110:267-70.
[34] Entzian P, Schlaak M, Seitzer U, et al. (1997) Antiinflammatory and antifibrotic properties of Colchicine: implications for idiopathic pulmonary fibrosis. Lung 175:41-51.
[35] Escalante A, Ehresmann GR, Quismorio FP (1991) Regression of reactive systemic amyloidosis due to ankylosing spondylitis following the administration of Colchicine. Arthritis Rheumatism 34:920-2.
[36] Espinoza LR, Cuéllar ML (1998) Psoriatic arthritis: Management. In: Rheumatology, Second Edition, Klippel JH, Dieppe PA (eds.), 6/23.1-23.6.
[37] Fak AS, Ozener C, Akoglu E (1992) Colchicine and secondary amyloidosis (letter). Ann Intern Med 117:795-6.
[38] Fam AG (1998) Gout in the elderly. Clinical presentation and treatment. Drugs Aging 13:229-43.
[39] Ferron GM, Rochdi M, Jusko WJ, Scherrmann JM (1996) Oral absorption characteristics and pharmacokinetics of Colchicine in healthy volunteers after single and multiple doses. J Clin Pharmacol 36:874-83.
[40] Floreani A, Lobello S, Brunetto M, et al. (1998) Colchicine in chronic hepatitis B: a pilot study. Aliment Pharmacol Ther 12:653-6.

[41] Gerster JC, Fallet GH (2000) Chondrokalcinose. In: Rheumatologie in Praxis und Klinik. Miehle, Fehr, Schattenkirchner, Tillmann (eds.), Seite 834-843, Thieme, Stuttgart, New York.

[42] Gertz MA, Kyle R (1991) Secondary systemic amyloidosis: response and survival in 64 patients. Medicine 70:246-56.

[43] Ghate JV, Jorizzo JL (1999) Behçet's disease and complex aphthosis. J Am Acad Dermatol 40:1-18.

[44] Goldfinger SE (1972) Colchicine for familial mediterranean fever. N Engl. J Med 287:1302.

[45] Graham W, Robert JB (1953) Intravenous Colchicine in the management of gouty arthritis. Ann Rheum Dis 12: 16-9.

[46] Gröbner W, Zöllner N (1996) Hyperurikämie. Urologe A 35:263-77.

[47] Gruberg L, Har-Zahav Y, Agranat O, Freimark D (1999) Acute myopathy induced by Colchicine in a cyclosporine treated heart transplant recipient: possible role of the multidrug resistance transporter. Transplant Proc 31:2157-8.

[48] Guindo J, Rodriguez de la Serna A, Ramio J et al. (1990) Recurrent Pericarditis. Relief with Colchicine. Circulation 82:1117-20.

[49] Guindo J, Adler Y, Spodick DH, et al. (1997) Colchicine for recurrent pericarditis: 51 patients followed up for 10 years. Circulation 96 (suppl I):1-29 (abstract).

[50] Haimov-Kochman R, Ben-Chetrit E (1998) The effect of Colchicine treatment on sperm production and function: a review. Human Reproduct 13:360-2.

[51] Harris MD, Siegel LB, Alloway JA (1999) Gout and hyperuricemia. Am Fam Physician 1999; 59:925-34.

[52] Harris ED, Krane SM (1971) Effects of Colchicine on collagenase in cultures of rheumatoid synovium. Arthritis Rheum 14:669.

[53] Hazen PG, Michel B (1979) Management of necrotizing vasculitis with Colchicine. Arch Dermatol 115:1303-6.

[54] Hueston JT (1992) Regression of Dupuytren's contracture. J Hand Surg Br 17B:453-7.

[55] Hueston JT, Tubiana R (1974) Dupuytren's disease. Churchill Livingston, Edinburgh, London.

[56] Kaklamani VG, Vaiopoulos G, Kaklmanis PG (1998) Behçet's disease. Semin Arthritis Rheum 27:197-217.

[57] Kaplan MN, Alling DW, Zimmermann HS, et al. (1986) A prospective trial of Colchicine in primary biliary cirrhosis. N Engl J Med 315:1448-54.

[58] Kelly SJ, Uri AJ, Freeland HS, et al. (1995) Effect of Colchicine on IgE-mediated early and late airway reactions. Chest 102:985-91.

[59] Kershenobich D, Uribe M, Suarez GI, et al. (1979) Treatment of cirrhosis with Colchicine. A double-blind randomized trial. Gastroenterology 77:532-6.

[60] Kershenobich D, Varga F, Garcia Tao G, et al. (1988) Colchicine in the treatment of cirrhosis of the liver. N Engl J Med 318:1709-13.

[61] Kot TV, Day RO, Brooks PM (1993) Preventing acute gout when starting allopurinol therapie. Colchicine or NSAIDs? Med J Austr 159:182-4.

[62] Krause I, Uziel Y, Guedj D, et al. (1997) Colchicine treatment in Behçet‘s disease: diverse efficacy in adults and children Arthritis Rheum 40 (suppl 9):67.

[63] Kuwertz-Bröking E, Koch HG, Schulze Everding A, et al. (1995) Colchicine for secondary nephropathic amyloidosis in cystic fibrosis. Lancet 345:1178-9 (letter).

[64] Lascaratos J (1995) ‚Arthritis‘ in Byzantium (AD 324-1453): unknown information from non-medical literature sources. Ann Rheum Dis 54:951-7.

[65] Levy M, Spino M, Read SE (1991) Colchicine: a state-of-the-art review. Pharmacotherapy 11:196-211.

[66] Lin DY, Sheen IS et al. (1996) A prospective randomized trial of Colchicine in prevention of liver cirrhosis in chronic hepatitis B patients. Aliment Pharmacol Ther 10:961-6.

[67] Lindor KD, Wiesner RH et al. (1991)The combination of prednisone and Colchicine in patients with primary sclerosing cholangitis. Am J Gastroenterol 85: 57-61.

[68] Livneh A, Langevitz P, Zemer D, Padeh S, Migdal A, Sohar E, Pras M (1996) The changing face of familial Mediterranean fever. Semin Arthritis Rheum 26:612-27.

[69] Matzumara N, Mizushima Y (1975) Leucocyte movement and Colchicine treatment in Behçet’s disease. Lancet 2:813.

[70] Merlini G (1995) Treatment of primary amyloidosis. Sem Hematol 32:60-79.

[71] Miettinen TA, Farkkila M et al. (1995) Serum cholestanol, cholesterol precursors, and plant sterols during placebo-controlled treatment of primary biliary cirrhosis with ursodesoxycholic acid and Colchicine. Hepatology 21:1261-8.

[72] Millaire A, De Groote P, Decoulx E, et al. (1994) Treatment of recurrent pericarditis with Colchicine. Europ Heart J 15:120-4.

[73] Milne ST, Meek PD (1998) Fatal Colchicine overdose: report of a case and review of the literature. Am J Emerg Med 16:603-8.

[74] Mizushima Y, Matsumara N, Mori M, et al. (1977) Colchicine in Behçet’s disease. Lancet 2:1037.

[75] Muramatsu C, Tanabe E (1985) Urticarial vasculitis: response to dapsone and Colchicine. J Am Acad Dermatol 13:1055.

[76] Nicod LP (1995) Traitement des fibroses pulmonaires idiopathiques. Schweiz Med Wschr 125:483-8.

[77] Nicod LP (1998) Recognition and treatment of idiopathic pulmonary fibrosis. Drugs 55:555-62.

[78] Ozen S, Karaaslan Y, Ozdemir O, et al. (1998) Prevalence of juvenile chronic arthritis and familial mediterranean fever in Turkey: a field study. J Rheumatol 25:2445-9.

[79] Peterson TC, Isbrucker RA, Hooper ML (1994) In vitro effect of platelet-derived growth factor on fibroproliferation and effect of cytokine antagonists. Immunopharmacology 28:259-70.

[80] Pittman JR, Bross MH (1999) Diagnosis and management of gout. Am Fam Physician 59:1799-1810.

[81] Pitts FN jun (1995) Colchicine therapy for palmar fibromatosis. N Engl J Med 333:393.

[82] Plantin P, Le Guillou S, Le Roux P, Guillet G (1987) Syndrome de sweet – 2 cas d'origine probablement infectieuse. Presse med 16:1333.

[83] Plotnick S, Hippert AS, Kantor G (1989) Colchicine and leucocytoclastic vasculitis. Arthritis Rheumatism 32:1489-90.

[84] Putterman C, Ben-Chetrit E, Caraco Y, Levy M (1991) Colchicine intoxication: clinical pharmacology, risk factors, features, and management. Sem Arthritis Rheum 21:143-55.

[85] Raghu G (1997) Idiopathic pulmonary fibrosis: a need for treatment with drugs other than corticosteroids – a role for antifibrotic agents? (editorial). Mayo Clin Proc 72:285-7.

[86] Rajan KT (1966) Lysosomes and gout. Nature 5039:559-60.

[87] Roberts WN, Liang MH, Stern SH (1987) Colchicine in acute gout: reassessment of risks and benefits. J Am Med Assoc 257:1920-2.

[88] Rochdi M, Sabouraud A, Girre C, et al. (1994) Pharmacokinetics and absolute bioavailability of Colchicine after i.v. and oral administration in healthy human volunteers and elderly subjects. Eur J Clin Pharmacol 46:351-4.

[89] Rodriguez de la Serna A, Guindo J, Marti V, Bayes de Luna A (1987) Colchicine for recurrent pericarditis. Lancet 2:1517 (letter).

[90] Ross DC (1999) Epidemiology of Dupuytren's disease. Hand Clin 15:53-62.

[91] Sabouraud A, Rochdi M, Urtizberea M, et al. (1992) Pharmacokinetics of Colchicine: a review of experimental and clinical data. Z Gastroenterol 30:35-9.

[92] Sadjadi SJ, Moshir M (1998) Treatment od Acne vulgaris with Colchicine. Acta Derm Venerol (Stockh) 78:388 (Letter).

[93] Sais G, Vidaller A, Jucgla A, et al. (1995) Colchicine in the treatment of cutanous leucocytoclastic vasculitis. Arch Dermatol 131:1399-402.

[94] Samuels J, Aksentijevich I, Torosyan Y, et al. (1998) Familial mediterranean fever at the millennium. Clinical spectrum, ancient mutations, and a survey of 100 american referrals to the National Institutes of Health. Medicine Baltimore 77:268-97.

[95] Sander HM, Randle HW (1986) Use of Colchicine in Behçet's syndrome. Cutis 37:344-8.

[96] Sarica K, Suzer O, Gurler A, et al. (1995) Urological involvement of Behcet patients and the effect of Colchicine on fertility. Eur Urol 27:39-42.

[97] Schattenkirchner M & Gröbner W (2000) Arthropathia urica. In: Rheumatologie in Praxis und Klinik. Miehle, Fehr, Schattenkirchner, Tillmann (eds.), Seite817-834, Thieme, Stuttgart, New York.

[98] Seegenschmiedt MH, Keilholz L (1998) Bei Dupuytren-Kontraktur in frühem Stadium hilft oft eine Strahlentherapie. Ärzte-Zeitung 16. Febr.:18.

[99] Seideman P, Fjellner B, Johannesson A (1987) Psoriatic arthritis treated with oral Colchicine. J Rheumatol 14:777-9.

[100] Speeg AU, Maldonado AL, Liaci J, Muirhead D (1992) Effect of cyclosporine n Colchicine secretion by a liver canalicular transporter studied in vivo. Hepatology 15:899-903.

[101] Speeg KV, Maldonado AL, Liaci J, Muirhead D (1992) Effect of cyclosporine on Colchicine secretion by the kidney multidrug transporter studied in vivo. J Pharmacol Exp Ther 261:50-5.

[102] Sterry W (1984) Kolchizin in der Dermatotherapie. Der Hautarzt 35:65-7.

[103] Su WPD, Fett DC, Gibson LE (1995) Sweet's Syndrome: acute febrile neutrophilic dermatosis. Semin Dermatol 14:173-8.

[104] Sudeck H, Horstmann R (1999) Gentest ermöglicht Diagnose des Familiären Mittelmeerfiebers. Dt Ärztebl 96:1002-4.

[105] Sullivan TP, King LE Jr, Boyd AS (1998) Colchicine in dermatology. J Am Acad Dermatol 39:993-9.

[106] Tateishi T, Soucek P, Caraco Y, et al. (1997) Colchicine biotransformation by human liver microsomes. Identification of CYP3A4 as the major isoform responsible for Colchicine demethylation. Biochem Pharmacol 53:111-16.

[107] Torres MD, Furst DE (1990) Treatment of generalized systemic sclerosis. Rheum Dis Clin North Am 16: 217-41.

[108] Vuoristo M, Farkkila M ert al. (1995) A placebo-controlled trial of primary biliary cirrhosis. Treatment with Colchicine and ursodeoxycholic acid. Gastroenterology 108:1470-8.

[109] Wallace SL, Singer JZ (1988) Review: systemic toxicity associated with intravenous administration of Colchicine – guidelines for use. J Rheumatol 15:495-9.

[110] Wang YH, Lee SD et al. (1994) A double-blind randomized controlled trial of Colchicine in patients with hepatitis B virus-related postnecrotic cirrhosis. J Hepatol 21:872-7.

[111] Warnes TW, Smith A, Lee F, et al. (1984) A controlled trial of Colchicine in primary biliary cirrhosis. Hepatology 4:1022 (abstract).

[112] Wechsler B, Piette JC (1992) Behçet's diesease. Br Med J 304:1199-2000.

[113] Weinzierl G, Flügel M, Geldmacher J (1993) Fehlen der Effektivität der alternativ nicht-chirurgischen Behandlungsverfahren bei Morbus Dupuytren. Chirurg 64:492-4.

[114] Werni R, Schwarz T, Gschnait F (1986) Colchicine treatment of urticarial vasculitis. Dermatologica 172:36-40.

[115] Wiles JC, Hansen RC, Lynch PJ (1985) Urticarial vasculitis treated with Colchicine. Arch Dermatol 121:802-5.

[116] Williams FM, Cohen PR, Arnett FC (1998) Accelerated cutaneous nodulosis during methotrexate therapy in a patient with rheumatoid arthritis. J Am Acad Dermatol 39(2 Pt 2):359-62.

[117] Wise CM, Agudelo CA (1998) Diagnosis and management of complicated gout. Bull Rheum Dis 47:2-5.

[118] Yazici H, Yurdakul S, Hamaryudan V (1995) Behçet's disease: How should we treat it? Clin Immunother 3:102-7.

[119] Yazigi A; Abou-Charaf LC (1998) Colchicine for recurrent pericarditis in children. Acta-Paediatr 87:603-4.

[120] Zabel P (1995) Pathogenese interstitieller Lungenveränderungen bei Kollagenosen – Folgerungen für die Therapie. Immun Infekt 23:97-106.

[121] Zemer D, Pras M, Sohar E, et al. (1986) Colchicine in the prevention and treatment of the amyloidosis of familial Mediterranean fever. N Engl J Med 314:1001-5.

[122] Zemer D, Livneh A, Danon ,YL, et al. (1991) Long-term Colchicine treatment in children with familial mediterranean fever, Arthritis Rheum 34:973-7.

[123] Zemer D, Livneh A, Langevitz P (1992) Reversal of the nephrotic syndrome by Colchicine in amyloidosis of familial mediterranean fever. Ann Int Med 116:426.

In: Arthritis Research: Treatment and Management
Editor: F. Columbus, pp. 81-105
ISBN 1-59033-984-3


*Chapter IV*

# Aquatic Exercise in the Treatment of Rheumatoid Arthritis and Juvenile Idiopathic Arthritis

***Else Marie Bartels*, Hans Lund[1] and Bente Danneskiold-Samsøe[1]***

*The Danish National Library of Science and Medicine,Copenhagen

[1]The Parker Institute, Frederiksberg, DK

## Abstract

Rheumatoid arthritis is a chronic inflammatory disease affecting the joint, and as the disease develops it may cause severe disability. The disease shows periods of active inflammation and periods of no inflammation. Apart from treatment of the inflammatory condition, it is important to keep the patients at the best obtainable functional level, both during inflammation and in the periods with no inflammation. This article examines aquatic exercise, also known as pool therapy, hydrotherapy, and sometimes in earlier literature even balneotherapy, which is treatment in water involving, for the patient specially designed, aquatic exercises. Pool therapy has many advantages for both rheumatoid-arthritis and juvenile-idiopathic-arthritis patients where all training has to take these patients' special joint condition into consideration, and where the changed condition in water will allow training which cannot be achieved on land.

## Introduction

Rheumatoid arthritis is a chronic inflammatory disease affecting the joint, and as the disease develops it may cause severe disability. The disease shows periods of active inflammation and periods of no inflammation [1]. Apart from treatment of the inflammatory condition, it is important to keep the patients at the best obtainable functional level, both during inflammation and in the periods with no inflammation [2].

Since the joints are affected, and since the joints may be very painful, there is a snowball effect on the functional level of the muscles involved with movements of the affected joints. Furthermore, the inflammation causes damage to the joints which may cause pain even when not inflamed. The pain and joint condition will lead to a decrease in the use of muscles connected with the affected joints, and will following create both changes in the electrical activity, and atrophy of these muscles, where these two factors are not directly correlated [3]. One must keep in mind though, that inflammation of the muscle is hardly ever found in rheumatoid arthritis [4], and all muscle wasting or damage may therefore be considered a secondary effect of the disease. In addition, joint deformities and pain might indirectly lead to reduction in strength by arthrogeneous muscle inhibition [5]. The overall effect may soon be crippling for the patients and lead to a life with high dependence on relatives or home help and a negative effect on their quality of life [6,7].

Juvenile rheumatoid arthritis or juvenile idiopathic arthritis is a disease affecting children [8], and it presents itself as inflammation of the joints. The cause is unknown, and the disease is not necessarily chronic, but in many cases the problems caused by the joint inflammation and the treatment of the disease are similar to the problems seen in rheumatoid arthritis and the treatment of this disease [9]. Very little research has been carried out in the use of pool therapy for this group of patients, and we have therefore decided to include the little knowledge available on the matter in this chapter.

Although no cure has been found for either rheumatoid arthritis or juvenile idiopathic arthritis, the new disease-modifying drugs like metotrexate alone, or this drug in combination with others, seem to lower the disease activity and, in particular, do limit or stop the erosion of the joints during inflammation [10]. With this major step forward, it is even more important to keep the arthritis patients fit and mobile and develop the physical-therapy part of the treatment to match this development in the medical side of the treatment.

For both rheumatoid arthritis and juvenile idiopathic arthritis, a sole treatment of the inflammatory condition is therefore only to some degree useful, if it is not combined with a focussed effort to keep the arthritis patient physically active enough to prevent a lowering of the patient's functional level further than cannot be prevented by the caused joint damage [7]. It is, furthermore, important to keep patients who are waiting for joint replacement as fit as possible with the best possible level of muscle strength to make a joint replacement successful.

The aim of physical-therapy treatment of rheumatoid-arthritis and juvenile-idiopathic-arthritis patients is therefore to give the patients an improved physical capacity, increased muscle strength, improved balance and coordination of movements, improved pain control, and better joint mobility [11].

Strength training of muscle in rheumatoid-arthritis and juvenile-idiopathic-arthritis patients is challenging due to the painful and fragile joints. It is not possible to put too much load on the joints, and even in light exercise, it is not wise to take the pain away with drugs, since the same pain has to stop a movement if this movement puts too much strain on the joint. With more joint damage, it may not be possible to carry out a whole range of exercises, normally possible on land, with an arthritis patient.

Aquatic exercise, also known as pool therapy, hydrotherapy, and sometimes in earlier literature even balneotherapy, is treatment in water involving, for the patient specially designed, aquatic exercises. Pool therapy has many advantages for both rheumatoid-arthritis and juvenile-idiopathic-arthritis patients where all training has to take these patients' special joint condition into consideration, and where the changed condition in water will allow training which cannot be achieved on land.

Use of hot-water treatment has been known for several thousand years [12,13], and warm-water treatment alone is known to ease pain, decrease stiffness and cause muscle relaxation [14,16], and this has been further developed with various forms of salt and/or sulphur treatment [17,20], mud packs [21,22], and jet streams [22].

In pool therapy the hot-water element is included, and the pool is usually at a higher temperature than normally found in swimming pools, most frequently between 32° and 36 °C [23]. Hot-water treatment alone gives the arthritis patients decrease in pain sensation, decreases stiffness of the muscular-skeletal system, and causes muscle relaxation [14, 16]. Hot-water treatment is therefore a much better base on which to start training of arthritis patients than a similar training on land. Hot-water treatment in itself does not create long-term improvement, but it has an instant short-term effect which motivates the patients for further participation [13,14,17,18]. The overall aims of the treatment are to increase the joint mobility, improve the aerobic capacity, improve muscle strength, and improve coordination and balance [24, 27].

The physics of water may be used in various ways during aquatic training. The buoyancy of the water will take some of the load off the involved joints and make it possible to train joints which must not be load-bearing. The buoyancy combined with the warm water does also give the patient a feeling of being able to move more easily than on land and thereby make training more feasible. It is possible to achieve the same physical capacity by training emerged in water, compared to training on land, which again helps achieving the goal of increasing the physical capacity of the arthritis patients [28]. Furthermore, the larger heat transfer in water affects the energetic conditions during exercise [29,30].

Water has a density not much higher than that of man, but very much higher than the density of air. This is seen as a resistance to all movement in water and, used correctly, creates ideal conditions for strength and balance training [31], other aims when training rheumatoid arthritis patients. Water walking alone has also proved effective to improve cardio-respiratory fitness and is recommended in cases where weight-bearing activities as jogging are not possible [32].

The higher hydrostatic pressure, a person is exposed to when immersed in water, will increase the pumping of venous blood towards the heart and will also affect breathing, when a person is immersed to the neck. This will again help when training physical capacity [33].

In pool therapy there are different schools with more or less described principles and exercise patterns. The clearly described methods are Halliwick [34], Bad Ragaz [35, 36], and WATSU [37, 38]. The pool therapy carried out in a particular place may be true to one of these methods, a mixture of these, or a patient-focussed set of exercises, either for the individual patient or for a particular patient group [15].

What seems uniform for most of the described studies [39, 48], and for programmes [49, 50] known in Denmark, is that the treatment is only taking place for very short time intervals of 3-12 weeks, and only for 1-3 times per week. A problem in a lot of studies assessing the use of pool therapy in treatment of rheumatoid arthritis is also that the design does not lend itself to give an evidence-based assessment of the study.

Based on the aims for an applied treatment, it is important to make certain that the chosen parameters, used to measure if the effects of the treatment, are good and reliable measures for achieving their aims, and that it is physiologically possible to fulfil the aims in the defined period of time and with the defined exercise programme.

It has been shown that physical training has a positive effect in keeping and even improving the functional level of rheumatoid-arthritis patients [39, 40]. Another study [51] has shown an increase in isokinetic muscle strength of m. quadriceps of rheumatoid-arthritis patients following only three weeks of training. Since rheumatoid arthritis patients usually are unfit both in terms of physical capacity, muscle strength, and mobility of joints, a programme of physical training is expected to have a measurable improvement of at least physical capacity and joint mobility after a couple of weeks, as is found in healthy groups. If, on the other hand, one wants to look at increase of muscle fibre diameter and substantial increase of muscle strength, it will take longer, since even training of athletes will not show an effect on these parameters in less than 8 weeks, while a change in the nervous stimulation of muscles takes place earlier [52].

Despite of a large collection of studies concerning pool therapy, there are still very few studies giving a clear assessment of the effect of this treatment on rheumatoid-arthritis and juvenile-idiopathic-arthritis patients. The aim of this chapter is to give an evaluation of pool therapy used in the treatment of rheumatoid-arthritis patients and in the treatment of juvenile-idiopathic-arthritis patients. Although the short-term effect of immersion in hot water could be added, the concern here is if the method improves one, some, or all of the following:

- Physical capacity
- Joint mobility
- Muscle strength
- Balance and coordination
- Pain management.

Possible negative side effects of the treatment will also be discussed.

## Inclusion Criteria for Pool Therapy Studies

Only studies concerning rheumatoid-arthritis patients or juvenile-rheumatoid/idiopathic-arthritis patients are included with the exception, that mixed studies are acceptable if the data on rheumatoid-arthritis patients can be separated from data from other patient groups. With the juvenile-idiopathic-arthritis, mixed patient groups never seem to be a problem.

Not all included studies will necessarily look at physical capacity, joint mobility, muscle strength, and balance and coordination, but as long as a study does deal with one of these physiological entities, a study has been included.

Another inclusion/exclusion criterion is that there must be a clear programme of aquatic exercises.

To find the studies, searches have been carried out in the bibliographic databases Medline (1966-2003), EMBASE (1980-2003), Cinahl (1982-2003) and Web of Science (1945-2003), and the Cochranedatabase has also been consulted. Since pool therapy for many years was not part of the methods exposed to studies leading to publications in peer-reviewed journals, the Danish National Library of Science and Medicine's catalogue was searched to reveal if more unknown studies of aquatic exercise existed in older monographs, and reference lists were checked for studies not found in the bibliographic databases.

## Description of Selected Studies

Table 1 shows the selected studies on effect of pool therapy on rheumatoid arthritis. The patient groups in the studies are all clearly defined as rheumatoid arthritis, and in most studies the age group spans from early to late fifties. The choice seems to be patients in functional class II-III, although some class I do participate in a few studies. The reason for this may possibly be that class II and III are mobile enough to participate on a regular basis in the training programmes, and their disease is severe enough to motivate to keep or improve the functional level.

Where drug treatment is mentioned, it is continued as before the study during the period of pool therapy, and can be said to represent a patient group which is stabilised in terms of medical treatment.

The pool therapy is lasting from 3-12 weeks in all studies, except for two, and the treatment takes place either every day (3 weeks therapy) or from 1-3 times a week. For the two studies lasting for two years with therapy once a week except for holidays, one study suffers from such a high drop-out rate [55], that nothing can be concluded from the study, while the other manages to keep the participants and show a long-lasting beneficial effect [54].

Not all studies are controlled, and the controlled studies may only have a small group of patients in each group, which in modern evidence-based medicine is a problem. Likewise, some studies are randomised, but with small groups and some patients dropping out, it may be questioned, if such a study ought to be included, were there plenty to choose between. There is an ethical aspect of this too. One pilot study finds an overpowering effect of hydrotherapy on muscle strength [45] which makes it difficult to defend keeping an untreated control group, if this group is not offered the therapy during a fairly short time span following the study.

Exercises in water may be anything from swimming or moving in water to a very structured programme. The few studies available do not make it possible to compare the effects of various types of water exercise, and it is therefore only possible to give an overall description of measured effect of pool therapy.

**Table 1. Studies of the Effect of Pool Therapy on Rheumatoid Arthritis Patients**

| Authors/ year | Randomised (R)/ Controlled (C)/ No Controls(NC) | Patient-Category/ number/ Sex/ Age | Drug treatment | Treatment type/ Length of treatment/ Frequency of treatment/ Length of session | Effect parametres | Results | Conclusion |
|---|---|---|---|---|---|---|---|
| C. Dial, R.A. Windsor 1985 [44] | NC | RA functional class II or III<br>Average disease duration 6.5 years<br>12 patients, 5♀, 7♂<br>Average age 59 | Not reported | Training programme in pool for a group for 8 weeks, twice a week for one hour, including ROM exercises, water ambulation, kicks and water games | - Pain<br>- Mobility<br>- Tenderness<br>- Joint movements<br>- Functional ability<br>- Activity of daily living (ADL) | Significant improvement of mobility and functional ability, as well as a subjective favourable impact due to social support during therapy sessions. | Pool therapy have a positive effect on functional ability, but lack of controls and randomisation weakens the results |
| B.Danneskiold-Samsøe, K.Lyngberg, T.Risum, M.Telling 1987 [45] | NC | RA functional class II or III.<br>No acute inflammation<br>Average disease duration 14 years<br>8 patients, 6♀, 2 ♂.<br>Average age 54 years | Not reported | Training programme in hot pool for two months, twice a week for 45 minutes.<br>Individual training and group training, mainly various types of leg exercises. | - Muscle strength<br>- Aerobic capacity test (Åstrand) | A significant improvement of both muscle strength and aerobic capacity was found following the pool therapy treatmernt. | Pool therapy shows a positive effect on the physical ability of rheumatoid arthritis patients, but randomised, controlled studies are needed to confirm this. |

**Table 1. Studies of the Effect of Pool Therapy on Rheumatoid Arthritis Patients (Continued)**

| Authors/ year | Randomised (R)/ Controlled (C)/ No Controls(NC) | Patient-Category/ number/ Sex/ Age | Drug treatment | Treatment type/ Length of treatment/ Frequency of treatment/ Length of session | Effect parametres | Results | Conclusion |
|---|---|---|---|---|---|---|---|
| M. Minor, J.E.Hewett, R.R.Webel, S.K.Anderson, D.R.Kay 1989 [39] | R, C | RA and OA<br>40 RA patients, all categories, average age 54.3 years.<br>80 OA patients, average age 63.8 years | Drug treatment continued as before pool therapy during the therapy period, varied according to the need of each particular patient. | Three types of physical training, out of which one is the control group. 12 weeks of training, 3 times a week with one hour training, and follow up after one year.<br><br>Aerobic walking (group 1), aerobic exercises in pool (group 2) and 'range of motion' (ROM)-exercises (control group) | - Aerobic capacity test (Naughton)<br>- "Sit-and-reach test"<br>- Joint movements in shoulder and ankle<br>- Joint assessment (pain and swelling)<br>- Grip strength<br>- Walking test<br>- Pain<br>- Length of morning stiffness<br>- Arthritis Impact Measurement Scale (AIMS)<br>- Tennesse Self Concept Scale (The physical ability part) | Pool therapy showed fewer active joints, decrease in morning stiffness, improved walk, larger grip strength, improved 'sit-and-reach test', as well as improved AIMS for physical activity, fear and depression. | Only 70% in all groups completed the full programme and were measured after 3 months and after a year from the end of the treatment. Of these 70%, all had got an interest in staying fit and were equal when comparing effect parametres related to the diseases. Directly after the finished treatment, pool therapy showed most improvement, then aerobic walking, and to a lesser degree ROM. None of the training programmes caused any increase in desease activity or other side effects. |

**Table 1. Studies of the Effect of Pool Therapy on Rheumatoid Arthritis Patients (Continued)**

| Authors/ year | Randomised (R)/ Controlled (C)/ No Controls(NC) | Patient- Category/ number/ Sex/ Age | Drug treatment | Treatment type/ Length of treatment/ Frequency of treatment/ Length of session | Effect parametres | Results | Conclusion |
|---|---|---|---|---|---|---|---|
| C.H.Stenström, B.Lindell, E.Swanberg, P.Swanberg, K. Harms-Ringdahl, R.Nordemar 1991 [54] | C | RA functional class II Average disease duration 12 years (therapy group) and 14 years (controls). 60 patients, 8♂. and 52 ♀. Average age 52 years. 30 exposed to pool therapy, and 30 as controls. The two groups comparable in terms of age, sex, and disease duration. | Not reported | Exercises in pool for two years, once a week 40 minutes, with two months break in summer and two weeks break over Christmas. Groups of 6 patients in each session. Exercises described Control group without training. Effect measurements blinded. | - (Ritchie Articular Index)RAI - Grip sterngth - Radiological assessment - Erythrocyte sedimentation rate, haemoglobin and Waaler-Rose's test - Pain in 6 different functional situations - Structured interviews (social and psychological aspects) | Pool therapy group: Better grip strength and higher level of physical activity. Significantly higher number admitted to hospital from the control group compared to the pool group. | The different needs between the patients in an RA group seems to be met in pool therapy. The result is that the therapy group improves their level of physical activity. Intensive pool therapy does not show any aggravation of the disease. There is a significant positive effect two years after completion of the pool therapy when the therapy group is compared to the control group. |

**Table 1. Studies of the Effect of Pool Therapy on Rheumatoid Arthritis Patients (Continued)**

| Authors/ year | Randomised (R)/ Controlled (C)/ No Controls(NC) | Patient-Category/ number/ Sex/ Age | Drug treatment | Treatment type/ Length of treatment/ Frequency of treatment/ Length of session | Effect parametres | Results | Conclusion |
|---|---|---|---|---|---|---|---|
| R.B.M.Landewé , R.Peeters, R.L.P.Verreuss, B.A.Masek, H.S.Goeithe, 1992 [46 ] | C | RA functional class II or III<br>No acute inflammation<br>27 patients in hot mineral –water pool and 19 patients (controlgroup) in hot pool<br>The groups were mathched for age, sex and disease duration | Not reported | Both test and control group did exercises in pool for 12 weeks, once a week for 30 minutes.<br>Exercises described. | - Morning stiffness<br>-Ritchie's index<br>- Pain (VAS)<br>- Erythrocyte counting<br>- Activity of daily living (ADL)<br>- Psychological aspects of RA | No differences found between pool therapy carried out in a mineral water and in a tap water pool.<br>Pool therapy gives a significant improvement on morning stiffness and on the subjective, but not on the objective parameters. | The type of water does not make a different when applying pool therapy, but the therapy has a positive effect on morning stiffness and on the subjective, but not on the objective parameters. |

**Table 1. Studies of the Effect of Pool Therapy on Rheumatoid Arthritis Patients (Continued)**

| Authors/ year | Randomised (R)/ Controlled (C)/ No Controls(NC) | Patient- Category/ number/ Sex/ Age | Drug treatment | Treatment type/ Length of treatment/ Frequency of treatment/ Length of session | Effect parametres | Results | Conclusion |
|---|---|---|---|---|---|---|---|
| T.M.Hansen, G.Hansen, A.M.Langgaard, J.O.Rasmussen 1993 [55] | R,C | RA. Functional class I or II.<br>49♀ and 26 ♂.<br>Average age 52 years.<br>10 patients left the study, leaving 65 patients in total. | Patients continued earlier prescribed drugs during the study. | Paticipants distributed in 5 groups. The control group had no instructions concerning training. The other 4 groups had a described programme for 15 minutes followed by aerobic training on land or in a pool for 15-30 minutes.<br>Two years training once a week instructed by a physiotherapist.<br>Patients encouraged to train at least three times a week and best every day.<br>Exercises described.<br>Effect assessing blinded. | - Duration of morning stiffness<br>- joint pain (VAS)<br>- number of swollen joints<br>- use of prescribed drugs<br>- Health Assessment Questionnaire (HAQ)<br>- Erythrocyte sedimentation rate<br>- Aerobic capacity test (Åstrand)<br>- Functional score<br>- Isometric muscle strength | No difference found between the groups on any assessed parameter | It is impossible to conclude anything from this study despite a well-set-up procedure due to a very low patient number in each group and a high drop-out percentage. |

Table 1. Studies of the Effect of Pool Therapy on Rheumatoid Arthritis Patients (Continued)

| Authors/ year | Randomised (R)/ Controlled (C)/ No Controls(NC) | Patient-Category/ number/ Sex/ Age | Drug treatment | Treatment type/ Length of treatment/ Frequency of treatment/ Length of session | Effect parametres | Results | Conclusion |
|---|---|---|---|---|---|---|---|
| J.Hall, S.M.Skevington , P.J.Maddison, K.Chapman 1996 [40] | R,C | RA, functional class II-III<br>139 patients in 4 groups. | Only patients with a stable use of prescribed drugs included. | Treatment for four weeks, twice a week for 30 minutes. One group treated with relaxation, one with relaxation in pool at a water temperature of 36 °C, one with exercises on land, and one with aquatic exercises. All training was guided by physiotherapists. Exercises described. | - Ritchie Articular Index (RAI)<br>- Morning stiffness<br>- Grip strength<br>- Joint mobility<br>- C-reactive protein<br>- McGill pain questionnaire<br>- The Beliefs in Pain Control Questionnaire<br>- Arthritis Impact Measuremennt Scale (AIMS2) | The pool-therapy group showed a significantly higher positive effect on RAI right after training. Training-on-land group showed a stronger effect on RAI three month following training. The pool therapy showed a significant improvement on knne-joint mobility. This group did also show a shigher positive effect at followup in "Affect" in AIMS2. Training on land showed a significantly positive effect on pain following training. | Pool therapy and exercises on land give a significantly higher measurable improvement than the relaxation control groups. There were no negative side effects of the training. All four treatments had some positive effects on the patients. |

**Table 1. Studies of the Effect of Pool Therapy on Rheumatoid Arthritis Patients (Continued)**

| Authors/ year | Randomised (R)/ Controlled (C)/ No Controls(NC) | Patient-Category/ number/ Sex/ Age | Drug treatment | Treatment type/ Length of treatment/ Frequency of treatment/ Length of session | Effect parametres | Results | Conclusion |
|---|---|---|---|---|---|---|---|
| P.Rintala, H.Kettunen, J.A.McCubbin 1996 [41] | R,C | RA funktional class I-II<br>Average disease duration 10.4 years.<br>29 ♀, 5♂.<br>Average age 48 ±10 years.<br>Matched groups. | All patients stable concerning drug treatment (gold, sulfasalazine, prednisone, methotrexate, D-penicillamine) | Training programme in pool with a water temperature of 30 ° C. 12 weeks training, twice a week for 45 minutes during the first two weeks, then increasing to 60 minutes for the last two weeks. Average participation (out of 24) 22 times, minimum 20 times. 9 paticipants per session.<br>Exercises described. | - Aerobic capacity test<br>- Muscle strength and endurance<br>- Joint mobility<br>- Pain (+/- & VAS) | Pool –therapy group significantly improved concerning strength and joint mobility. | Pool therapy is a treatment which gives RA patients improved strength and mobility without any negative effect on disease activity. |

**Table 1. Studies of the Effect of Pool Therapy on Rheumatoid Arthritis Patients (Continued)**

| Authors/ year | Randomised (R)/ Controlled (C)/ No Controls(NC) | Patient- Category/ number/ Sex/ Age | Drug treatment | Treatment type/ Length of treatment/ Frequency of treatment/ Length of session | Effect parametres | Results | Conclusion |
|---|---|---|---|---|---|---|---|
| S.Sanford Smith, M.MacKay-Lyons, S.Nunes-Clement 1998 [42] | R,C | RA funktional class II or III.<br>Pool-therapy group: 9♀ and 3♂.<br>Average age 61.9 years.<br>Average disease duration 20.2 years<br>Range-of-motion (ROM) Group: 10♀ and 2♂.<br>Average age 54.9 years.<br>Average disease duration 11.6 years. | Prescribed drugs unchanged during the period of pool therapy or ROM-therapy. | Pool therapy at 36 °C for 10 weeks, three times per week for one hour. Five patients per session.<br>Exercises described and instructed thruogh the whole programme by physiotherapist.<br>ROM-group : ROM-evxercises targetting shoulders, hands and knees. Isometric strenthening exercises, and if no active joint, isotonic exercises.<br>Exercises instructed individually at the beginning of the programme, and then continued at home, repeating the exercise sequence 2-3 times a day.<br>Control by physiotherapist every three weeks. | - Count of active joints<br>- Grip strength<br>- Duration of morning stiffness<br>- Erythrocyte-sedimentation rate<br>- HAQ<br>- Aerobic capacity test | No differences found between the pool-therapy group and the ROM-exercise group.<br>Both groups showed improved exercise tolenrance and improved joint mobility. | Both pool therapy and exercises on land create improvements in jojnt mobility and in exercise tolerance.<br>Neither type of exercise had any negative effects on the activity of the disease. The lack of diffent effects of the different type of exercise training may be due to the low number of participants in this study and to the reported low participation rate. |

**Table 1. Studies of the Effect of Pool Therapy on Rheumatoid Arthritis Patients (Continued)**

| Authors/ year | Randomised (R)/ Controlled (C)/ No Controls(NC) | Patient-Category/ number/ Sex/ Age | Drug treatment | Treatment type/ Length of treatment/ Frequency of treatment/ Length of session | Effect parametres | Results | Conclusion |
|---|---|---|---|---|---|---|---|
| M.Yurtkuran, M.A.Yurtkuran, K.Dilek, M.Güllülü, Y.Karakoc, L.Özbek, Ü.Bingöl, 1999 [43] | R,C | RA<br>Functional class II and III.<br>Pool-therapy group: 26♀ and 6♂.<br>Average age 44 years.<br>Average disease duration 15.5 years.<br>Drug therapy group: 21♀ and 4♂.<br>Average age 39 years.<br>Average disease duration 12 years. | None of the participants were treated with DMARD or glucocorticoids during the two months period prior to the study. None of the patients took NSAIDs or any physical therapy. The control group/drug therapy group was treated with 3.5 mg/kg CsA daily during the two months study. | The pool-therapy group was given relaxing exercises in a 35° C pool for three weeks, every day for 30 minutes.<br>The drug-therapy group was treated as described. | - pain on VAS<br>- Grip strength<br>- Morning stiffness<br>- Number of tender joints<br>- Haemoglobin (Hb)<br>- Erythrocyte sedimentation rate(ESR)<br>- C-reactive protein at baseline (CRP) | Reduction in pain was seen in both groups, but at a higher level in the pool-therapy group.<br>Both groups showed an improved grip strength.<br>Both groups showed a reduction in morning stiffness.<br>Hb, ESR and CRP did not change during treatment in the two groups.<br>No negative side effects in the pool-therapy group. Nephrotoxicity, hirsutism,gastrointestinal disturbance and gingival hyperplasia were seen in the drug-therapy group. | Improvement in clinical symptoms of RA was seen earlier in the pool-therapy group than in the drug-therapy group, although they both showed similar effects. The pool-therapy group showed no side effect from the treatment while the drug therapy had some not trin´vial negative effects. |

Despite the above mentioned weaknesses, there is one very strong point going through all the studies: Not one study has reported a worsening of the patients' condition, and no negative side effects have been seen. This is expressed most forcefully in the study by Yurtkuran et al [43], where pool therapy is compared to cyclosporin A treatment. The improvements in clinical symptoms in this study are the same following either of the two treatments, but the drug treatment shows some unwanted side effects (nephrotoxicity, hepatotoxidity, and hirsutism).

The advantage of hydrotherapy, according to all the studies, is that it is possible to meet the individual patient´s training needs while working with a smaller group.

As an overall result, pool therapy improves the physical ability and activity, both in terms of strength and joint mobility, and probably also morning stiffness. It may have a longer-lasting effect on pain, but this is not certain. From the two years study by Stenström [54], it is seen that the effect of the therapy is still there two years after the completion of the therapy, and the therapy group showed less need for hospitalisation compared to the control group, a strong indication of the beneficial effect of pool therapy.

As a final outcome of the aquatic exercise therapy, there are several reports of enjoyment of the therapy which motivates for further participation, a parameter not easily measured or evaluated.

When looking at the studies concerning juvenile idiopathic arthritis, the number of patients in each study is generally small, and the studies, apart from Takken 2003, may be classified as pilot studies.

The age groups studied vary in the range of 4 to 18 years, but the groups are mainly characterised by consisting of growing children with a strong need to develop and keep their muscle mass, and to keep their joint movement as close to normal angle as possible. The functional class of the participating children are only described in some studies, and it varies from I-V.

Several of the children have active joints which are swollen or hot, but in terms of drug treatment they are generally stable and continuing the drug course planned in their medical treatment.

The therapy periods vary from two days to 6 months, and the intensity varies from every day for several hours to one hour sessions once a week. One included study is not directly therapy, but a questionnaire trying to map use of various exercise types to improve the fitness of juvenile-idiopathic-arthritis children.

The variation between studies in terms of intensity and exercises is therefore as great as seen for the rheumatoid arthritis patients, but the very important positive result in all studies is that none of the pool therapies applied show a worsening of the patients' condition, and there are no negative side effects of the treatment. The children all enjoyed the pool therapy and looked forward to the therapy sessions, both for social reasons and due to not experiencing more pain during the exercises.

**Table 2. Pooltherapy Studies for Juvenile Idiopathic Arthritis**

| Authors/ year | Randomised (R)/ Controlled (C)/Crossover (CO)/ Questionnaire (Q) | Patient Category/number/ sex/age | Drug treatment | Treatment type/ Length of treatment/ Frequency of treatment/ Length of session | Effect para-metres | Results | Conclusion |
|---|---|---|---|---|---|---|---|
| J. Baldwin 1972 [56] | CO | 12 patients. Age 9-18 years. 2 boys, 10 girls. Two groups matched for age and severity of disease, varying from grade II (slow) to V,(impossible) | No information | Pool therapy in groups. Home exercises adjusted to the individual patient.Movements of limbs in all exercises. One group: 20 weeks mainly pool therapy, then 9 weeks break followed by home exercises instructed by physiotherapist. Another group this programme in reverse. | - Strength measurements<br>- Mobility of joint<br>- Soreness and swelling<br>- Personal and parent's assessment of condition<br>Measurements 0.5, 7 and 12 months following start of programme. | Both pool therapy and exercises on land improve strength and mobility of joints and the general personal evaluation of the disease. Pool therapy gives a longer-lasting effect than exercises on land. | Both types of exercise therapy has a positive effect on the patients physical and mental condition, and pool therapy has a longer-lasting effect. Pool therapy is experienced as more enjoyable and less painful than exercises on land. |

**Table 2. Pooltherapy Studies for Juvenile Idiopathic Arthritis (Continued)**

| Authors/ year | Randomised (R)/ Controlled (C)/Crossover (CO)/ Questionnaire (Q) | Patient Category/number/ sex/age | Drug treatment | Treatment type/ Length of treatment/ Frequency of treatment/ Length of session | Effect para-metres | Results | Conclusion |
|---|---|---|---|---|---|---|---|
| U. Latzka, N. Böhler, G. Lukeschnitsch, I. Pilz 1982 [48] | - | 25 patients. Age 6-16 years. 8 systemic, 11 polyarticular, and 6 oligoarticular. | Drug treatment kept as prescribed by own doctor during the therapy period (one or more of the following prescribed: NSAIDS, gold, D-pennicil-amin, azathioprin, corticoids) | 4 weeks residential summercamp with a substantial part of aquatic exercise. Every day: Aquatic exercise for 1 hour in a 29°-32 °C warm pool either with one-to-one or with group instuction by physiotherapist. The aquatic exercise was followed by exercises on land aiming at mobilising joints. Last occupational therapy in use of tools. Sports activity during spare time mainly swimming. | - Mobility (Neutral-0-method)<br>- Number of active joints<br>- Walking time for 15 metres<br>- Joint mobility<br>- Erythrocyte sedimentation rate (ESR)<br>- C-reactive protein (CRP)<br>- Rheumafactor<br>- Haemoglobin (Hb) | Mobility of joints improved (measured by angle). Number of active joints decreased. ESR improved. No change in CRP or rheumafactor. Hb increased. No negative effects of the training was reported. | Only 4 weeks intensive training with mainly aquatic exercises improves functional level and reduces number of active joints. Pool therapy is the ideal therapy for juvenile iddiopathic arthritis because it does not give any discomfort or worsening of the condition, and it is reported to be experienced as enjoyable by the children. |

**Table 2. Pooltherapy Studies for Juvenile Idiopathic Arthritis (Continued)**

| Authors/ year | Randomised (R)/ Controlled (C)/Crossover (CO)/ Questionnaire (Q) | Patient Category/number/ sex/age | Drug treatment | Treatment type/ Length of treatment/ Frequency of treatment/ Length of session | Effect para-metres | Results | Conclusion |
|---|---|---|---|---|---|---|---|
| M.Vostrej S.R. Hollister 1985 [57] | CO | Unknown number of patients. Age 7-12 years. | Not known | One group aerobic exercises in pool programme aiming at improving range of movement (ROM) in 88°F water, and another group free swimming in 88°F warm pool. One day's session of 45 minutes for both. Crossover of the two groups on another day. | -Range of motion (ROM) | ROM improved after both types of training, but the effect was significantly greater after pool therapy than after free swimming. | Warm-water exercise is an effective way of improving ROM in juvenile idiopathic arthritis. Pool therapy is superior to free swimming. Study preliminary and ought to be followed by a larger, controlled study. |
| M.C Bacon, C.Nichol-son, H.Binder, P.H.White [47] | - | 11 patient, 7 girls and 4 boys. 4 polyarticular, 4 oligoarticular and 3 systemic. Age 4-13 years. Functional class I-III. At least one lower extremity joint involved. No acute flare during the last 3 months. | All continued drugs prescribed prior to the therapy period during the time of therapy. | 6 weeks pool therapy in 82-83 °F warm water, twice a week for one hour. The programme consisted of 45 minutes structured exercises followed by 15 minutes free play, all led by physiotherapist. Exercises aiming at improving range of motion (ROM) and strength of the lower extremities. Exercises described. | - ROM<br>- Gait<br>- Balance<br>- Functional mobility of lower extremities<br>- Tolerance to and recovery from vigorous exercise. | Increase in bilateral internal and external hip rotation and hip flexion with knee extension. No improvement in balance or in time tasks. Faster recovery from vigorous exercise. No extra discomfort or negative effects of the pool therapy. | Improvement in ROM, combined with no negative effect of and a lot of enjoyment from pool therapy makes it recommendable for juvenile idiopathic arthritis. |

**Table 2. Pooltherapy Studies for Juvenile Idiopathic Arthritis (Continued)**

| Authors/ year | Randomised (R)/ Controlled (C)/Crossover (CO)/ Questionnaire (Q) | Patient Category/number/ sex/age | Drug treatment | Treatment type/ Length of treatment/ Frequency of treatment/ Length of session | Effect para-metres | Results | Conclusion |
|---|---|---|---|---|---|---|---|
| J.C. Kirschheimer, AWanivenhaus, A. Engel 1993 [58] | Q | 62 patients.<br>Average age 10.9 years.<br>Duration of disease:<br>GroupI 0-5 years;<br>GroupII 5.1-15 years. | No information | Paticipation in sports over the last 8 years. | Longitudinal study of joints, and overall functional ability | Swimming helps the juvenile idiopathic arthritis children to keep reasonably fit, and have no damaging effects on joints. No special care has to be taken here. Cycling has also an entirely positive effect on the functional ability, but joint protection is recommended. | Swimming is, due to lack of damaging effects, recommendable for juvenile idiopathic arthritis patients as a mean of keeping fit and participating in a sport on equal terms with healthy children. |
| T.Takken, J.van der Net, P.J.M. Helders 2001 [59] | - | 10 patients, all girls.<br>4 oligoarticular, 3 polyarticular, and 3 systemic.<br>Age 5-12 years.<br>Duration of disease 4-7.8 years.<br>All except one had active joints.<br>Attendance 85%. | All except one was given one or more of the following drugs: Prednison, methotrexate, NSAID, DMARD, cyclosporin.<br>The medication was kept the same during the training period as just before. | 15 weeks aerobic aquatic training programme in groups of 2-4 patients supervised by a physiotherapist and an exercise physiologist. Water temperature was 32 °C. One session per week for 60 minutes. | - Number of active joints<br>- Mobility (Pediatric Escola Paulista de Medicina Range of Motion Scale (pEPMROM))<br>-Child Health Assessment Questionnaire (CHAQ)<br>- 6 minutes walking test<br>- Juvenile Arthritis Quality of life Questionnaire (JAQQ) | Improvement in overall quality of life score.<br>No discomfort or worsening of condition. | The chosen effect parametres are probably too complicated and not very well suited to measure improvements of physical and psychosocial function in a small pilot study. The improvement of the overall quality of life score and the lack of negative effects of the therapy calls for a larger controlled and randomised study. |

**Table 2. Pooltherapy Studies for Juvenile Idiopathic Arthritis (Continued)**

| Authors/ year | Randomised (R)/ Controlled (C)/Crossover (CO)/ Questionnaire (Q) | Patient Category/number/ sex/age | Drug treatment | Treatment type/ Length of treatment/ Frequency of treatment/ Length of session | Effect para-metres | Results | Conclusion |
|---|---|---|---|---|---|---|---|
| T.Takken, J.van der Net, W.Kuis, P.J.M. Helders 2003 [60] | R, C | 54 patients, 38 girls and 16 boys. Stratified to disease subclasses oligoarticular and polyarticular. 27 in pool therapy group, average age 8.9 ±1.9 years, consisting of 16 girls and 11 boys. 27 in the control group, average age 8.7±2.3 years, consisting of 24 girls and 4 boys. Randomisation according to disease and age. | All received one or more of the following drugs: NSAIDs, DMARD, immunosup-pression medication, steroids in the 6 months prior to inclusion and continued usual medication during the study. | The pool therapy group was exposed to training over a 6 months period, 20 sessions in all with breaks for school holidays, pool maintenance and similar. One session per week, 2-4 patients with physiotherapist, for 60 minutes. Water temperature 30-33 °C. Exercises described. | - Child Health Assessment Questionnaire (CHAQ)<br>- Functional ability<br>- Juvenile Arthritis Functional Assessment Scale (JAFAS)<br>- Juvenile Arthritis Quality of life Questionnaire (JAQQ)<br>- Number of active joints<br>- Maximal Exercise Test (MXT) using bicycle ergometer<br>- 6 minutes walking test | Joint status and physical fitness similar in the therapy and in the control group at start of therapy. Small, but not significant improvements in the pool-therapy group compared to the control group. No worsening in condition seen in the therapy group. | Pool therapy does not show a significant improvement on the condition of the juvenile idiopathic arthritis patients, although most parameters improve compared to the control group. Exercise in water has no negative effects on the patients condition. |

All studies report improvement in strength and particularly in joint movement. Some report a decrease in active joints. The larger randomised and controlled study does, on the other hand, not report a significant effect of pool therapy, although improvement is seen for nearly all parameters [60]. The reason for this may simply be that this study is not very intensive with only 20 sessions of 1 hour each spread over 6 months. The more intensive therapy schemes may get the children to an acceptable level of physical ability to allow a more active life.

The questionnaire study concerning preferred sports for juvenile-idiopathic-arthritis patients concludes furthermore, that water exercise is the preferred type of keeping fit due to that no special care has to be taken with the arthritis children, and they may participate on equal terms with their healthy peers.

# Conclusion

In the two arthritis groups considered here, the overwhelming problem is reduction of functional level which will lead to disability of a degree where constant help in daily living tasks is needed. All patients suffer pains, cannot be exposed to excessive strain on their joint, and experience reduction of muscle strength. Quality of life can quickly be reduced, if the right treatment at the right time is not available. Medical treatment is very important, but only one side of keeping the arthritis patients as physically active as possible. Physical therapy is the other part, and the preferential type for the arthritis patients at any given time may vary as much as the drug treatment may.

When looking at pool therapy, it must be seen as part of the physical-therapy package. The advantage is, of course, the pain-diminishing effect of the warm water, and the possibility of moving without damaging joints with weight-bearing exercise at times where the joints are active. The other advantage is the possibilities in using the water as gentle resistance in training due to the fact, that the patients are able to adjust the speed of movement against the force, and thereby may train weaker muscles without overloading. Exercises in warm water seem to have a pleasure value not found in exercises on land, which in itself motivates the patients to continue the treatment. However, it is important to limit the intensity and duration of the aquatic-exercise therapy to prevent damage to the joints. The decrease in pain may make the patient train harder, and the pain response following training must therefore be followed carefully. It is also important to bear in mind that Chlorine evaporates at much higher rate from the water when the temperature rises beyond 32°C. This will affect the water quality and make it harder to keep the pool clean. Hygiene is therefore an important matter in pool therapy.

Overall, aquatic exercises is a useful physical therapy which must be recommended as part of the physical-therapy programme designed for rheumatoid-arthritis and juvenile-idiopathic-arthritis patients, both during periods where other exercise may not be possible due to active joints, and when wanting to give the patients a boost and quickly see improvement in physical ability, which most often leads to more physical activity and believe in being able to cope, and with the emotional effect of feeling better.

In a time where evidence-based medicine is the law, and where treatment can only be justified if a clear effect is shown, it will be necessary to carry out larger randomised and controlled studies, comparing pool therapy with both medical and physical therapy treatments. It will then be possible to compare effect and cost of various combinations of medical and physical therapy. Based on these studies, it will be possible to prescribe aquatic exercises to the individual at the right intensity and duration as part of the total package of drug treatment and various types of physical therapy.

# References


[1] Masi, A. T., Feigenbaum, S. L., and Kaplan, S. B. Articular patterns in the early course of rheumatoid arthritis. *American journal of Medicine*1983; 75(suppl.6A):16-26.

[2] Wolfe, F. and Carthey, M. A. The assessment and prediction of functional disability in rheumatoid arthritis. *Journal of Rheumatology*1991; 18:1298-1306.

[3] Lieber RL. Skeletal Muscle Adaption to Decreased Use. In: Lieber RL, editor. *Skeletal Muscle Structure, Function, and Plasticity*. Baltimore: Lippincott Williams and Wilkins, 2002: 225-286.

[4] Danneskiold-Samsoe B, Grimby G. Muscle morphology and enzymes in proximal and distal muscle groups of lower limb from patients with corticosteroid treated rheumatoid arthritis: the relationship to maximal isokinetic muscle strength. *Clin Sci (Colch )* 1986; 71(6):685-691.

[5] Helliwell PS, Jackson S. Relationship between weakness and muscle wasting in rheumatoid arthritis. *Ann Rheum Dis* 1994; 53(11):726-728.

[6] Pincus, T. and Callahan, L. F. Predictive values for quantitative physical and questionnaire measures of functional status for 9 years morbidity in rheumatoid arthritis. *Journal of Rheumatology*1992; 19(7):1051-1057.

[7] Hazes JM. Determinants of physical function in rheumatoid arthritis: association with the disease process. *Rheumatology (Oxford)* 2003; 42 Suppl 2:ii17-ii21.

[8] Ansell, B. M. Joint manifestations in children with juvenile chronic arthritis. *Arthritis & Rheumatism*1977; 20:204-206.

[9] Cassidy JT. Juvenile chronic arthritis. Management. In: Klippel JH, Dieppe P, editors. *Rheumatology*. Philadelphia: Mosby, 1994: 20.1-20.10.

[10] Jarrett, S., Quinn, M. A., and Emery, P. The evidence for early intervention in rheumatoid arhtritis. *Advances in Rheumatology*2003; 1(2):42-52.

[11] Hicks JE, Gerber LH. Rehabilitation of the patient with arthritis and connective tissue disease. In: DeLisa J.A., editor. *Rehabilitation Medicine*. Philadelphia: Lippincott-Raven, 1998: 1502-1504.

[12] Cosh, J. A. and Kersley, G. D. Rheumatism Treatment Centres in Britain - Bath Ancient and Modern. *Annals of Physical Medicine*1969; 10:167-174.

[13] Whitelock, H. When to Use Hydrotherapy and How it Works. *Rheumatology Review*1994; 3:187-191.

[14] Glass, J. Physical Medicine in Rheumatology. *Australian and New Zealand Journal of Medicine*1978; 8(suppl 1):168-170.

[15] Ferrell, K. M. Aquatics for People with Arthritis. *Lippincott's Primary Care Practice*1998; 2:102-104.

[16] Jetter JKN. *Arthritis and Back Pain Exercises for the Bath.* London: Bantam, 1987.

[17] Sukenik S, Flusser D, Codish S, Abu-Shakra M. Balneotherapy at the Dead Sea area for knee osteoarthritis. *Israel Medical Association Journal: IMAJ* 1999; 1(2):83-85.

[18] Sukenik S, Neumann L, Flusser D, Kleiner-Baumgarten A, Buskila D. Balneotherapy for rheumatoid arthritis at the Dead Sea. *Isr J Med Sci* 1995; 31(4):210-214.

[19] Sukenik S, Neumann L, Buskila D, Kleiner-Baumgarten A, Zimlichman S, Horowitz J. Dead Sea bath salts for the treatment of rheumatoid arthritis. *Clin Exp Rheumatol* 1990; 8(4):353-357.

[20] Rutner, M. and Sommer, F. Einsparung von NSAR durch die Kombination mit einen medizinischen Rheumabad. *Zeitschrift für Allgemein Medizin*1990; 66:210-212.

[21] Sukenik S, Buskila D, Neumann L, Kleiner-Baumgarten A, Zimlichman S, Horowitz J. Sulphur bath and mud pack treatment for rheumatoid arthritis at the Dead Sea area. *Ann Rheum Dis* 1990; 49(2):99-102.

[22] Svarcova J, Hofta T, Kouba A, Trnavsky K, Zvarova J. Beeinflussung der Schmerzsymtomatik im Fussbereich bei Patienten mit Rheumatoid-Arthritis durch Unterschiedliche Physiotherapiemittel. *Zeitschrift fur Physiotherapie* 1990; 42(2):109-112.

[23] Risum T. Hydroterapi - træning i vand. Copenhagen: 1998.

[24] Smith, R. Water Works: Aquatic Therapy and the Arthritis Patient. *Rehabilitation Management*1997; 10:54-58, 115.

[25] Goland, A. Basic Hydrotherapy. *Physiotherapy*1981; 67:258-268.

[26] Hall, J. The Physiology of Immersion. *Physiotherapy*1990; 76:517-521.

[27] Bates AHN. *Aquatic Exercise Therapy.* Philadelphia: W.B.Saunders Company, 1996.

[28] Ritchie SE, Hopkins WG. The intensity of exercise in deep-water running. *Int J Sports Med* 1991; 12(1):27-29.

[29] Becker, B. E. The Biological Aspect of Hydrotherapy. *Journal of Back and Musculoskeletal Rehabilitation*1994; 4:255-264.

[30] Cureton KJ. Physiological Responses to Water Exercise. In: Ruoti RG, editor. *Aquatic Rehabilitation.* Philadelphia: Lippincott, 1981: 39-56.

[31] Eitner D. Exercise in water. In: Kuprian W, editor. *Physical therapy for sports.* Philadelphia: W.B.Saunders, 1995: 153-162.

[32] Whitley, J. D. and Schoene, L. L. Comparison of heart rate responses. *Physical Therapy*1987; 67:1501-1504.

[33] Sheldahl, L. M., Tristani, F. E., Clifford, P. S., Hughes, C. V., Sobocinski, K. A., and Morris, R. D. Effect of head-out water immersion on cardio-respiratory response. *JACC*1987; 10(6):1254-1258.

[34] Martin, J. The Halliwick Method. *Physiotherapy*1981; 67:288-291.

[35] Boyle, A. M. The Bad Ragaz Ring Method. *Physiotherapy*1981; 67:265-268.

[36] Garrett G. Bad Ragaz Ring Method. In: Ruoti RG, editor. *Aquatic Rehabilitation.* Philadelphia: Lippincott, 1997: 289-304.

[37] Dull H. WATSU: *Freeing the Body.* Middletown: 1993.

[38] Dull H. WATSU. In: Ruoti RG, Morris DM, Cole AJ, editors. *Aquatic Rehabilitation.* Philadelphia: Lippincott, 2001: 333-352.

[39] Minor MA, Hewett JE, Webel RR, Anderson SK, Kay DR. Efficacy of physical conditioning exercise in patients with rheumatoid arthritis and osteoarthritis. *Arthritis Rheum* 1989; 32(11):1396-1405.

[40] Hall J, Skevington SM, Maddison PJ, Chapman K. A randomized and controlled trial of hydrotherapy in rheumatoid arthritis. *Arthritis Care Res* 1996; 9(3):206-215.

[41] Rintala P, Kettunen H, McCubbin JA. Effects of a Water Exercise Program for Individuals with Rheumatoid Arthritis. *Sports Medicine Training and Rehabilitation* 1996; 7:31-38.

[42] Sanford Smith SM-LMN-CS. Therapeutic Benefit of Aquaaerobics for Individuals with Rheumatoid Arthritis. *Physiotherapy Canada* 1998; 50(1):40-46.

[43] Yurtkuran M, Yurtkuran MA, Dilek K, Güllülü M, Karakoc Y, Özbek L et al. A randomized, controlled study of balneotherapy in patients with rheumatoid arthritis. *Phys Rehab Kur med* 1999; 9:92-96.

[44] Dial C, Windsor RA. A formative evaluation of a health education - water exercise program for class II and III adult rheumatoid arthritis patients. *Patient Education and Counseling* 1985; 7:33-42.

[45] Danneskiold-Samsoe B, Lyngberg K, Risum T, Telling M. The effect of water exercise therapy given to patients with rheumatoid arthritis. *Scand J Rehabil Med* 1987; 19(1):31-35.

[46] Landewé, R. B. M., Peeters, R., Verreussel, R. L. P., Masek, B. A., and Goeithe, H. S. Geen verschil in effectiviteit gemeten tussen behandeling in een thermaalbad en in een oefenbad bij patiënten met reumatoïde artritis. *Nederlands Tijdschrift voor Geneeskunde*1992; 136(4):173-176.

[47] Bacon MC, Nicholson C, Binder H, White PH. Juvenile rheumatoid arthritis. Aquatic exercise and lower-extremity function. *Arthritis Care Res* 1991; 4(2):102-105.

[48] Latzka, U., Böhler, N., Lukeschitsch, G., and Pilz, I. Östereichische Therapiferien für Kinder mit juveniler chronischer Arthritis. *Östereichische Ärzezeitschrift*1982; 37(23):1561-1564.

[49] Lauridsen I. Varmtvandsmotion: Vejledning for brugere af varmtvandsbassiner. Brøndby: Dansk Handicap Idrætsforbund, 1989.

[50] Bretler U. Bassinterapi. Copenhagen: Interessegruppen for bassinterapi i Storkøbenhavn, 1991.

[51] Lyngberg KK, Ramsing BU, Nawrocki A, Harreby M, Danneskiold-Samsoe B. Safe and effective isokinetic knee extension training in rheumatoid arthritis. *Arthritis Rheum* 1994; 37(5):623-628.

[52] Kraemer, W. J., Fleck, S. J., and Evans, W. J. Strength and power training: Physiological mechanism of adaption. *Exercise and sport sciences reviews*1996; 24:363-397.

[53] Danneskiold-Samsoe, B., Lyngberg, K., Risum, T., and Telling, M. The Effect of Water Exercise Therapy Given to Patients with Rheumatoid Arthritis. *Scandinavian journal of rehabilitation medicine*1987; 19:31-35.

[54] Stenström, C. H., Lindell, B., Swanberg, E., Swanberg, P., Harms-Ringdahl, K., and Nordemar, R. Intensive Dynamic Training in Water for Rheumatoid Arthritis Functional Class II - a Long-term Study of Effects. *Scandinavian Journal of Rheumatology*1991; 20:358-365.

[55] Hansen TM, Hansen G, Langgaard AM, Rasmussen JO. Long term physical training in rheumatoid arthritis. A randomized trial with different training programs and blinded observers. *Scand J Rheumatol* 1993; 22(3):107-112.

[56] Baldwin, J. Pool therapy compared with individual home exercise therapy for juvenile rheumatoid arthritic patients. *Physiotherapy*1972; 58(7):230-231.

[57] Vostrejs, M. and Hollister, J. R. The effectiveness of an aquanastic program: A controlled study. *Arthritis & Rheumatism*1985; 28(4):S150.

[58] Kirchheimer, J. C., Wanivenhaus, A., and Engel, A. Does sport negatively influence joint scores in patients with juvenile rheumatoid arthritis - An 8-year prospective study. *Rheumatology International*1993; 12:239-242.

[59] Takken, T., van der Net, J., and Helder, P. J. M. Do juvenile idiopathic arthritis patients benefit from an exercise program? A pilot study. *Arthritis Care and Research*2001; 45:81-85.

[60] Takken, T., van der Net, J., Kuis, W., and Helder, P. J. M. Aquatic fitness training for children with juvenile idiopathic arthritis. *Rheumatology*2003; 42:1-7.

In: Arthritis Research: Treatment and Management
Editor: F. Columbus, pp. 107-126
ISBN 1-59033-984-3


*Chapter V*

# Exercise for Children with Arthritis

***Tim Takken,* Janjaap van der Net and Paul J.M. Helders***
Department of Pediatric Physical Therapy, Wilhelmina Children's Hospital,
University Medical Center Utrecht, Utrecht, The Netherlands

## Abstract

In the first part of this chapter the physical fitness levels of children with Juvenile Arthritis (JA) are reviewed. The majority of the studies indicate that JA patients do have an impaired physical fitness (for example muscle strength, muscle bulk, anaerobic and aerobic fitness) compared to healthy children. These results will be discussed in the light of the paradigm of *rheumatoid cachexia*. In the second part of this Chapter the available clinical trials on exercise training for juvenile arthritis patients are reviewed. These observations from the literature indicate a need for a randomized controlled trial with adequate sample size and objective measures of functional ability and quality of life. Summarizing this literature, 172 children with Juvenile Arthritis patients have been trained in eleven different studies. However, most of the studies have methodological weaknesses. The results of the first, recently conducted, randomized-trial which evaluated the effects of an aquatic aerobic physical training program in JIA patients are discussed and directions for futures research are described.

Although the evidence-base is small, the current research indicate that it is save for children with JA to participate in physical activities and (adapted) sports activities. Also

* Address of correspondence: Dr Tim Takken, MSc PhD, Exercise Physiologist, Department of Pediatric Physical Therapy, Wilhelmina Children's Hospital, University Medical Center Utrecht, Room KB2.056.0, PO Box 85090, NL 3508 AB Utrecht, The Netherlands, +31 30 2504030 (phone); +31 30 2505333 (fax), Email: t.takken@wkz.azu.nl, Http://www.kinderfysiotherapiewkz.nl

for children with JA, the era of inactivity and bed rest for treating their disease seems past and the need to become physical active has become evident.

## Introduction

In general, physical fitness consists of different components such as body composition, flexibility, strength, speed, and endurance. However, currently physical fitness has become synonymous with cardio-respiratory fitness (maximal oxygen uptake; $VO_{2peak}$). Physical fitness is dependent on both lifestyle factors such as physical activity levels and nutritional habits, as well as genetic factors.

More and more evidence comes available indicating that physical active subjects have a lower mortality rate compared to sedentary persons. Already in 1953 Jeremy Morris described the relationship between physical activity and coronary heart disease and physical activity levels in London transit workers. Morris et al [1] reported that conductors working on London,s double-decker buses experienced less than half the incidence of heart attacks as the sedentary drivers. (The conductors climbed around 600 stairs per working day; the drivers sat for 90% of their shift; [1]). Another well-known researcher in this field is Ralph Paffenberger Jr. He described this phenomenon in the now "almost classic" Harvard Alumni Study and showed that physical activity levels and other lifestyle factors could be related to mortality in graduate students of the University of Pennsylvania and Harvard University [2]. In the years after these publications many studies confirmed this finding.

The U.S. Centers for Disease Control and Prevention reviewed the literature a few years ago in their landmark report "Physical Activity and Health: A Report of the Surgeon General" [3]. This report showed that a low physical fitness is associated with a higher mortality rate, a higher risk in certain forms of cancer, obesity, decreased mental health, hypertension and a lower quality of life

Most of the studies performed were based on exercise behaviors assessed using questionnaires. Recently Myers and colleagues examined 6213 consecutive men referred for treadmill exercise testing for clinical reasons during 6.2 years follow-up. The results indicated that every increase of physical fitness leads to a reduction in overall mortality in a clinical, adult male population [4]. Moreover studies from the Cooper Institute for Aerobics Research indicated that physical fitness is of comparable importance in cardiovascular mortality with that of diabetes mellitus and other cardiovascular disease risk factors like smoking, cholesterol and hypertension [5].

For children and adolescents with a disability or chronic disease, physical fitness is equally important [6]. Maintaining and improving physical fitness can assure that children and adolescents with a chronic disease will enter adulthood with a sound basis for their future health.

# Age Related Decline in Physical Fitness

A literature review on North-American and European studies on aerobic physical fitness clearly showed the improvement in $VO_{2peak}$ during childhood and the age related decline in $VO_{2peak}$ in both men and women [7]. This decline started approximately at the age of 20 with a mean rate of 41 $ml \cdot kg^{-1} \cdot min^{-1}$, irrespectively of gender. Additionally, women do have lower initial levels of $VO_{2peak}$ (± 30%) when entering adulthood. This is not only the effect of a higher body fat mass in woman, but also in absolute values, men out perform women. Thus women with a chronic disease with a pediatric onset such as juvenile arthritis, are at risk for a low $VO_{2peak}$, which can lead to an early disability when $VO_{2peak}$ values reach critical thresholds for activities of daily living [8, 9](see also [10])

**Table 1. Comparison of Physical Fitness Variables betweenJuvenile Arthritis Patients and Controls**

| Study | Assessed Variable | Used Method | Number of patients | Finding s |
|---|---|---|---|---|
| [11] | Skeletal muscle strength | Hand held dynamometer | 20 | ↓ |
| [12] | | Hand held dynamometer | 20 | ↓ |
| [13] | | Hand held dynamometer | 11 | ↓ |
| [14] | | Computerized dynamometer | 28 | ↓ |
| [15] | | NA | 9 | = |
| [12] | Muscle bulk | Ultrasound | 20 | ↓ |
| [16] | | Femoral muscle circumference | 32 | ↓ |
| [17] | Pulmonary function | Standard pulmonary function tests | 31 | ↓ |
| [18] | Anaerobic performance | WaNT | 31 | = |
| [19] | | WaNT | 13 | ↓ |
| [20] | | 50-meter run | 20 | ↓ |
| [21] | | 50-meter run | 32 | ↓ |
| [22] | Body composition | Skin folds | 20 | = |
| [18] | | Skin folds | 31 | = |
| [22] | Submaximal Endurance | 9 min run walk test | 20 | ↓ |
| [23] | | Heart rate during sub-maximal exercise | 30 | ↑ |
| [18] | Aerobic exercise capacity | VO2peak determined using maximal bicycle exercise test. | 30 | = |
| [24] | | VO2peak determined using maximal treadmill exercise test. | 45 | ↓ |
| [23] | | VO2peak determined using maximal bicycle exercise test. | 30 | ↓ |
| [25] | | VO2peak determined using maximal bicycle exercise test. | 23 | ↓ |
| [26] | | VO2peak determined using maximal bicycle exercise test. | 16 | ↓ |
| [10] | | Systematic review | 144 | ↓ |

WaNT: Wingate anaerobic test; ↓: decreased compared to healthy controls; =: no difference between JA patients and controls; ↑: increased compared to healthy controls, $VO_{2peak}$: maximal oxygen uptake, NA: not available.

# Physical Fitness Levels in Patients with Juvenile Arthritis

Numerous studies have been performed to investigate the physical fitness levels of juvenile arthritis (JA) patients and compared these results to reference values or with values from healthy control subjects. The most important findings from the physical fitness studies in JA are summarized in Table 1. From these findings one can conclude that the physical fitness levels of JA patients are diminished at least in the domain of muscle strength, muscle bulk, pulmonary function, anaerobic performance, sub-maximal endurance and $VO_{2peak}$.

# Physiology

In this paragraph the physiological background of the impaired physical fitness (e.g. $VO_{2peak}$) will be reviewed. $VO_{2peak}$ is the product of cardiac output (heart rate x stroke volume) and the arterio - mixed venous oxygen difference (the Fick equation)[27]. Three studies [23-25] provided peak heart rate data. These studies show that peak heart rate is on average 6 beats minute$^{-1}$ (95% CI -10, - 2.8) lower than in healthy controls during a maximal exercise test, indicating that some of the JA patients terminated the exercise test before reaching the maximum capacity of their cardiovascular system. If the cardiovascular system was the limited factor in the exercise capacity of JA patients, the heart rate would be taxed to a maximum, since stroke volume already reaches its maximum level at approximately 50-70 % of $VO_{2peak}$ [28].

Another cause of the impaired $VO_{2peak}$ might be a lower stroke volume of the heart. It is known from the literature that inactivity in children causes a decrease in stroke volume [29]. However it is not clear whether this is the limiting step in oxygen transport in untrained children, because a decrease in stroke volume can be compensated at submaximal intensities by an increased heart rate. As previously mentioned, the peak heart rate during a maximal exercise test is lower in JA patients compared to healthy children. This indicates that the cardiovascular system is not the limiting factor in oxygen uptake of JA patients.

It is more likely, the limiting step is on the non-hemodynamic side of the Fick equation. Many possible causes can be distinguished with respect to this side of the equation. Pulmonary function abnormalities have also been reported JA patients (see Table 1)[17], caused by weakness of the respiratory muscles. However, this was only found in effort-dependent tests (e.g. forced vital capacity and peak expiratory flow). It is not likely that an impaired lung function is the cause of the lower $VO_{2peak}$.

Muscular atrophy is also a common finding in JA patients who have lower muscle bulk compared to healthy subjects [11, 12, 16]. This is still evident after some years without disease flares, and is more pronounced in children with a disease onset before the age of 3 [16].

A lower muscle mass implies a smaller muscle mass to consume oxygen. Also a patient experiences fatigue at an earlier workload and will terminate the test earlier compared to healthy subjects. Suggestions for the cause of the lower muscle bulk are inactivity, medication and disease activity.

Muscular biopsy studies in children with JA are, to our knowledge, not performed. Available evidence from studies with adult Rheumatoid Arthritis patients, suggests an atrophy in both type I and type II muscle fibers. The atrophy is most pronounced in the type II muscle fibers and can not be fully explained by disuse. It is suggested that muscle fibers are directly involved in the inflammation process [30]. Data from short-term and long-term training studies in RA patients and a training study in JA patients [15] show that this muscular atrophy in both muscle fiber types can be reduced by dynamic exercise training [31, 32]. Thus, a part of the impairment in physical fitness might be caused by hypoactivity, the other part might be caused by medication and/or high levels of inflammatory parameters, and particularly tumor necrosis factor alpha [33](TNF alpha; See Figure 1). This muscular atrophy has been called "*Rheumatoid Cachexia*" (34]. A study in adult RA patients [35] showed a significant relationship between plasma TNF alpha levels and protein breakdown. Early treatment of JA patients with TNF alpha blocking agents, such as Infliximab or Etanercept, might reduce the TNF alpha induced muscular atrophy. A recent study found also very promising effects of a TNF alpha blocking agent on disease activity and functional ability in patients with a persistent JA [36]. There are also indications that Methotrexate treatment could prevent this protein breakdown, at least in adult RA patients [35]. Early treatment of all JA patients with Methotrexate or TNF alpha blocking agents might give a better outcome for physical performance and functional ability in JIA patients. The long-term risks and benefits of these agents are still not well documented in patients with JA. Also the efficacy and required dose of these therapies for the treatments of the cachexia are unknown. These kinds of therapies can only be initiated in JIA patients, when additional studies have been performed.

Exercise training has been shown its value in adult RA patients [37], also during episodes of active disease [38]. In children, there are no well-controlled studies researching rheumatoid cachexia. However exercise studies in adults with RA using resistance training, are promising in preventing the loss in muscle mass [35].

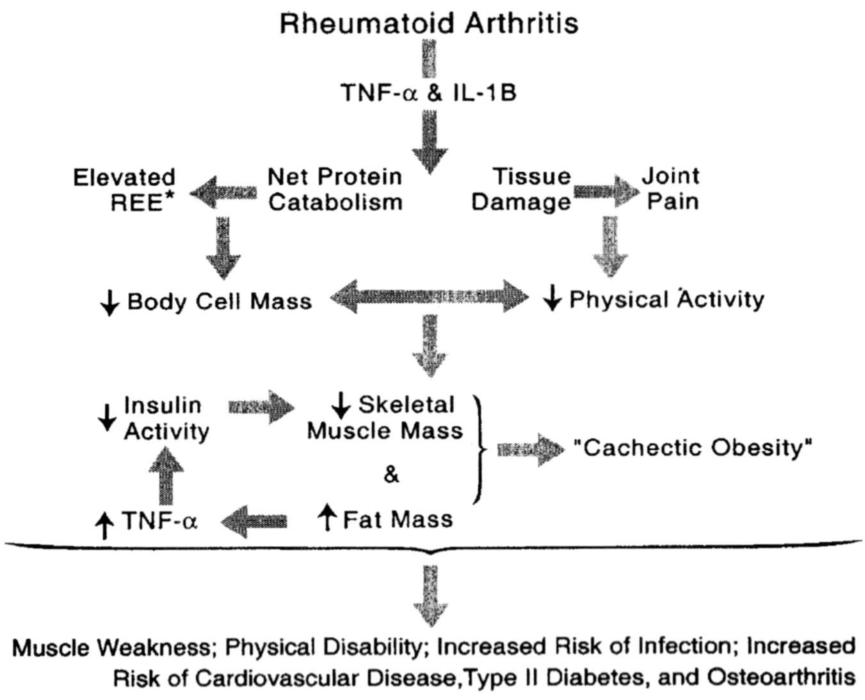


Figure 1. Summary of the metabolic consequences of rheumatoid arthritis. The increased levels of inflammatory parameters leads to a loss of body cell mass, predominantly skeletal muscle mass, and reduced physical activity, which reinforce each other and lead to further losses of skeletal muscle mass and predispose to fat gain. *Resting energy expenditure (REE) is elevated in active rheumatoid arthritis. Redrawn from Walsmith and Roubenoff [33].

## Trainability of Children with Juvenile Arthritis

It is believed in the past that young children were not trainable in terms of improvements in $VO_{2peak}$. Some researchers found no improvements while others did [39]. Payne & Morrow systemically reviewed the literature and performed a meta-analysis on these data. They found that in healthy, active, children exercise training generates small to moderate effects (± 8%) on physical fitness ($VO_{2peak}$ ) [39]. Rowland et al. [40] found for instance an improvement of 6.5 % in $VO_{2peak}$ in healthy children after an exercise program (3 x week 30 min vigorous treadmill running). Patients with a chronic disease have low physical activity levels and are more detrained compared to healthy children [27, 41]. Thus, in theory they have more potential to train (no ceiling effect as is often proposed for the lower training effect in healthy children). However, disease activity (inflammatory parameters) and medication (for example the effects of Cyclosporine A [42] and prednisone [43]) might diminish the trainability of the chronically ill child. Rowland [44] proposed that exercise training programs aiming to improve physical fitness for healthy children should incorporate adult guidelines for exercise intensity and duration (3 x week 30 min at 60 of heart rate reserve). The question arises whether adult guidelines are appropriate for chronically ill children? Klepper and Giannini proposed some general guidelines for the training of children with juvenile arthritis and even described an example of a typical exercise training program [45].

One of the often-asked questions is when to start a training program for children with juvenile arthritis. Klepper & Giannini [45] recommend children with chronic arthritis to start an individualized exercise program soon after diagnosis [45]. But should children train during active disease episodes? Research on adults with mild to moderate active rheumatoid arthritis [38, 46] showed that exercise training did not increase disease activity. Fisher et al. [47] showed that immune parameters even improved with resistance training in children with JA. These reports suggest that exercise can be started even when arthritis is not in remission and that exercise can be continued during episodes of active disease.

## Exercise Immunology in Juvenile Arthritis

There is a growing interest in the area of exercise in relation to immunology. With the improvement of research techniques it will become easier, cheaper and quicker to analyze effects of exercise training and/or physical activity levels on immune status. In the field of arthritis research only a few reports have been published on this topic [46, 48], as most of the exercise studies focussed on improvement in exercise capacity, functional ability, range of motion etc. In adult RA a few papers have been published [46, 48] including 2 review papers [49, 50]. In Juvenile Idiopathic Arthritis only two research projects have become available from the University of Buffalo, NY. This work, to date only published as abstracts [47, 51-56], suggest that resistance exercise training can improve not only muscle function, but also immune function in patients with juvenile arthritis (see Table 2).

## Rationale for Exercise

In adults with RA the major reason for their low 'physical fitness' was originally thought to be the lack of physical activity (deconditioning) [57] due to soreness and pain in muscles and joints [58] and the availability of technology supporting a sedentary lifestyle. However, as dicussed above also high levels of inflammatory parameters could result in a loss in muscle mass. Adults stated that they better could perform activities of daily living after a physical training program [58], i.e. their functional status had been improved.

**Table 2. Training Intesventions in Juvenile Arthritis Patients**

| Study | No of Patients | Disease subclass | Age (years) | Duration | Program | Medium | Results |
|---|---|---|---|---|---|---|---|
| Klepper [66] | 25 | 25pJA | 8-17 | 8wks 3 sessions /wk | 2 sessions /week supervised, 1 session/wk @ home. Focussed on aerobic exercise (fitball) | Land-based | Joint count ↑; 9 min run walk ↑; Articular severity index =; pain =; swelling=; ROM=. |
| Baldwin [59] | 12 | NA | 8-18 mean 11.7 | 2 x 20 wks (cross-over study) | 2x 15 wks Pool: 2x15 min Land 30 min Focussed on strength & mobilisation hip and knee joints | 1 pool group, 1 land based group | Pool therapy: quadriceps strength ↑; Home therapy: mobility ↑; Parents & patients: pool therapy was more beneficial and enjoyable than home therapy |
| Bacon [79] | 11 | 4oJA, 4pJA, 3sJA | 4-13 | 6wks 2 sessions / wk | 45 min structured act, 15 min play | Pool T: 27-28C | Hip rotation & flexion ↑; HR recovery after exercise ↑; Balance tests & times tasks = Gait = |
| Oberg [15] | 10 | 5oJA, 3pJA, 1sJA, 1pso | 7-15, mean 10.4 | 3 months 2 sessions / wk | 40 min, gymnastics, pool, focussed on strength & endurance | Pool + land | Muscle strength quadriceps ↑; Muscle strength trapezius =; EMG ↑ (normalized towards control) |
| Feldman [80] | 9 | PJA | 8-11 | 12 weeks 1 or 2 sessions/week | NA | Pool + land | Efficiency of gait ↑; $VO_{2peak}$ =; Anaerobic performance ↑. |
| Klepper [61] | 5 | NA | 5-13 | 6 wks (13sessions) | 60 min/session, focussed on aerobics, strength and stretching | Land | Joint count V; Articular severity ↑; pain perception ↑; 9 min run walk ↑; sit-up test ↑; self esteem ↑. |
| Moncur [60] | 7 | 7pJA | NA | 12 wks | NA | Bicycle ergometer | Joint count ↑; abs $VO_{2peak}$ ↑; rel $VO_{2peak}$ ↑; exercise time ↑. |

**Table 2. Training Intesventions in Juvenile Arthritis Patients (Continued)**

| Study | No of Patients | Disease subclass | Age (years) | Duration | Program | Medium | Results |
|---|---|---|---|---|---|---|---|
| Fisher [51-54] | 10 | NA | 6-14 | 8 wks | Resistance training, 3/wk duration and intensity: NA | Land | Plasma lactate ↑, neutrophils ↑, inflammation ↑, quadriceps & hamstrings strength ↑, hamstrings & quadriceps endurance ↑, contraction speed ↑, $VO_{2peak}$ ↑, bloodpressure ↑, peakHR ↑, functional status ↑, pain ↑, disability ↑. |
| Fisher [47] | 19 | NA | Mean 11.3 | 8 wks | Resistance training, 3/wk duration and intensity: NA | Land | Strength ↑, endurance ↑, contraction speed ↑, EMG activity ↑, inflammatory mediators ↑. |
| Takken [62] | 10 | 3sja, 3 pja, 4oja | 5-12 | 15 wks | 60 min/wk, aquarobic training | pool | Functional ability =, Quality of life ↑, endurance =. |
| Takken [63] | 54 | 23 oja, 29 pja, 2 sja | 5-13 | 20wks | 60 min/wk, aquarobic training | pool | Functional ability =, Quality of life =, joint status ↑, $VO_{2peak}$ =, endurance =. |

oja, oligoarticular juvenile arthritis, pja, polyarticular idiopathic arthritis; sja, systemic juvenile arthritis; pso: psoriatric arthritis; NA: not available; PT: physical therapist; RN: registered nurse; ExPhys: exercise physiologist; EMG: electromyogram; peakHr: peak heartrate; ↑: $VO_{2peak}$: peak oxygen consumption; ROM: range of motion; ↑: improvement, = no improvement; ↓: worsening.

It is interesting to search for the rationale for an exercise program for children. For example Joan Baldwin [59] for the Hospital for Sick Children, Toronto, Canada reported the results of her training study for juvenile arthritis patients in 1972, three years before the first adult research from Stockholm, Sweden [57] was published. But Baldwin did not mention why she started the research. However, it shows that she did not start because of the promising results in the adult rheumatoid arthritis population, but the assumed a need for exercise and conditioning in this patient group. Moncur et al (1990) used the adult results as a rationale for their research [60], the same is true for the research of Susan Klepper [61].

# Clinical Trials: Training Interventions

We recently performed two studies on exercise training for children with Juvenile Arthritis [62, 63]. Before we conducted these two studies [62, 63], there were only a few papers on the topic of exercise training for children with arthritis. The training studies available in the literature to date, both full report publications and abstracts are summarized in Table 2. Compared to the available number of studies on adult RA patients [37], the body of evidence from pediatric studies on exercise training in Juvenile Arthritis is very small. Summarizing this literature, 172 children with Juvenile Arthritis patients have been trained in nine different studies. Currently, three other exercise intervention studies are being conducted in Europe (United Kingdom and Switserland) and one in Canada. The results will become available soon.

In general, three modalities can be distinguished: land-based training, aquatic training and bicycle ergonometer training. In all modalities effects have been found, however most studies used different outcome measures. For the sake of comparison, it shows the need for an established core set of variables for assessing the effectiveness of therapeutic interventions in JA. All studies included assessments in the domains of pathology and impairment within the disablement process, such as range of motion, pain and joint count. But performance variables (functional limitation and disability) are all measured using different methods. A standardized set of measures would facilitate the comparison of different studies and exercise interventions.

The previously published studies on the effects of physical training programs for JA patients were small pilot studies [15, 60, 62, 64], were not controlled by randomization [59, 65, 66], and had small sample. More over, the previous conducted studies on this topic in JA, the main focus was on improvements in physical fitness and on impairments like joint swelling and range of motion. None of the previous studies used contemporary, and recently validated, functional assessment tools (e.g. Childhood Health Assessment Questionnaire) as outcome measure for their study. As these instruments are more and more accepted as outcome measures in clinical trials in pediatric rheumatology, it is important for the comparison with other studies, to include these instruments as an outcome measure in an intervention study.

Therefore, we studied the effects of an aquatic training program, on physical fitness, functional ability, joint status, and health-related quality of life in a randomized-controlled design [63]. In this randomized trial, fifty-four patients (38 girls, 16 boys) diagnosed with JA were recruited from the pediatric rheumatology outpatient clinics of the Wilhelmina Children's Hospital, University Medical Center Utrecht, the Netherlands and the University Hospital Groningen, the Netherlands. Patients were stratified to disease subclass (two strata: an oligoarticular JA group and a polyarticular (with or without systemic onset) JA) and individually randomly assigned to the assessment only group (Con-group) or the training group (Exp-group). The investigators and the subjects were blinded for previous measurements at each stage of the evaluation; the investigators and subjects were not blinded for the group allocation of each subject.

All patients received the usual care and medical treatment during the study. The patients in the Exp-group received an aquatic group (2-4 children/group) exercise program, 1 hour a week, supervised by an instructed community physical therapist. If there was only one patient at a certain training location, the patient was allowed to bring a relative or friend to join the training program. The training took place in heated (30-33°C) community-based local pools at twenty different locations throughout The Netherlands. The training program was conducted within a half-year period. Due to holidays, seasonal holidays and pool maintenance, the program consisted of approximately twenty training sessions on the different locations. Training sessions were based on the same framework. The training started with a warm-up, followed by an aerobic conditioning part, a short rest period, again followed by a second conditioning part. The training ended with a cooling-down. The warm- up, rest, and cooling down periods consisted of low intensity swimming, aquarobics, play, flexibility exercises, or ball games. The conditioning parts consisted mainly of high intensity swimming, diving, walking through the water, aqua jogging, or splashing with the legs. The duration and intensity of both conditioning parts increased stepwise during the program. During the training sessions the heart rates of the patients were measured using a portable heart-rate monitor (Polar Accurex Plus, Polar Oy, Kempele, Finland) to monitor the training intensity.

## Outcomes

Functional ability was measured using the Dutch translation of the Childhood Health Assessment Questionnaire (CHAQ)[67] and the Juvenile Arthritis Functional Assessment Scale (JAFAS)[68]. Health-related quality of life was assessed with a Dutch translation of the Juvenile Arthritis Quality of Life Questionnaire (JAQQ)[69] and the Child Health Questionnaire (CHQ)[70]. Joint status was assessed by the number of tender and swollen joints and the range of motion. Joint mobility was scored on the Pediatric Escola Paulista de Medicina Range of Motion Scale (pEPMROM)[71]. The physical fitness (vo2peak) of the patients was assessed using a maximal bicycle exercise test to detemine the $VO_{2peak}$ and a sub maximal 6-minute walking test (6mwt). A more detailed description of the methods is available elsewhere [63].

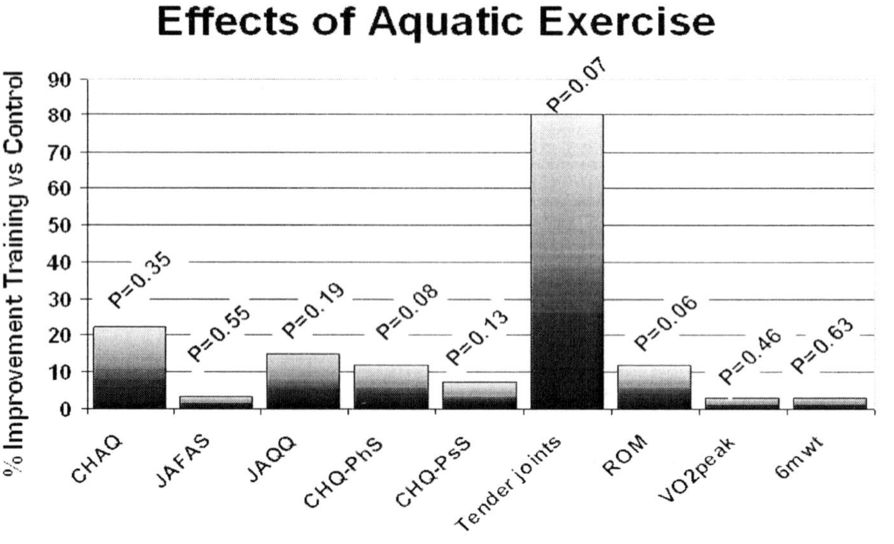


Figure 2. The effects of a 20-week Aquatic Exercise program for JA patients on selected functional outcome measures. Abbreviations: CHAQ: Childhood Health Assessment Questionnaire, JAFAS: Juvenile Arthritis Functional Assessment Questionnaire, JAQQ: Juvenile Arthritis Quality of Life Questionnaire, CHQ-PhS: Child Health Questionnaire physical summary, CHQ-PsS: Child Health Questionnaire Psycho-Social summary, Tender joints: Number of tender and swollen joints, ROM: range of motion measured on the pediatric Escola Paulista de Medicina Range of Motion Scale (pEPMROM), vo2peak: maximal oxygen uptake, 6mwt: Distance walked on the 6-minute walking test. Data from reference [63].

## Results and Discussion

In this trial we found no statistical significant effects of a 20-week aquatic training program for JA patients on functional ability, quality of life, joint status, and physical fitness (See Figure 2). However, there was a borderline-significant effect of an improved joint status (tender joints and joint range of motion) during the training program (p=0.07 and p=0.06 respectively) and CHQ-Physical Summary (p=0.08). The non-significant effects could be explained by the chosen outcome measures. We hypothesized the aquatic exercises would improve physical fitness. This increased physical fitness could result in a transfer to improved function ability, and an increase in health-related quality of life. However this transfer of the training effects seems very difficult. Numerous exercise studies in adult RA patients found improvements in physical fitness, joint pain, morning stiffness and fatigue, but no clear improvements in functional ability [37, 72]. In our study, the largest effects were found in the joint status domain.

The aquatic training did not improve the $VO_{2peak}$ of leg exercise on the bicycle ergometer, maybe an arm exercise protocol would have shown improvements, since as lot of exercises in the program were performed using both legs and arms.

Moreover, the used outcome instruments might have lacked the sensitivity to detect the training effects. The majority of the instruments (CHAQ, CHQ, JAFAS, pEPMROM, JAQQ) are developed and validated as discriminative instruments for disability, and not yet as an outcome for effect studies. However, in clinical practice they are used frequently for evaluative purposes, and the Pediatric Rheumatology International Trials Organization selected some of them for trial evaluation (CHAQ and CHQ). Van den Ende et al. [73] found a very limited sensitivity to change of the adult version of the CHAQ, the HAQ, in an exercise trial with adult RA patients. The value of the CHAQ for detecting changes due to an exercise-training program might be limited. However, there was a positive relationship between baseline CHAQ score and improvement after the intervention, indicating that patients with a higher level of disability benefited more from the aquatic training than the patients with a lower level of disability.

The lack of improvements in the current study could also be the result of a limited trainability of children with JA as discussed previously. Even in healthy children, some investigators have found no or small effects in physical fitness of exercise training programs [40], out data more or less confirm this finding for JA patients. A meta-analysis of all available exercise training programs showed on average an eight percent increase in physical fitness in healthy children [39]. Compared to adults, the degree of aerobic trainability is somewhat limited in children. Additionally, for detrained, chronically ill patients it might not be possible to adhere programs based on adult standards for intensity and duration. They might be compromised in their level of trainability.

For children with arthritis there are some guidelines available, however they are based on preliminary-evidence [45]. Moderate intensity exercise, as in our program, will facilitate most of the disease prevention and health promoting effects of exercise [74], however these are long-term effects of exercise training.

The current program lasted approximately a half-year; however, healthy peers will participate for years in certain sport activities like soccer, cycling, tennis, or athletics. A long-term exercise training study (> 2 years) would be of interest to performed in the current patient group. Our results clearly indicated however, that our program, as measured by joint status does not negatively influence the disease process. As parents and JA patients were highly interested to participate in adapted physical training programs, this study shows that an aquatic training program could be a valuable adjunct to the common medical care of children with JA.

Limited information is available concerning changes in physical fitness and functional ability in JA patients following an exercise-training program. Thus more research is needed in this area. From a practical point of view, it was not possible to increase the frequency of the training (i.e. two training sessions a week), busy family schedules and a limited pool access did not allow higher training frequencies. The inclusion of a home-based exercise part (land-based) should be considered in a future study. This might also support patients, and parents in achieving a more active lifestyle. Moreover, studies on healthy adults have shown that a higher exercise frequency (more than 3 days per week) is needed for an improvement in physical fitness [75]. However, one must bear in mind that JA patients do have a diminished load-bearing capacity because of their inflammatory disease and the immune suppressive medication. Exercise training might improve immune function [49], however a training load which is too large might easily lead to overreaching or overtraining, as is often seen in athletes with a compromised immune system [76].

The current exercise study tried to find a minimum level of exercise training, which could improve functional ability and fitness, but on the other hand did not impede the immune system.

The lack of significant improvements in the training group also shows the importance of an active life style for children with JA. The current research showed that it is very difficult to improve physical fitness. The sound bite "it is easier to maintain good health through proper exercise, diet and emotional balance than to regain it once it is lost" might be also true for JA patients.

## Directions for Future Research

Future studies should try to reveal the acute and long-term effects of exercise, both risks and benefits, on immunological status of JIA patients. The exercise immunology of fitness training programs for arthritis patients should become one of the main targets for new research. For children with a rheumatic condition, the effects of long-term interventions should be investigated. Current studies ranged from 6 weeks to almost 6 months. However, healthy peers participate for years in certain sport activities like soccer, cycling, tennis, or speed skating. A long-term exercise program (> 2 years) could be performed as a group training program as in the current study in the water, but also on land (fitness, resistance training or even an anaerobic exercise training program). Other possibilities are home-based exercise programs, a cybertraining program using internet, or a combination of all options. However one must bear in mind that an individualized approach is very important. Exercise intensity and exercise duration should be monitored by an educated specialist because of the risk of overtraining and overreaching. The intensity and duration should be well-matched with the disease to best meet the patients' need.

A long-term training program during childhood and adolescence increases adult values for physical fitness. In this respect, the prevention of age-related decline in physical fitness using angiotensin-converting enzyme inhibitors is promising for patients with a chronic disease [77]. However, medication can never replace exercise, a long-lasting exercise adherence might improve not only physical fitness, but also quality of life, psychosocial well-being and life expectancy [78]. These are very important "side effects" of physical training.

Because of the costs of a specialist supervised training program, patients who will be most at risk for a very low exercise capacity and who will benefit the most from the exercise program should be identified in the JIA patient population and should have priority in entering such a training program. Thus far, no studies are undertaken to investigate the differences in training-response in juvenile arthritis patients.

Tracking physical fitness, physical activity, immunological status, and functional ability of JA patients into adulthood will increase our understanding of functional ability in JA patients as well as in the underlying immunological, physical and physiological determinants in JA patients. This data might also reveal patient subgroups that are at risk for a low physical fitness when entering adulthood.

## Conclusion

With the advances in the medical treatment of JA patients using new and successful treatments the interest in adapted physical training programs is increasing. The effects of adapted training programs are not well investigated. The first randomized controlled trial found positive effects of an aquatic fitness-training program in children with JA. Since there were no signs for worsening in health status, one can conclude that this was a safe exercise program. As there are lot of different exercise modalities, effort should be invested to create and investigate the safety and effectiveness of exercise training programs for children with JA and explore the possibilities of a long-term exercise program.

## References

[1] Morris JN, Heady JA, Raffle PAB, Roberts CG, Parks JW. Coronary heart disease and physical activity of work. *Lancet* 1953;2:1053–1057, 1111–1120.

[2] Paffenbarger RS, Jr., Hyde RT, Wing AL, Hsieh CC. Physical activity, all-cause mortality, and longevity of college alumni. *N Engl J Med* 1986;314(10):605-13.

[3] US Department of Health and Human Services. *Physical Activity and Health: A Report of the Surgeon General.* Atlanta, GA: U.S.: Department of Health and Human Services, Centers for Disease Control and Prevention, National Center for Chronic Disease Prevention and Health Promotion.; 1996.

[4] Myers J, Prakash M, Froelicher V, Do D, Partington S, Atwood JE. Exercise capacity and mortality among men referred for exercise testing. *N Engl J Med* 2002;346(11):793-801.

[5] Wei M, Kampert JB, Barlow CE, Nichaman MZ, Gibbons LW, Paffenbarger RSJ, et al. Relationship between low cardiorespiratory fitness and mortality in normal-weight, overweight, and obese men. *Jama* 1999;282(16):1547-53.

[6] Goldberg B. Children, sports, and chronic disease. *The Physician and Sports Medicine* 1990;18(10):44-56.

[7] Shvartz E, Reibold RC. Aerobic fitness norms for males and females aged 6 to 75 years: a review. *Aviat Space Environ Med* 1990;61(1):3-11.

[8] Shephard RJ. Adapting physical activity to an aging population. *International Journal of Sports Cardiology* 1987;4(1):1-14.

[9] Takken T, Van der Net J, Helders PJ. Relationship between functional ability and physical fitness in juvenile idiopathic arthritis (JIA) patients. *Scand J Rheumatol* 2003;32(3):174-178.

[10] Takken T, Hemel A, Van der Net J, Helders PJM. Aerobic fitness in children with juvenile idiopathic arthritis: a systematic review. *Journal of Rheumatology* 2002;29(12):2643-2647.

[11] Lindehammar H, Backman E. Muscle function in juvenile chronic arthritis. *J Rheumatol* 1995;22(6):1159-65.

[12] Lindehammar H, Sandstedt P. Measurement of quadriceps muscle strength and bulk in juvenile chronic arthritis. A prospective, longitudinal, 2 year survey. *J Rheumatol* 1998;25(11):2240-8.

[13] Hedengren E, Knutson LM, Haglund-Akerlind Y, Hagelberg S. Lower extremity isometric joint torque in children with juvenile chronic arthritis. *Scand J Rheumatol* 2001;30(2):69-76.

[14] Giannini MJ, Protas EJ. Comparison of peak isometric knee extensor torque in children with and without juvenile rheumatoid arthritis. *Arthritis Care Res* 1993;6(2):82-8.

[15] Oberg T, Karsznia A, Gare BA, Lagerstrand A. Physical training of children with juvenile chronic arthritis. Effects on force, endurance and EMG response to localized muscle fatigue. *Scand J Rheumatol* 1994;23(2):92-5.

[16] Vostrejs M, Hollister JR. Muscle atrophy and leg length discrepancies in pauciarticular juvenile rheumatoid arthritis. *American Journal of Diseases of Children* 1988;142(3):343-5.

[17] Knook LM, de Kleer IM, van der Ent CK, van der Net JJ, Prakken BJ, Kuis W. Lung function abnormalities and respiratory muscle weakness in children with juvenile chronic arthritis. *Eur Respir J* 1999;14(3):529-33.

[18] Malleson PN, Bennett SM, MacKinnon M, Jespersen DK, Coutts KD, Turner SP, et al. Physical fitness and its relationship to other indices of health status in children with chronic arthritis. *J Rheumatol* 1996;23(6):1059-65.

[19] Takken T, van der Net J, Helders PJ. Short-term muscle power in juvenile idiopathic arthritis. *Physical Therapy* 2001;81(5):A77.

[20] Fan JS, Wessel J, Ellsworth J. The relationship between strength and function in females with juvenile rheumatoid arthritis. *J Rheumatol* 1998;25(7):1399-405.

[21] Wessel J, Kaup C, Fan J, Ehalt R, Ellsworth J, Speer C, et al. Isometric strength measurements in children with arthritis: reliability and relation to function. *Arthritis Care Res* 1999;12(4):238-46.

[22] Klepper SE, Darbee J, Effgen SK, Singsen BH. Physical fitness levels in children with polyarticular juvenile rheumatoid arthritis. *Arthritis Care Res* 1992;5(2):93-100.

[23] Giannini MJ, Protas EJ. Exercise response in children with and without juvenile rheumatoid arthritis: a case-comparison study. *Phys Ther* 1992;72(5):365-72.

[24] Golebiowska M, Brozik H, Bujnowski T. Aerobic and anaerobic metabolism in children with juvenile chronic arthritis in relation to some clinical data. In: Coudert J, editor. *Pediatric Work Physiology, Children and Exercise*. Paris: Masson; 1992. p. 175-177.

[25] Takken T, van der Net J, Helders PJM. Aerobic exercise testing in juvenile rheumatoid arthritis (JRA) patients. *Clinical Exercise Physiology* 2002;4(1):38-43.

[26] Giannini MJ, Protas EJ. Aerobic capacity in juvenile rheumatoid arthritis patients and healthy children. *Arthritis Care Res* 1991;4(3):131-135.

[27] Bar-Or O. Pathophysiological factors which limit the exercise capacity of the sick child. *Med Sci Sports Exerc* 1986;18(3):276-82.

[28] Åstrand P-O, Rodahl K. *Textbook of Work Physiology. Third Edition* ed. New-York.: McGraw-Hill; 1986.

[29] Eriksson BO, Engstrom I, Karlberg P, Lundin A, Saltin B, Thoren C. Long-term effect of previous swimtraining in girls. A 10-year follow-up of the "girl swimmers". *Acta Paediatr Scand* 1978;67(3):285-92.

[30] Edstrom L, Nordemar R. Differential changes in type I and type II muscle fibres in rheumatoid arthritis. A biopsy study. *Scand J Rheumatol* 1974;3(3):155-60.

[31] Nordemar R, Berg U, Ekblom B, Edstrom L. Changes in muscle fibre size and physical performance in patients with rheumatoid arthritis after 7 months physical training. *Scand J Rheumatol* 1976;5(4):233-8.

[32] Nordemar R, Edstrom L, Ekblom B. Changes in muscle fibre size and physical performance in patients with rheumatoid arthritis after short-term physical training. *Scand J Rheumatol* 1976;5(2):70-6.

[33] Walsmith J, Roubenoff R. Cachexia in rheumatoid arthritis. *Int J Cardiol* 2002;85(1):89-99.

[34] Roubenoff R, Roubenoff RA, Cannon JG, Kehayias JJ, Zhuang H, Dawson-Hughes B, et al. Rheumatoid cachexia: cytokine-driven hypermetabolism accompanying reduced body cell mass in chronic inflammation. *J Clin Invest* 1994;93(6):2379-86.

[35] Rall LC, Rosen CJ, Dolnikowski G, Hartman WJ, Lundgren N, Abad LW, et al. Protein metabolism in rheumatoid arthritis and aging. Effects of muscle strength training and tumor necrosis factor alpha. *Arthritis Rheum* 1996;39(7):1115-24.

[36] Lovell DJ, Giannini EH, Reiff A, Cawkwell GD, Silverman ED, Nocton JJ, et al. Etanercept in children with polyarticular juvenile rheumatoid arthritis. Pediatric Rheumatology Collaborative Study Group. *N Engl J Med* 2000;342(11):763-9.

[37] Van den Ende CH, Vliet Vlieland TP, Munneke M, Hazes JM. Dynamic exercise therapy in rheumatoid arthritis: a systematic review. *Br J Rheumatol* 1998;37(6):677-87.

[38] van Den Ende CH, Breedveld FC, le Cessie S, Dijkmans BA, de Mug AW, Hazes JM. Effect of intensive exercise on patients with active rheumatoid arthritis: a

[39] randomised clinical trial. *Annals of the Rheumatic Diseases* 2000;59(8):615-21.

[40] Payne VG, Morrow JRJ. Exercise and VO2 max in children: a meta-analysis. *Research Quarterly For Exercise And Sport* 1993;64(3):305-13.

[41] Rowland TW, Boyajian A. Aerobic response to endurance exercise training in children. *Pediatrics* 1995;96(4 Pt 1):654-8.

[42] Bar-Or O. *Pediatric sports medicine for the practitioner.* New York: Springer-Verlag; 1983.

[43] Biring MS, Fournier M, Ross DJ, Lewis MI. Cellular adaptations of skeletal muscles to cyclosporine. *J Appl Physiol* 1998;84(6):1967-75.

[44] Horber FF, Scheidegger JR, Grunig BE, Frey FJ. Evidence that prednisone-induced myopathy is reversed by physical training. *J Clin Endocrinol Metab* 1985;61(1):83-8.

[45] Rowland TW. Aerobic response to endurance training in prepubescent children: a critical analysis. *Med Sci Sports Exerc* 1985;17(5):493-7.

[46] Klepper SE, Giannini MJ. Physical conditioning in children with arthritis: Assessment and guidelines for exercise prescription. *Arthritis Care Res* 1994;7(4):226-36.

[47] Baslund B, Lyngberg K, Andersen V, Halkjaer Kristensen J, Hansen M, Klokker M, et al. Effect of 8 wk of bicycle training on the immune system of patients with rheumatoid arthritis. *J Appl Physiol* 1993;75(4):1691-5.

[48] Fisher NM, Venkatraman JT, O'Neil KM. The effects of resistance exercises on muscle and immune function in juvenile arthritis. *Arthritis Rheum* 2001;44(9 suppl):S276.

[49] Lyngberg K, Tvede N, Halkjaer Kristensen J, Andersen V, Pedersen BK. Physical exercise iduces modulation of the cellular immune system in patients with rheumatoid arthritis. *Scandinavian Journal of Medicine and Science in Sports* 1991;1(2):167-173.

[50] Shephard RJ, Shek PN. Autoimmune disorders, physical activity, and training, with particular reference to rheumatoid arthritis. *Exercise and Immunology Review* 1997;3:53-67.

[51] Pool AJ, Axford JS. The effects of exercise on the hormonal and immune systems in rheumatoid arthritis. *Rheumatology (Oxford)* 2001;40(6):610-4.

[52] Lin H, Venkatraman JT, Fisher N, O'Neil K, Gong P, Chu W. Effects of quantitative rehabilitation exercise (QPER) on biochemical indices in juvenile arthritis (JA). *FASEB J* 1999;13(8):A931,#687.

[53] Fisher NM, Venkatraman JT, O'Neil KM. Effects of resistance exercise on children with juvenile arthritis. *Arthritis Rheum* 1999;42(9 Suppl):S396.

[54] Venkatraman JT, Fisher NM, Lin H, O'Neil KM. Effects of resistance exercise on plasma levels and production of cytokines and lipid mediators in juvenile arthritis. *Arthritis Rheum* 1999;42(9 Suppl):S396.

[55] Velazquez V, Fisher NM, Venkatraman KM, O'Neil KM. Effect of lower extremity resistance exercise rehabilitation on interleukin-1b, interleukin-1RA, and interleukin-6 in juvenile arthritis. *Arthritis Rheum* 1999;42((9)Suppl):S185.

[56] Venkatraman JT, Fisher NM, Meksawan K, Krishnan A, Downie A. Effects of resistance exercise training (RET) on chemokine levels in juvenile arthritis (JA). *FASEB J* 2000;14(4):A526 #367.1.

[57] O'Neil KM, Fisher nm, Venkatraman jt. Immunologic effects of acute exercise on inflammatory mediators in children with juvenile idiopathic arthritis. *Arthritis Rheum* 2001;44(9):s339.

[58] Ekblom B, Lovgren O, Alderin M, Fridstrom M, Satterstrom G. Effect of short-term physical training on patients with rheumatoid arthritis I. *Scand J Rheumatol* 1975;4(2):80-6.

[59] Ekblom B, Lovgren O, Alderin M, Fridstrom M, Satterstrom G. Effect of short-term physical training on patients with rheumatoid arthritis. a six-month follow-up study. *Scand J Rheumatol* 1975;4(2):87-91.

[60] Baldwin J. Pool therapy compared with individual home exercise therapy for juvenile rheumatoid arthritic patients. *Physiotherapy* 1972;58(7):230-231.

[61] Moncur C, Marcus R, Johnson S. Pilot project of aerobic conditioning of subjects with juvenile arthritis. *Arthritis Care Res* 1990;3(2):S16.

[62] Klepper SE, Bleakney D, Donohoe M, Simpson GM, Singsen BH. Physical fitness in juvenile rheumatoid arthritis. *Arthritis Care Res* 1992;5(4):S20.

[63] Takken T, van der Net J, Helders PJ. Do juvenile idiopathic arthritis patients benefit from an exercise program? A pilot study. *Arthritis Rheum* 2001;45(1):81-5.

[64] Takken T, Van der Net J, Kuis W, Helders PJ. Aquatic fitness training for children with juvenile idiopathic arthritis. *Rheumatology* 2003;In Press(42).

[65] Vostrejs M, Hollister JR. The effectiveness of an aquanastics program: a controlled study. *Arthritis and Rheumatism* 1985;28(Suppl):S150.

[66] Bacon MC, White PH, Raiten DJ, Craft N, Margolis S, Levander OA, et al. Nutritional status and growth in juvenile rheumatoid arthritis. *Semin Arthritis Rheum* 1990;20(2):97-106.

[67] Klepper SE. Effects of an eight-week physical conditioning program on disease signs and symptoms in children with chronic arthritis. *Arthritis Care and Research* 1999;12(1):52-60.

[68] Singh G, Athreya BH, Fries JF, Goldsmith DP. Measurement of health status in children with juvenile rheumatoid arthritis. *Arthritis Rheum* 1994;37(12):1761-9.

[69] Lovell DJ, Howe S, Shear E, Hartner S, McGirr G, Schulte M, et al. Development of a disability measurement tool for juvenile rheumatoid arthritis. The Juvenile Arthritis Functional Assessment Scale. *Arthritis Rheum* 1989;32(11):1390-5.

[70] Duffy CM, Arsenault L, Duffy KN, Paquin JD, Strawczynski H. The Juvenile Arthritis Quality of Life Questionnaire-development of a new responsive index for juvenile rheumatoid arthritis and juvenile spondyloarthritides. *J Rheumatol* 1997;24(4):738-46.

[71] Wulffraat N, van der Net JJ, Ruperto N, Kamphuis S, Prakken BJ, Ten Cate R, et al. The Dutch version of the Childhood Health Assessment Questionnaire (CHAQ) and

the Child Health Questionnaire (CHQ). *Clin Exp Rheumatol* 2001;19(4 Suppl 23):S111-5.

[72] Len C, Ferraz MB, Goldenberg J, Oliveira LM, Araujo PP, Quaresma MR, et al. Pediatric Escola Paulista de Medicina Range of Motion Scale: a reduced joint count scale for general use in juvenile rheumatoid arthritis. *Journal of Rheumatology* 1999;26(4):909-13.

[73] Rall LC, Roubenoff R. Benefits of Exercise for Patients with Rheumatoid Arthritis. *Nutrition in Clinical Care* 2000;3(4):209-215.

[74] van den Ende CH, Breedveld FC, Dijkmans BA, Hazes JM. The limited value of the Health Assessment Questionnaire as an outcome measure in short term exercise trials. *J Rheumatol* 1997;24(10):1972-7.

[75] Sothern MS, Loftin M, Suskind RM, Udall JN, Blecker U. The health benefits of physical activity in children and adolescents: implications for chronic disease prevention. *Eur J Pediatr* 1999;158(4):271-4.

[76] Pollock ML, Gaesser GA, Butcher JD, Despres J-P, Dishman RK, Franklin BA, et al. ACSM Position Stand: the recommended quantity and quality of exercise for developing and maintaining cardiorespiratory and muscular fitness, and flexibility in healthy adults. *Med Sci Sports Exerc* 1998;30(6):975-991.

[77] Mackinnon LT. Chronic exercise training effects on immune function. *Med Sci Sports Exerc* 2000;32(7 Suppl):S369-76.

[78] Onder G, Penninx BW, Balkrishnan R, Fried LP, Chaves PH, Williamson J, et al. Relation between use of angiotensin-converting enzyme inhibitors and muscle strength and physical function in older women: an observational study. *Lancet* 2002;359(9310):926-30.

[79] Rejeski WJ, Brawley LR, Shumaker SA. Physical activity and health-related quality of life. *Exercise and Sport Science Reviews* 1996;24:71-108.

[80] Bacon MC, Nicholson C, Binder H, White PH. Juvenile rheumatoid arthritis. Aquatic exercise and lower-extremity function. *Arthritis Care Res* 1991;4(2):102-105.

[81] Feldman BM, Wright FV, Bar-Or O, Dent P. Rigorous Fitness Training and Testing for children with poliarticular arthritis: a pilot study. *Arthritis and Rheumatism* 2000;43(9 (suppl)):s120.

In: Arthritis Research: Treatment and Management
Editor: F. Columbus, pp. 127-145
ISBN 1-59033-984-3


*Chapter VI*

# Physical Function Assessment in Children with Rheumatic Diseases

***L. Nandini Moorthy[1*], Margaret G.E. Peterson[2], Karen B. Onel[3] and Thomas J.A. Lehman[4]***

[1]Assistant Professor of Pediatric Rheumatology, 100 Bayard Street, 3rd Floor, New Brunswick, NJ 08903

[2]Director Applied Statistics Core, Hospital For Special Surger, New York, NY 10021

[3]Assistant Professor of Pediatrics, Weill Medical College of Cornell University, Assistant Attending Pediatrician and Assistant Scientist, Hospital for Special Surgery, New York, NY 10021

[4]Attending Physician and Senior Scientist, Hospital for Special Surgery, Professor of Clinical Pediatrics, Weill Medical College of Cornell University Chief, Division of Pediatric Rheumatology, Hospital for Special Surgery, New York, NY 10021

## Abstract

Pediatric rheumatic diseases with predominantly arthritic involvement such as juvenile idiopathic arthritis (JIA) can cause considerable physical functional impairment and significantly affect the children's quality of life (QOL). Physical function, QOL, health-related QOL (HRQOL) and health status are personal constructs used as outcomes to estimate the impact of these diseases and often used as proxies for each other. The chronic, fluctuating nature of these diseases differs within and between patients, and

* Contact: L. Nandini Moorthy, MD MS, Mailing address: 413 Copperfield Lane, Metuchen, NJ 08840, Email: LNMoorthy@mac.com; Phone: (732) 906 9794 (Home); (732) 906 9378 (Work)

complicates the measurement of these outcomes. In children, additional dimensions such as their growing needs and expectations, limited use of age-specific questionnaires, and the use of proxy respondents further obscure this evaluation. This article will briefly review the different constructs inclusive of and related to physical function, and the different scales used for measuring them. An understanding of these instruments will enable assessment of outcomes in clinical studies of children with rheumatic diseases, measure the impact of the disease and treatments on their lives, and guide us in formulating appropriate interventions to improve their overall well being.

## Introduction

Pediatric rheumatic diseases causing arthritis, fatigue, muscle weakness and blindness are associated with significant functional impairment. In some cases, physical functional ability is often the chief determinant of their quality of life (QOL). QOL, health-related QOL (HRQOL), physical function and health status scales are all used as outcome measures in children with significant musculoskeletal involvement, and account for varying degrees of patient-perceived state of physical ability/and or impact of physical disability on overall well being. For the purposes of this chapter, these constructs will be termed collectively as "outcome measures." Monitoring the impact of these diseases on children's overall well being with standardized instruments is therefore crucial in order to evaluate their outcomes.

The World Health Organization QOL group defined QOL as "individuals' perceptions of their position in life in the context of the culture and value systems in which they live and in relation to their goals, expectations, standards and concerns. It is a broad ranging concept affected in a complex way by the person's physical health, psychological state, level of independence, social relationships, and their relationships to salient features of their environment" [1]. Calman et al has presented a "goal-oriented" model where QOL measures the difference between a person's expectations and current position at a certain time [2]. Recent scientific advances have increased life span, often at the expense of increased medication use and commensurate drug-related complications, more frequent medical visits and evaluation, all of which can lead to significant emotional and lifestyle changes. QOL emerges as a critical issue in this regard and becomes a primary consideration for the improvement in modern medicine.

Specifically for patients with chronic diseases, health primarily impacts the overall QOL. HRQOL is defined as "optimum levels of mental, physical, role and social functioning, including relationships, and perceptions of health, fitness, life satisfaction and well-being" [3]. Implicit in HRQOL is the "assessment of patient's satisfaction with treatment, outcome and health status and with future prospects" [3]. Health status usually refers to general physical and mental health and is often weighted towards symptoms and physical function. Sometimes, disease-specific measures of impact on organ systems are used to denote health status. In clinical studies, there is considerable overlap between QOL, HRQOL and health status. Since QOL, HRQOL, and health status are distinct constructs measuring different patient-specific information, all three deserve appropriate consideration in clinical outcome studies [4].

# Pediatric Rheumatic Diseases Causing Physical Functional Impairment

Physical ability is a very relevant outcome in children with predominantly musculoskeletal involvement such as juvenile idiopathic arthritis (JIA) [5-10]. Pediatric rheumatic diseases comprise a heterogeneous group of diagnoses that have different clinical features, complications and prognosis. An overview of these different diseases causing different types and extents of disability will illustrate the pleomorphic nature of the population studied and serve in evaluating the appropriateness of instruments used in the specific population.

## Juvenile Idiopathic Arthritis (JIA)

Juvenile Idiopathic Arthritis (JIA) is a chronic inflammatory disease causing erosive arthritis in children, often progressing to disability. JIA occurs in children of all races, with annual incidence ranging from 0.008-0.226 per 1000 children, and prevalence from 0.07-4.01 per 1000 children [11]. One of the most frequently occurring pediatric rheumatic diseases, JIA impacts bio-psychosocial aspects of patients and families, necessitating careful diagnosis and institution of appropriate treatment. JIA comprises of the following seven categories as per the new classification: 1) Oligoarticular onset JIA also termed as Pauciarticular onset JIA (PaJIA); 2) Polyarticular onset JIA (PoJIA RF+) with positive results on testing for Rheumatoid Factor (RF); 3) Polyarticular onset JIA (PoJIA RF-) with negative results on testing for RF; 4) Systemic onset JIA (SoJIA); 5) Psoriatic arthritis JIA; 6) Enthesis-related arthritis; and 7) Other arthritis undefined by above mentioned criteria [12]. Each subtype is associated with specific complications and disabilities.

PaJIA occurs in over half the children with JIA less than 5 years of age, and affects girls more than boys. Children with PaJIA present in the first six months with arthritis, and are characterized by the involvement of four or fewer joints, typically large ones such as knees, ankles, and elbows. About 20% of children with PaJIA, mostly ANA positive girls, may be afflicted with silent chronic anterior uveitis, which may result in irreversible damage and blindness if not managed appropriately [13]. Most children with PaJIA have good functional outcome, although few evolve to chronic destructive polyarticular type of disease, with significant debilitation. Long-standing cases of PaJIA often exhibit limb-length discrepancy requiring orthotic or surgical correction.

PoJIA encompasses approximately one-third of the diagnoses of JIA, affects girls more frequently, and is characterized by gradual involvement of five or more joints during the first six months [14, 15]. Children may experience morning stiffness, fatigue, and pain due to arthritis and/ or tenosynovitis. The arthritis may be intermittent or persistent, affecting the large joints of knees, elbows, ankles and wrists, as well as the cervical spine, temporomandibular joints, and small joints of hands and feet. Late-onset PoJIA in RF-positive girls has a similar clinical course to adult Rheumatoid Arthritis (RA) [14]. Children with rapidly progressive destructive synovitis, early involvement of small joints of hands and feet, unrelenting inflammation, subcutaneous nodules, and RF positivity are at significant risk for long-term disability [14]. Many children develop severe erosive hip disease along with other joint involvement, resulting in contractures, joint destruction and ankylosis, often necessitating joint replacements. About 5% of children may develop chronic uveitis, which often adds another layer of disability upon an already diminished functional state [16]

SoJIA comprises nearly 10-20% of JIA diagnoses throughout childhood, equally affecting both genders [17]. Children with SoJIA present with high spiking fevers, arthritis, transient erythematous, macular rash, and may have other systemic features such as anorexia, arthralgias, and hepatosplenomegaly, and lymphadenopathy. Arthritis may occur concurrently with the systemic symptoms or may occur years after the initial presentation. Although about half of the children may improve significantly, the rest may remain persistently ill with varying degrees of systemic involvement and /or chronic erosive polyarthritis, micrognathia, cervical spine fusion and destructive hip resulting in severe functional disability [18, 19]. Children with long-standing disease may have significant growth retardation including short stature and failure to thrive. Uveitis is rare in these children.

Children with psoriatic arthritis may have skin involvement, uveitis, and often experience a progressive chronic course similar to PoJIA. Varying degrees of arthritis, enthesitis, sacroiliac joint tenderness, inflammatory spinal pain or both, and acute anterior uveitis characterize spondyloarthropathy. Back pain, heel pain, and morning stiffness are primary symptoms, which may worsen to severe functional limitation if the disease progresses to ankylosing spondylitis.

Severe erosive disease can cause significant loss of joint motion, an important determinant of functional disability in children [20]. Depending upon the severity and extent of disease involvement, children often experience significant pain and disability, which impede the execution of ordinary activities. [21]. Since JIA has such widespread impact on physical function, functional ability has been included as one of the core set of outcome variables for the assessment of children with JIA and these core response variables are also valuable in defining flare in them [22, 23]. Aggressive treatment along with physical and occupational therapy remain the keystones of managing severe disease..

## Dermatomyositis

Dermatomyositis is a rare chronic inflammatory disease causing significant weakness of the proximal muscles associated with characteristic skin rash. Muscle involvement causing motor weakness hinders children from performing routine activities such as walking, getting up from bed, combing hair and eating food. Generalized fatigue, fever and muscle pain and weakness could worsen functional status. Children with persistent inflammatory disease may exhibit diminished muscle mass due to atrophy, calcific nodules and flexion contractions that cause substantial functional impairment. Physical function is a core set-outcome criterion for measuring clinical outcome and assessing clinical improvement in children with myositis [24].

### Other Rheumatic Diseases

Other inflammatory vasculitic diseases cause functional impairment due to fatigue, arthritis, myositis, rash, and organ damage. In some instances these may be disfiguring and lead to blindness, paralysis or cognitive impairment. Children with scleroderma may experience skin tightening that is significant enough to cause contractures. In cases of severe morphea, the involvement of the skin may be so profound that it may involve bony tissue, possibly leading to complete non-use of the affected limb.

### Medication-related Morbidity

In addition to the disease-related causes of functional limitation, many children with the above-mentioned rheumatic diseases suffer consequences of long-term steroid use, such as avascular necrosis of the joints,severe osteoporosis which makes bones prone to frequent fracturing, requiring surgical joint repair and /or replacement to improve function. Moreover, children on steroids are prone to infection and experience delayed healing of wounds due to their compromised immune status thus complicating their post-operative course. Steroid-related side-effects include obesity, cushingoid features, acne and growth retardation leading to low self-esteem in children, that in addition to the disease-related morbidity may reduce their motivation to participate in physical activities.

For children with rheumatic disease, functional impairment encompasses physical, visual and cognitive limitation, and is complicated by the psychosocial impact of having a chronic disease. As pain and fatigue significantly influence children's well being, these should be critical considerations in the measurement of physical ability.

## Problems Encountered in Assessing Outcomes in Children

The heterogeneity of rheumatic diseases causing functional impairment, children's changing cognitive skills, needs and expectations, limited availability of questionnaires during the transition from childhood to adulthood, overlap in the constructs measured by these scales, as well as the use of proxy respondents are all factors that complicate measurement of physical function, health status, QOL and HRQOL in children [25-29]. Many instruments modified from adult scales may not take into account a specific phase of children's development which impacts cognitive function, autonomy, body image, expectations, level of independence and recall [30]. Age and language-adjusted formats with items relevant for each age group are ideal for the evaluation of physical function and related outcomes in children over a broad age-range. As most rheumatic diseases are chronic, frequently progressing into adulthood, it is essential to address the lack of instruments to measure physical function, QOL, HRQOL and health status through this phase of growth. Appropriate transitional measures can enable prospective follow-up from childhood to adulthood and facilitate the formulation of both clinically and methodologically accurate comparisons.

Although physical function scales are considered as objective measures of children's ability, their items often measure impact on domains other than physical such as social and emotional. For example, items in the CHAQ such as "run and play" and "run errands and shop" are composite, involving not only physical ability but also motivation to be with friends, energy, social impetus, and potential exposure to sunlight, all of which may be impacted by the systemic disease. In some cases, children with significant disease may not have any friends, or have very low self-esteem to even meet friends. Additionally, there may be logistic issues that preclude children from running errands or shopping. Frequently, a particular physical activity is the final translation of an action motivated by necessity, or interest, which is influenced by social, emotional, logistic, economic and school-related factors in children, and therefore the assessment should be reviewed critically for the existing interconnectedness. Therefore, refinement of measures is necessary to measure physical ability alone.

Given the chronic, fluctuating nature of many rheumatic illnesses and the importance of obtaining self-perceived report of physical ability and QOL/HRQOL, child-reports appear to be the ideal solution. However, children's health, memory, mood and communication skills may affect their reports, making them flawed, and often invalid for our purposes. In such cases, parents' reports may be more useful, although it is important to bear in mind that their assessments are uniquely affected by their own health status, individual expectations and personal experiences [27]. Moreover, a parent's perception of the child's QOL greatly influences the probability of seeking health care for the child, thus creating a selection bias [31]. Despite these concerns, proxy respondents are widely used and the level of agreement with child self-report has varied widely [26, 28, 32, 33].

The level of parent-child agreement in children with arthritis and other conditions appears to vary for disability, pain, QOL, and HRQOL. Greater correlation between child and parent reports has been noted in the more objective domains such as physical function as compared to the social and emotional domains. Brunner et al examined agreement 58 child-parent dyads from Rheumatology clinics and found good agreement for scores of the Childhood Health Assessment Questionnaire (CHAQ), Juvenile Arthritis Quality of life Questionnaire (JAQQ) and moderate agreement for Pediatric Quality of Life inventory

(PedsQL), visual analog scale of wellbeing, and the standard gamble utilities [34]. Loonen et al in his study of over 80 children with inflammatory bowel disease and parents, found that children reported a higher HRQOL than their parents [32]. Parents adequately rated their objective components of their children's HRQOL such as body complaints and motor functioning, but seemed more deficient in rating subjective domains [32]. Despite good agreement regarding HRQOL scores between parents and adolescent with cancer, parents reported the disease having a greater impact on the children [33]. Finally, greater agreement was found in cases of non-depressed and non-divorced parents as compared to those who were depressed and divorced, implicating psychosocial aspects of parents as a major determinant in their rating of children's HRQOL [32, 33].

In contrast to Loonen et al's findings, a Dutch study showed parents who rated children as having a higher HRQOL in the areas of physical complaints, motor functioning, autonomy, cognitive functioning and positive emotions scales than the children themselves [26]. Chambers et al found that parents underestimated their child's pain around their surgery and that correlations between child and parent's ratings of pain were not representative of the relationships of the reports [35]. Wagner et al explored the function of children's illness-related cognitive assessments in the parent-child adjustment relationships specific to the context of juvenile arthritis, and found that increased parental distress and child illness intrusiveness were related to increased depressive symptoms in the child [36]. These findings stress the need to explore the relationship between the child and parent factors in child adjustment, since their influence upon parent responses to questionnaires subject them to cautious interpretation. The level of child-parent agreement therefore varies with child's physical and health status, parent's physical and emotional well being, domain assessed, instrument used, and the construct measured. A stronger effort to obtain child-reports in conjunction with parent-reports and further exploratory studies will contribute to the constructive examination ofthe determinants of concordance.

## Commonly Used Outcome Measures in Pediatric Rheumatic Diseases

Pediatric studies typically use descriptive health status scales, which explore various domains and their relationship with each other, instead of utilities or preference-based measures, which quantitatively assess individual preferences. With utility scales, results have been variable in case of children with musculoskeletal diseases, and therefore the account will focus on descriptive measures [37]. The choice of the instrument is dependent upon the extent of the impact and type of pediatric rheumatic disease, since there are some scales that focus on measuring the impact of physical function alone and others that assess physical function as a part of the assessment of a more global construct such as health status or QOL.

## Steinbrocker Classification

Developed over 5 decades ago, the Steinbrocker classification divides patients into four functional classes based on their abilities to perform activities of daily living, and is used to evaluate short- and long-term functional outcome of patients with JIA [38]. There is a wide range of disability included in these classes and strict delineation between subgroups is often not possible. With the advent of newer instruments that integrate evaluation of physical, social and mental domains, this instrument is used less often.

## Childhood Health Assessment Questionnaire (CHAQ)

The Childhood Health Assessment Questionnaire (CHAQ), a widely used valid and reliable measure of physical function in children with rheumatic diseases is adapted from the Health Assessment Questionnaire (HAQ) [10, 39-41]. The HAQ, used widely in adults, takes into account drug side effects, death and dollar costs in addition to disability, discomfort and pain, although the commonly used components for outcome studies are the disability index, discomfort and pain scales. The CHAQ consists of both child- (8-19 years) and parent-reports (2-19 years), takes less than 10 minutes to complete, easy to administer, score and interpret, with main areas of focus being disability and discomfort. The CHAQ domains estimating disability index and the pain scales and scoring are analogous to those in the HAQ. The CHAQ does not take into account drug side effects, death and dollar costs. The 30 items relating to disability pertain to problems or limitations in the past week attributable to illness in the eight domains of dressing and grooming, arising, eating, walking, hygiene, reach, grip, and activities. The answers are in the form of a 4-point Likert scale with an additional option "not applicable." Disability index, estimated as the mean of the eight domain scores ranges from 0-3, where zero indicates no disability and three translates to severe disability. The score accounts for the aids or devices used, and assistance needed to perform the listed activities. Doubly anchored visual analog scales evaluate Discomfort and Global assessment [10].

When originally developed in 1994, the CHAQ was found to have excellent psychometric properties including test-retest reliability, convergent validity, and good correlations with other scales measuring related constructs such as the Steinbrocker's functional class, active joint count, disease activity and degree of morning stiffness and subsequently has been found to be responsive [10, 42]. However, Ruperto et al compared the relative responsiveness of outcome measures in children with oligoarticular juvenile chronic arthritis which included physician and parent global assessments, functional ability as assessed by the CHAQ, articular variables, and laboratory markers of systemic inflammation.

The most responsive measures were the physician global assessment of disease activity, and articular variables such as the active joint count, global articular severity score, and the number and score of swollen joints. Among the least responsive measures were the CHAQ, morning stiffness, and laboratory indicators of systemic inflammation [43].

The CHAQ has been extensively used in assessing functional outcome in children with arthritis and has been translated into several languages and cross-culturally adapted in a number of countries [44]. The minimal clinically important improvement and deterioration has been calculated for the CHAQ scores to follow long–term outcomes in children with JIA [45]. CHAQ is also valid, internally reliable, and responsive in assessing physical function in children with idiopathic inflammatory myositis and is used as an important measure of functional outcome in clinical trials [46].

## Juvenile Arthritis Functional Assessment Scale (JAFAS) and Juvenile Arthritis Functional Assessment Report (JAFAR)

The Juvenile Arthritis Functional Assessment Scale (JAFAS) assesses physical function in children aged 7-16 years in clinic settings. It is a comprehensive measure of physical function, which requires standardized equipment and entails administration by a trained health professional, physical or an occupational therapist, who times the child's performance on 10 tasks [8]. The JAFAS is reliable and valid, but its responsiveness has not been established. It has been used along with the CHAQ as a measure of functional ability in a study examining the relationship between joint impairment and physical function [20]. The JAFAS has been used as a standard measure of physical function in a study to evaluate the reliability and validity of a Spanish version of the CHAQ [47].

The Juvenile Arthritis Functional Assessment Report (JAFAR), a reliable and valid 23-item scale evaluating physical functional ability has both child- and parent- reports [9]. The responses are in the form of 3-point scales, and total scores range from 0-46, where lower scores indicate better function. Both these versions have good construct validity, reliability and responsiveness [9] [48]. The JAFAR has been used in multiple clinical studies to assess physical function in children with JIA [36]. While measuring convergent validity of the Childhood Myositis Assessment Scales (CMAS), JAFAR was one of the standard measures of physical function [49]. The content for both scales JAFAS and the JAFAR was derived from the HAQ, AIMS, and the McMaster Health Index Questionnaire [50]. The greatest limiting feature for both scales is that they cannot be used in children under 7 years of age. Additionally, JAFAS requires a skilled trained professional for test administration.

# Juvenile Arthritis Functional Status Index (JASI)

Juvenile Arthritis Functional Status Index (JASI) evaluates activities of daily living and functional mobility in children with JIA between 8-18 years of age [5, 6]. Items for JASI were generated rigorously after interviews of children, parents, teachers, clinicians, and subsequently consolidated on priority basis. JASI part I is composed of 100 functional items divided into 5 groups that include self-care, domestic, mobility, school, and extracurricular. Responses are in the form of 7 point rating Likert scale. JASI Part II is more patient-specific, where the child delineates up to five tasks that are difficult to perform and these are assessed on subsequent follow-up on an individualized basis. The JASI has excellent reliability and construct validity, but its responsiveness has not been established. Despite good measurement properties, its use is limited because of the longer time taken to administer the test (over 40 minutes) and the lack of validity in children less than 8 years of age.

# Childhood Arthritis Impact Measurement Scales (CHAIMS)

The Childhood Arthritis Impact Measurement Scales (CHAIMS), adapted from Arthritis Impact Measurement Scales (AIMS) used in adults, was the first disease-specific measure developed for children with JIA [7, 51]. Despite measuring physical function and discomfort in children, this scale has not gained in popularity [7, 52, 53]. Some limitations include lack of robust psychometric properties for all dimensions, non-applicability of many scales for younger children, and lack of published studies demonstrating the use of this instrument [7, 54].

# Functional Status Measure FSII (R)

The Functional Status measure FSII (R), evaluates health status of children aged 0-16 years with chronic diseases that predominantly affect physical function [55]. The FSII (R) is a validated general health status measure in children between ages of 0 to 16 with 47-item (long form) and 14-item (short form) parent-reports. The FSII (R) addresses the areas of eating, sleeping, play behavior and emotional health, and has been demonstrated to have good convergent validity and internal consistency. The FSII (R) has not yet been used to assess a homogenous population of children with arthritis. In a sample of children undergoing clubfoot surgery, the FSII (R) was not found to be sensitive to the problems encountered by the children [56]. The use of this questionnaire is limited by the lack of validity for older children and the lack of a child version.

## Childhood Myositis Assessment Scale (CMAS)

The Childhood Myositis Assessment Scale (CMAS) has been designed as a 14-item quantitative functional assessment tool used for evaluating axial and proximal muscle function in the context of strength and endurance in children with idiopathic inflammatory myopathies [57, 58].

## Juvenile Arthritis Quality of Life Questionnaire (JAQQ)

The Juvenile Arthritis Quality of Life Questionnaire (JAQQ) was developed as a valid and responsive disease-specific measure of physical and psychosocial function in children afflicted with JIA, including spondyloarthropathies [59-62]. Children and their parents completed a questionnaire addressing physical and psychosocial function, and general symptoms and rated items based on the frequency of occurrence and importance. This method of item-generation ensured content relevance. Subsequently, the experts rated these items for their potential responsiveness and grouped them into four categories including gross motor function, fine motor function, psychosocial function and general symptoms. Although the JAQQ has excellent psychometric properties, and measures overall disease-specific HRQOL, its discriminative ability is not as robust, thus limiting comparison between groups [54].

## Childhood Arthritis Health Profile (CAHP)

The Childhood Arthritis Health Profile (CAHP) was developed to evaluate the global physical and psychosocial health status of children over 13 years with JIA. It is a parent-report comprising the following domains: physical functional status, psychosocial functioning, behavior, general health perceptions, and family functioning and impact of disease [63, 64]. This scale consists of the CHQ as the core general health status measure and additionally consists of a module focused on juvenile arthritis [65, 66]. The domains of CAHP are relevant to children with arthritis, but due to lack of sufficient studies published using the CAHP, lack of parallel child-report, and inapplicability in children under 13 years of age limits its use.

## Pediatric QOL Inventory (PedsQL)

The Pediatric QOL Inventory (PedsQL) 4.0 generic module is a brief, valid and reliable measure of QOL in healthy and sick children between 2-18 years [25, 67-69]. PedsQL4.0 has both parent- and child-reports with separate language-adjusted formats for the various age-groups [25]. Both versions comprise of 23 items that address the following four domains: physical, emotional, social, and school functioning. The total, physical and psychosocial summary scores (average of emotional, social and school functioning scores) are calculated on a 0-100 scale, with higher score indicating better QOL. Varni et al showed that the PedsQL appeared to influence clinical decision-making leading to increases in HRQOL in rheumatology clinic, and was sensitive to changes in clinical status over time in the orthopedic clinic [70]. The PedsQL Rheumatology module, designed similar to the generic module has 22 items grouped into five domains of pain and hurt, daily activities, treatment, worry, and communication. The parent-version for children between 2-4 years does not include the worry and communication domains since previous exploratory interviews revealed that these constructs cannot be precisely assessed in toddlers [69]. Together the generic and rheumatologic modules take about 10-15 minutes to complete and have shown to be reliable, valid, and responsive in pediatric rheumatic diseases [69].

## Short-Form General Health Survey SF-36 and Short Form-20 (SF-20)

The Short-Form General Health Survey SF-36 and Short Form-20 (SF-20) are widely used health status measures used in clinical studies of healthy and diseased adults and older adolescents including those with SLE and other rheumatic diseases [71-81]. Being reliable, valid and responsive, the SF-36 consists of multi-item scales that measure eight domains: physical functioning, role limitations due to physical health and emotional problems, bodily pain, social functioning, general mental health covering psychological distress and well-being, vitality, energy or fatigue, and general health perceptions [72, 73, 82]. The major limitation of studies using SF-36 or SF-20 is that they claim to be measuring QOL when they are actually using an instrument derived to measure health status. Therefore a cautious review of studies using these instruments is critical.

## Child Health Questionnaire (CHQ)

The Child Health Questionnaire (CHQ), adapted form the SF-36, evaluates the child's overall health status through following domains: general health perceptions, physical functioning, general behavior, mental health, emotional or time impact, on the parent, family cohesion, change in health, bodily pain, limitations in school, work, and activities with friends due to physical problems and due to emotional and behavioral difficulties, behavior, mental health, and self-esteem, and limitations in family activities [65]. There are both parent-(above 5 years) and child-reports (above 10 years), but the reports are not parallel. The CHQ has been found to be sensitive to clinical changes in children with JIA [83].

## Others

The Child Health and Illness Profile, largely used for adolescent research, is a valid and reliable general health status measure for children between ages 11 and 17 years [84-89]. The EuroQOL, a generic health utility index extensively used in adult studies, has been shown to have validity in assessing QOL in children with JIA [90]. The TNO AZL Children's Quality of Life questionnaire (TACQOL) is a generic parent- report of HRQOL in children aged 6-15 years [27]. The Quality of My Life Visual Analog Scale has been used for measuring the overall QOL and HRQOL in children [4].

## Conclusion

Although various tools are available for examining physical function and related outcomes in children with pediatric rheumatic diseases, they pose several limitations that complicate their efficacy, including the lack of a parallel child or parent report, non applicability in younger children, lack of clinical studies to establish all the psychometric properties, increased length and problems with administering them. The CHAQ, CHQ, JAQQ and the PedsQL are excellent scales for evaluating children with chronic rheumatic diseases. Since QOL, HRQOL, health status and physical function are all relevant constructs in children with chronic rheumatic diseases, it may be necessary to use different measures in conjunction while evaluating them. Given the close relationship between QOL and physical function, it is essential to recognize the subjective nature of assessment, and therefore child-reports should be obtained wherever possible.

The focus of scale development has been in the area of JIA and juvenile dermatomyositis. It is crucial to take into account the disabling effects of uveitis, while evaluating physical function. Additionally, other pediatric systemic diseases, albeit not as common than JIA, are also associated with physical functional impairment, even if only as a part of a widespread systemic process. Therefore, the validation of these instruments in children with systemic vasculitides would enable assessment of physical function and HRQOL in clinical and research contexts.

Physical ability remains very important in children for the development of their motor skills, self-esteem and independence. Therefore, further refinement of existing instruments, and the examination of their relationship with cognitive skills, self-esteem and other markers of development would contribute to a greater understanding of the impact of physical disability in this population..

# References

[1] World Health Organization, *Health Promotion Glossary*. 1998, World Health Organization, Geneva.

[2] Calman, K., Quality of life in cancer patients--an hypothesis. *Journal of Medical Ethics.*, 1984. 10(3): p. 124-7.

[3] Bowling, A., *Health-Related Quality of Life: Conceptual Meaning, Use and Measurement, in Measuring disease: A review of disease-specific quality of life measurement scales*. 2001, Open University Press: Buckingham, Philadelphia, PA. p. 1-22.0

[4] Feldman, B., et al., Distinction of quality of life, health related quality of life, and health status in children referred for rheumatologic care. [see comments.]. *Journal of Rheumatology*, 2000. 21(1): p. 226-33.

[5] Wright, F., et al., The Juvenile Arthritis Functional Status Index (JASI): a validation study. *Journal of Rheumatology*, 1996. 23(6): p. 1066-79.

[6] Wright, F., et al., Development of a self-report functional status index for juvenile rheumatoid arthritis. *Journal of Rheumatology.*, 1994. 21(3): p. 536-44.

[7] Coulton, C., et al., Assessment of the reliability and validity of the arthritis impact measurement scales for children with juvenile arthritis. *Arthritis and Rheumatism.*, 1987. 30(7): p. 819-24.

[8] Lovell, D., et al., Development of a disability measurement tool for juvenile rheumatoid arthritis. The Juvenile Arthritis Functional Assessment Scale. *Arthritis and Rheumatism*, 1989. 32(11): p. 1390-5.

[9] Howe, S., et al., Development of a disability measurement tool for juvenile rheumatoid arthritis. The Juvenile Arthritis Functional Assessment Report for Children and their Parents. *Arthritis and Rheumatism*, 1991. 34(7): p. 873-80.

[10] Singh, G., et al., Measurement of health status in children with juvenile rheumatoid arthritis. *Arthritis and Rheumatism*, 1994. 37: p. 1761-1769.

[11] Manners, et al.,Worldwide prevalence of juvenile arthritis why does it vary so much? *Journal of Rheumatology*, 2002. 29(7): p. 1520-30.

[12] Petty, R., Southwood TR. Baum J. Bhettay E. Glass DN. Manners P. Maldonado-Cocco J. Suarez-Almazor M. Orozco-Alcala J. Prieur, AM., Revision of the proposed classification criteria for juvenile idiopathic arthritis: Durban, 1997.[comment]. *Journal of Rheumatology*, 1998. 245(10): p. 1991-4.

[13] Lehman, T.J.A., Pauciarticular Juvenile Rheumatoid Arthritis, in *UpToDate*, B. Rose, Editor. 2003, UpToDate: Wellesley.

[14] Lehman, T.J.A., Polyarticular unset juvenile rheumatoid arthritis, in *UptoDate*, B. Rose, Editor. 2003: Wellesley.

[15] Brewer EJ Jr., B.J., Baum J, Cassidy JT, Fink C, Jacobs J, Hanson V, Levinson JE, Schaller J, Stillman JS., Current proposed revision of JRA Criteria. JRA Criteria Subcommittee of the Diagnostic and Therapeutic Criteria Committee of the American

Rheumatism Section of The Arthritis Foundation. *Arthritis and Rheumatism*. 20(2 Suppl):195-9, 1977 Mar., 1977. 20(2 Suppl): p. 195-9.

[16] Cassidy, J.T., Petty, R. E., Juvenile Rheumatoid Arthritis, *in Textbook of Pediatric Rheumatology,* J.T. Cassidy, and Petty, R. E., Editor. 2001, Saunders. p. 218-321.

[17] Lehman, T.A., Systemic onset juvenile rheumatoid arthritis, in *UptoDate*, B. Rose, Editor. 2003: Wellesley.

[18] Minden K, N.M., Listing J, Biedermann T, Bollow M, Schontube M, Zink A., Long-term outcome in patients with juvenile idiopathic arthritis. *Arthritis and Rheumatism*, 2002. 46(9): p. 2392 -- 401.

[19] Svantesson H, A.A., Eberhardt K, Elborgh R., Prognosis in juvenile rheumatoid arthritis with systemic onset. A follow-up study. *Scandinavian Journal of Rheumatology*., 1983. 12(2): p. 139 -- 44.

[20] Bekkering, W., et al., The relationship between impairments in joint function and disabilities in independent function in children with systemic juvenile idiopathic arthritis. *Journal of Rheumatology*, 2001. 28(5): p. 1099-105.

[21] Schanberg, L., et al., Daily pain and symptoms in children with polyarticular arthritis. *Arthritis and Rheumatism*, 2003. 48(5): p. 1390-7.

[22] Giannini, E., et al., Preliminary definition of improvement in juvenile arthritis.[comment]. *Arthritis and Rheumatism*, 1997. 40(7): p. 1202-9.

[23] Brunner, H., et al., Preliminary definition of disease flare in juvenile rheumatoid arthritis. *Journal of Rheumatology*, 2002. 29(5): p. 1058-64.

[24] Rider, L., et al., Defining Clinical Improvement in Adult and Juvenile Myositis. [Review] [72 refs]. *Journal of Rheumatology*, 2003. 30(3): p. 603-17.

[25] Varni, J., M. Seid, and P. Kurtin, PedsQL 4.0: reliability and validity of the Pediatric Quality of Life Inventory version 4.0 generic core scales in healthy and patient populations. *Med Care*, 2001. 39(8): p. 800-12.

[26] Theunissen, N., et al., The proxy problem: child report versus parent report in health-related quality of life research. *Quality of Life Research*, 1998. 7(5): p. 387-97.

[27] Vogels, T., et al., Measuring health-related quality of life in children: the development of the TACQOL parent form. *Quality of Life Research*., 1998. 7(5): p. 457-65.

[28] Eiser, C. et al., Can Parents rate their child's health-related Quality of life? Results of a systematic review. *Quality of Life Research*, 2001. 10: p. 347-357.

[29] Eiser, C., et al., Health-related quality-of-life measures for children. *Int J Cancer*, 1999. S12: p. 87-90.

[30] Eiser C, M.R., Quality-of-life Measures in Chronic Diseases of childhood, *in Health Technology Assessment*. 2001, Department of Psychology, University of Sheffield, Sheffield, UK. p. 1-156.

[31] Varni, J., M. Seid, and P. Kurtin, Pediatric Health-Related Quality of Life Measurement Technology: A Guide for Health Care Decision Makers. *JCOM*, 1999. 6(4): p. 33-40.

[32] Loonen, H., et al., Are parents able to rate the symptoms and quality of life of their offsprings with IBD? *Inflammatory Bowel Disease*, 2002. 8(4): p. 270-276.

[33] Sawyer M, A.G., Toogood I, Rice M., A comparison of parent and adolescent reports describing the health-related quality of life of adolescents treated for cancer. *International Journal of Cancer*, 1999. 12: p. 39-45ss.

[34] Brunner, H.I., et al., *Are parents good proxy reporters for children with chronic musculoskeletal disprders (MSKD)?* ACR 65th Annual Meeting, San Francisco, CA, 2001.

[35] Chambers, C., et al., Agreement between child and parent reports of pain. *Clinical Journal of Pain,* 1998. 14(4): p. 336-42.

[36] Wagner, J., et al., The influence of parental distress on child depressive symptoms in juvenile rheumatic diseases: the moderating effect of illness intrusiveness. *Journal of Pediatric Psychology*, 2003. 28(7): p. 453-62.

[37] Brunner, H. et al., Preference-based measurement of health-related quality of life (HRQL) in children with chronic musculoskeletal disorders (MSKDs). *Medical Decision Making*, 2003. 23(4): p. 314-22.

[38] Steinbrocker, O., C. Traeger, and R. Batterman, Therapeutic criteria in rheumatoid arthritis. *JAMA*, 1949. 140(8): p. 659-662.

[39] Fries, J., The assessment of disability: from first to future principles. *Br J Rheumatol*, 1983. 22(Suppl): p. 48-58.

[40] Fries, J., et al., Measurement of patient outcome in arthritis. *Arthritis and Rheumatism*, 1980. 23: p. 137-145.

[41] Ramey, D., J.-P. Raynaud, and J. Fries, The Health Assessment Questionnaire 1992: status and review. *Arthritis Care and Research*, 1992. 5: p. 119-129.

[42] Singh, G., B. Bown, and B. Athreya, Functional status in juvenile rheumatoid arthritis: senstivity to change of the Childhood Health Assessment Questionnaire. *Arthritis Rheum,* 1991. 34: p. S81.

[43] Ruperto, N., et al., Responsiveness of clinical measures in children with oligoarticular juvenile chronic arthritis. *Journal of Rheumatology*, 1999. 26(8): p. 1827-30.

[44] Ruperto N, R.A., Pistorio A, Malattia C, Cavuto S, Gado-West L, Tortorelli A, Landgraf JM, Singh G, Martini A, Paediatric Rheumatology International Trials Organisation., Cross-cultural adaptation and psychometric evaluation of the Childhood Health Assessment Questionnaire (CHAQ) and the Child Health Questionnaire (CHQ) in 32 countries. Review of the general methodology. *Clinical and Experimental Rheumatology.*, 2001. 19(4 Suppl 23): p. S1-9.

[45] Dempster H, P.M., Young N, Feldman BM., The clinical meaning of functional outcome scores in children with juvenile arthritis. *Arthritis and Rheumatism.*, 2001. 44(8): p. 1768-74.

[46] Huber AM, H.J., Lachenbruch PA, Perez MD, Zemel LS, Rennebohm RM, Wallace CA, Lindsley CB, Passo MH, Ballinger SH, Bowyer SL, Reed AM, White PH, Katona IM, Miller FW, Rider LG, Feldman BM. Juvenile Dermatomyositis Disease Activity

Collaborative Study Group., Validation of the Childhood Health Assessment Questionnaire in the juvenile idiopathic myopathies. Juvenile Dermatomyositis Disease Activity Collaborative Study Group. *Journal of Rheumatology*, 2001. 28(5): p. 1106-11.

[47] Goycochea-Robles, M., et al., Validation of a Spanish version of the Childhood Health Assessment Questionnaire.[Comment]. *Journal of Rheumatology*, 1997. 24(11): p. 2242-5.

[48] Giannini, E., et al., Intravenous immunoglobulin in the treatment of polyarticular juvenile rheumatoid arthritis: a phase I/II study. Pediatric Rheumatology Collaborative Study Group.[comment]. *Journal of Rheumatology*, 1996. 23(5): p. 919-24.

[49] Lovell DJ, L.C., Rennebohm RM, Ballinger SH, Bowyer SL, Giannini EH, Hicks JE, Levinson JE, Mier R, Pachman LM, Passo MH, Perez MD, Reed AM, Schikler KN, Smith M, Zemel LS, Rider LsG., Development of validated disease activity and damage indices for the juvenile idiopathic inflammatory myopathies. II. The Childhood Myositis Assessment Scale (CMAS): a quantitative tool for the evaluation of muscle function. The Juvenile Dermatomyositis Disease Activity Collaborative Study Group. *Arthritis and Rheumatism*, 1999. 42(10): p. 2213-9.

[50] Chambers, L., et al., The McMaster Helath Index Questionnaire as a measure of the quality of life for patients with rheumatoid disease. *Journal of Rheumatology*, 1982. 9: p. 780.

[51] Meenan, R., P. Gertman, and J. Mason, Measuring health status in arthritis: the Arthritis Impact Measurement Scales. *Arthritis Rheum*, 1980. 23: p. 14.

[52] Duffy, C. and K. Duffy, Health assessment in the rheumatic diseases of childhood. [Review] [49 refs]. *Current Opinion in Rheumatology*, 1997. 9(5): p. 440-7.

[53] Duffy, C., L. Tucker, and R. Burgos-Vargas, Update on functional assessment tools. [Review] [31 refs]. *Journal of Rheumatology.*, 2000. 27(Suppl58): p. 11-4.

[54] Duffy, C. and D. Lovell, Assessment of Health Status, Function, and Outcome, *in Textbook of Pediatric Rheumatology,* J.T.a.P. Cassidy, Ross E, Editor. 2001, W.B. Saunders Company. p. 178-187.

[55] Stein, R. and D. Jessop, Functional status II(R). A measure of child health status. [erratum appears in Med Care 1991 May;29(5):following 489.]. *Medical Care*, 1990. 28(11): p. 1041-55.

[56] Roye, B.D., et al., Patient-Based Outcomes After Clubfoot Surgery. *Journal of Ped iatric Orthopedics,* 2001. 21(1): p. 42-49.

[57] Rider, L., et al., Development of validated disease activity and damage indices for the juvenile idiopathic inflammatory myopathies. I. Physician, parent, and patient global assessments. *Arthritis Rheum*, 1997. 40: p. 1976-83.

[58] Lovell, D., et al., Development of validated disease activity and damage indices for the juvenile idiopathic inflammatory myopathies. II. The Childhood Myositis Assessment Scale (CMAS): a quantitative tool for the evaluation of muscle function. *Arthritis Rheum,* 1999. 42: p. 2213-9.

[59] Duffy, C., et al., The Juvenile Arthritis Quality of Life Questionnaire--development of a new responsive index for juvenile rheumatoid arthritis and juvenile spondyloarthritides. *Journal of Rheumatology*, 1997. 24(4): p. 738-46.
[60] Duffy, C., et al., Validity and sensitivity to change of the Juvenile Arthritis Quality of Life Questionnaire (JAQQ). *Arthritis and Rheumatism*, 1993. 37: p. S144.
[61] Duffy, C., et al., Relative sensitivity to change of the Juvenile Quality of Life Questionnaire following a new treatment. *Arthritis and Rheumatism*, 1994. 37: p. S196.
[62] Duffy, C., et al., Relative sensitivity to change of the Juvenile Arthritis Quality of Life Questionnaires on sequential followup. *Arthritis and Rheumatism*, 1995. 38: p. S178.
[63] Tucker, L., et al., The Childhood Arthritis Health Profile (CAHP): validity and reliability of the condition specific scales. *Arthritis and Rheumatism*, 1995. 38: p. S178.
[64] Tucker, L., B. DeNardo, and J. Schaller, The Childhood Arthritis Health Profile: Correlation of juvenile rheumatoid arthritis specific scales with disease severity and activity. *Arthritis and Rheumatism*, 1996. 39: p. S57.
[65] Landgraf, J., L. Abetz, and J. Ware, *The Childhood Health Questionnaire: A user manual.* 1996, Boston, New England Medical Center, The Health Institute.
[66] Tucker, L., Outcome measures in childhood rheumatic diseases. [Review] [32 refs]. *Current Rheumatology Reports*, 2000. 2(4): p. 349-54.
[67] Varni, J., M. Seid, and R. CA., The PedsQL: measurement model for the pediatric quality of life inventory. *Med Care*, 1999. 37(2): p. 126-39.
[68] Varni, J., et al., The PedsQL in pediatric cancer: reliability and validity of the Pediatric Quality of Life Inventory Generic Core Scales, Multidimensional Fatigue Scale, and Cancer Module. *Cancer*, 2002. 94(7): p. 2090-106.
[69] Varni, J., et al., The PedsQL in pediatric rheumatology: reliability, validity, and responsiveness of the Pediatric Quality of Life Inventory Generic Core Scales and Rheumatology Module. *Arthritis and Rheumatism*, 2002. 46(3): p. 714-25.
[70] Varni, J., et al., The PedsQL 4.0 Generic Core Scales: sensitivity, responsiveness, and impact on clinical decision-making. *Journal of Behavioral Medicine*, 2002. 25(2): p. 175-93.
[71] Ware, J. and C. Sherbourne, The MOS 36-item Short-Form Health Survey (SF-36) I. Conceptual framework and item selection. *Med Care*, 1992. 30: p. 473-483.
[72] Ware, et al., General Health Status and Quality of life, in *Measuring Health - A Guide To Rating Scales and Questionnaires,* Ian McDowell and Claire Newell, Editors. 1996, Oxford University Press: New York, Oxford. p. 446-456.
[73] Ware, J., et al., *SF-36 Health Survey: manual and interpretation guide*. 1993, Boston, MA: The New England Medical Center.
[74] Thumboo, J., et al., A prospective study of factors affecting quality of life in systemic lupus erythematosus. *Journal of Rheumatology*, 2000. 27(6): p. 1414-20.

[75] Karlson, E., et al., The relationship of socioeconomic status, race, and modifiable risk factors to outcomes in patients with systemic lupus erythematosus. *Arthritis and Rheumatism.*, 1997. 40(1): p. 47-56.
[76] Perez-Cuevas, J., et al., A quality of life study in women with systemic lupus erythematosus and its relation to disease activity[Spanish]. *Anales de Medicina Interna,* 1999. 16(9): p. 457-60.
[77] Sutcliffe, N., et al., Associates of health status in patients with systemic lupus erythematosus. *Journal of Rheumatology*, 1999. 26(11): p. 2352-6.
[78] Fortin, P., et al., Impact of disease activity and cumulative damage on the health of lupus patients. *Lupus*, 1998. 7(2): p. 101-7.
[79] Gilboe, I., T. Kvien, and G. Husby, Health status in systemic lupus erythematosus compared to rheumatoid arthritis and healthy controls. *Journal of Rheumatology*, 1999. 26(8): p. 1694-700.
[80] Vu, T. and A. Escalante, A comparison of the quality of life of patients with systemic lupus erythematosus with and without endstage renal disease. *Journal of Rheumatology*. 26(12):2595-601, 1999 Dec., 1999. 26(12): p. 2595-601.
[81] Stoll, T., et al., Prediction of depression in systemic lupus erythematosus patients using SF-36 Mental Health scores. *Rheumatology*, 2001. 40(6): p. 695-8.
[82] Beaton, D., C. Bombardier, and S. Hogg-Johnson, Choose your tool: a comparison of the psychometric properties of fie generic health status instruments in workers with soft tissue injuries. *Qual Life Res,* 1994. 3: p. 50-56.
[83] Selvaag, A., et al., Measuring health status in early juvenile idiopathic arthritis: determinants and responsiveness of the child health questionnaire . *Journal of Rheumatology,* 2003. 30(7): p. 1602-10.
[84] Starfield, B., et al., Adolescent health status measurement: development of the Child Health and Illness Profile. *Pediatrics.*, 1993. 91(2): p. 430-5.
[85] Starfield, B., et al., The adolescent child health and illness profile. A population-based measure of health. *Medical Care*, 1995. 33(5): p. 553-66.
[86] Starfield, B., et al., Health status of well vs ill adolescents. *Archives of Pediatrics and Adolescent Medicine*, 1996. 150(12): p. 1249-56.
[87] Feigelman, S., et al., Psychosocial and environmental correlates of violence perpetration among African-American urban youth. *Journal of Adolescent Health.*, 2000. 27(3): p. 202-9.
[88] Forrest, C., et al., The health profile of incarcerated male youths. *Pediatrics.*, 2000. 105(1 Pt3): p. 286-91.
[89] Altshuler, S. and J. Poertner, The child health and illness profile-adolescent edition: assessing well-being in group homes or institutions. *Child Welfare.*, 2002. 81(3): p. 495-513.
[90] Brooks, R., EuroQol: the current state of play. [Review] [32 refs]. *Health Policy*, 1996. 37(1): p. 53-72.

In: Arthritis Research: Treatment and Management
Editor: F. Columbus, pp. 147-184
ISBN 1-59033-984-3


*Chapter VII*

# Management of Osteoarthritis

***Jiri Chard***
Medical Research Council – Health Services Research Collaboration, Department of Social Medicine, University of Bristol, Whiteladies Road, Bristol BS8 2PR, UK

## Abstract

### Introduction

Osteoarthritis (OA) is the most prevalent form of arthritis, and represents a major burden on individuals, health systems and societies. In this chapter the issues relating to the successful management of OA are discussed, these include epidemiology, diagnosis, treatment and service provision.

### Methods

Literature searches were conducted on ISI – Web of Science, Medline, Embase and Cochrane Collaboration Library for all years up to 2003 for articles relating to the management of Osteoarthritis. In addition, the bibliographies of existing review articles were searched for further relevant articles. No restrictions were placed in type of publication included in the review. The literature identified was then incorporated within a general discussion of the management of osteoarthritis. Primary data from qualitative interviews and focus groups, and quantitative questionnaire surveys was also included.

### Results

The results of the searches show that a large research base is available on OA, but unfortunately this research is concentrated on pharmaceutical and surgical interventions, and furthermore research is concentrated on mono-therapy rather than poly-therapy or service delivery. However, the research that is available demonstrates that successful management is possible, and an attempt is made at outlining a management strategy and service structure for OA. Unfortunately, published data on service organisation for OA is very limited, but the primary data sources allow an evidence-based service structure for OA to be outlined.

### Discussion

OA is a complex condition with a number of factors influencing disease progression and so need for treatment and services. Treatment is split between non-surgical patient self-managed treatment and surgical health professional managed treatment. This split means that different health professionals need different skills when dealing with OA patients and the patient has to expect different types management styles at different points in disease progress. The effectiveness of treatments varies enormously and is influenced by a number of factors, such patient compliance. It is also clear that many of the more effective treatments are associated with potential harm or only short-term benefit, which has to be taken into account with any treatment decision. It appears that a formal service structure could improve the quality of service for OA. The one area that appears to be lacking in the research literature is identifying which packages of care are most effective on which patients. However, successful management of OA is possible, in spite of the issues outlined above.

## Introduction

Osteoarthritis (OA) is the most prevalent form of arthritis, and represents a major burden on individuals, health systems and societies. In this chapter I will provide an overview of the issues relating to the successful management of osteoarthritis. This includes sections on the epidemiology of osteoarthritis, diagnosis of OA, effectiveness of treatment for OA and provision of services for OA. This will hopefully provide the reader with a greater insight into the successful management of OA than it is possible to provide in a short journal review article.

# Methods & Data sources

## Literature Search

Results from previous literature searches undertaken by the author were used as the basis for this article [1 2]. However additional literature searches were undertaken on Medline, Embase, Cochrane Collaboration Library and ISI – Web of Science for all years up to and including 2003 to identify articles published since these searches were undertaken, and identify literature on areas not covered by the existing searches. The bibliographies of identified review articles were also searched for additional articles. It was only possible to review articles written in the English language. The search strategy was designed to identify any article relating to the any treatment or service for osteoarthritis in any joint. There was no restriction (such as RCTs only) on the type of publication selected.

This chapter is not a systematic review, though articles were systematically identified. However, the aim has been to provide evidence on treatments and services where it exists and to highlight where evidence is currently deficient.

# Primary Data Sources

Survey and interview data from a number of studies undertaken by the author into issues surrounding service delivery for osteoarthritis are also included in the chapter. This provides the basis for the discussion on service delivery issues at the end of the chapter.

# What is Osteoarthritis?

Osteoarthritis (OA) is a common, age-related condition of synovial joints characterised pathologically by localised areas of loss of articular cartilage associated with overgrowth of bone at the joint margins (osteophytosis), changes in the subchondral bone, fibrosis of the joint capsule, and variable degrees of mild synovitis. These pathological changes, when severe, appear on a radiograph as joint space narrowing and osteophyte formation, and it is the radiograph that is generally used to diagnose the condition. The pathology may also be associated with pain and functional impairment that are major causes of disability in older people. However, there is evidence that the association between joint space narrowing and clinical symptoms is not linear [3].

OA can develop in any synovial joint in the body, but some sites are much more likely to be affected than others. It is commonest in the distal interphalangeal joints of the fingers, the base of the thumb, the apophyseal joints of the cervical and lumbar spine, the medial tibio-femoral and lateral patello-femoral compartments of the knee joint, the superior pole of the hip, and the base of the big toe. Symptomatic OA is uncommon in the ankle or elbow [4].

# Epidemiology of Osteoarthritis

Epidemiological evidence shows OA is a highly prevalent condition [5 6 7]. Radiographic features are practically universal in at least some joints in people aged over 60 years, but significant clinical disease probably affects 10-20% of people in this age group, and knee disease is about twice as prevalent as hip disease in people aged over 60 (about 10% *v* 5%) [8 9 10]. We also know the impact that osteoarthritis has on the individual: pain, stiffness and functional problems (Table 1), and OA has also been associated with depression and anxiety, though these are the results of the physical symptoms, rather than being cause directly by the disease. So an individual's disease severity is based on the interaction of physiological, psychological and environmental factors [10 11 12]. In addition to the physical and psychological impacts of the disease, OA also has serious social and economic consequences. Research shows that people being severely financially and socially disadvantaged as a result of OA [10 13 14]. The recent World Health Organisation (WHO) review of the impact of diseases noted that musculoskeletal disorders are the fourth commonest cause of disability-adjusted life years (DALYs), with OA making the greatest contribution [15]. This relates to a massive burden on the individual, health systems and society. The financial burden for OA in the USA alone is estimated to $65 billion per year. And this burden is only likely to grow with the increase in prevalence of the main risks factors associated with OA, namely an ageing and obese population.

**Table 1- The Heterogeneity of Osteoarthritis**

| | Hip | Knee | Hand |
|---|---|---|---|
| Selected risk factors | | | |
| 1. Age | + | ++ | ++ |
| 2. Gender | F=M | F>M | F>>M |
| 3. Obesity | + | +++ | + |
| 4. Trauma | +/- | + | + |
| Selected outcomes | | | |
| 1. Pain | +++ | ++ | + |
| 2. Disability | ++ | ++ | +/- |
| 3. Likely to progress | ++ | + | +/- |
| 4. May stabilise or regress | + | +/- | ++ |

Strength of the associations summarised as none (-), weak (+/-), moderate (+), strong (++) or very strong (+++). (from Dieppe *et al*, 2003) [160]

Note: Different Features and Associations of OA of Three of the Commonest Joint Sites to be Affected.

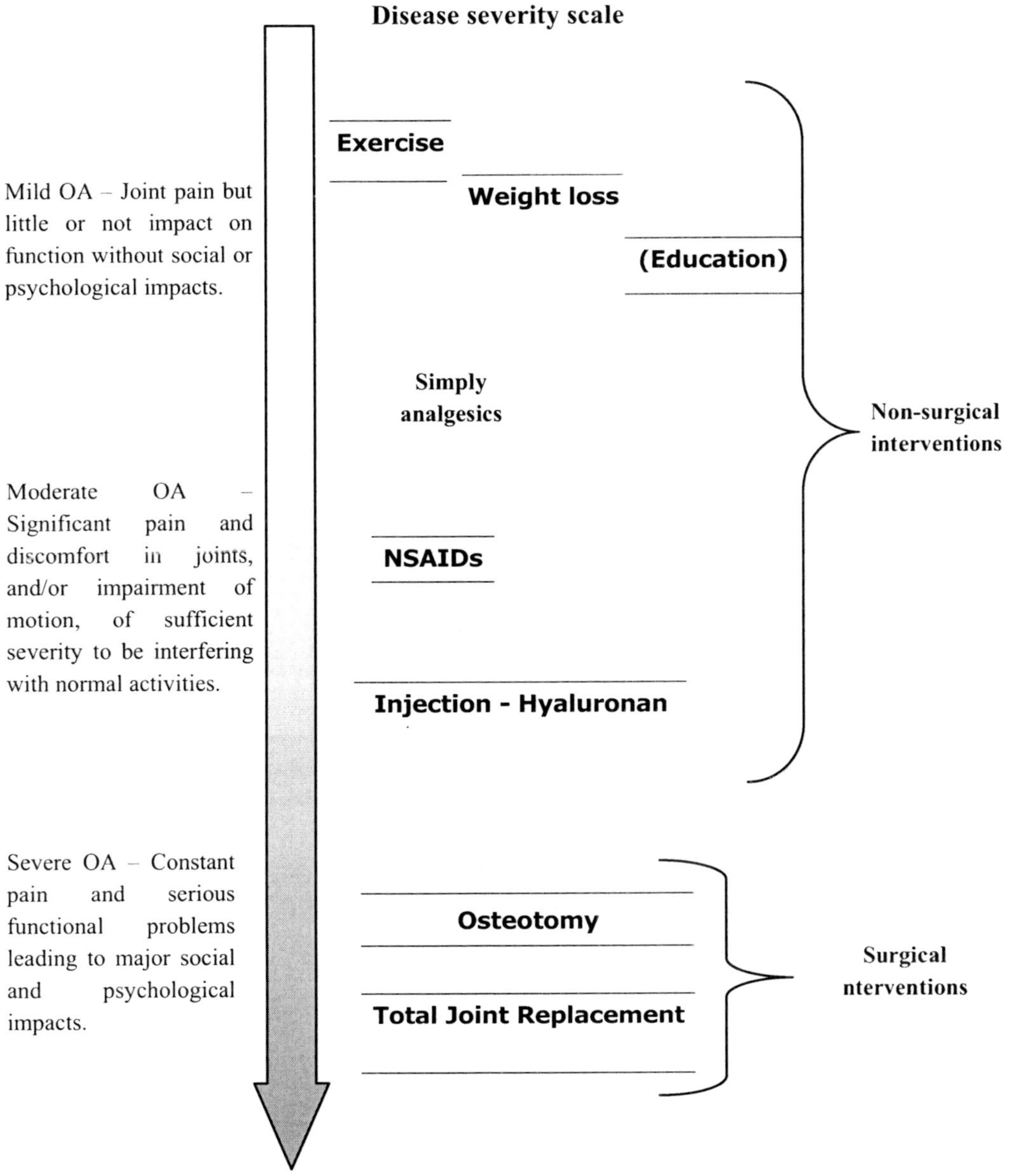


Figure 1. Treatments for Osteoarthritis.

**Notes:**

- Each intervention is introduced – dependent on any contra-indications – based on severity.
- Treatments are cumulative, with more treatments being added to the management plan as and when required.
- Here only treatments with a proven adequate level of efficacy are shown, but patients can use additional treatments – such as dietary supplements.

## Diagnosis

Diagnosis of OA is often based on radiographic findings of joint abnormalities, but as was stated earlier the link between radiographic findings and physical symptoms is not linear, and this says nothing about any links between radiographic findings and social and psychological disease impact [3]. The American College of Rheumatology has classification criteria for reporting OA of the hand, hip and knee that includes physical abnormalities and pain (Table 2) [16 17 18 19 20]. The main value of these criteria is for research – to aid reporting of patients and entry criteria to studies; they are not diagnostic criteria. However, they do provide us with insights into the main features of the disease that separate it from other rheumatic diseases (Table 2). Some of these features, such as pain made worse by joint use and at the end range of movement, are common to all joints, others, such as palpable crepitus at the knee, are site specific. In addition to the above criteria are a number of standard self-report instruments used to assess the severity of OA for research studies, the best known of which is the Western Ontario McMaster Osteoarthritis Index (WOMAC) [21] which measures pain, stiffness and functional difficulties. It may be possible to apply such measures to routine clinical use, but at present this is not the case. So, in the assessment of the severity of OA, in addition to joint damage, the following factors have to be taken into account - pain, function, social, psychological factors and quality of life.

## Factors Influencing Available Research on Treatment of OA

Review evidence shows that a large amount of research has been undertaken on the treatment of osteoarthritis [22], but the amount and quality of evidence available for each specific intervention varies considerably – with a massive amount of pharmaceutical research available, but very little research on alternatives such as education [22 23]. The reasons for these differences include:

- The different regulatory requirements for their approval and use – pharmaceuticals are required by law to be RCT tested before approval for use is given, but there is no similar requirement on educational interventions or many complementary therapies.
- The different commercial interests involved. – pharmaceutical and surgical prosthesis companies are amongst the largest in the world, and spend billions on research and development of products, in contrast physiotherapy does not have such corporate structure and so research and development is on a much smaller scale.
- The relative difficulty of undertaking high quality research on complex interventions in comparison with drug trials – placebo control drug trials are

relatively simply, placebo controlled education trials are far more difficult. The result is research on complex interventions is often limited to observational studies rather than more complex research designs.

- Different research traditions between health professions. – The medical profession has a long tradition of research whilst physiotherapists do not. This impacts on the level of research conducted within health services with physicians dominating research to the exclusion of other health professionals.

**Table 2 – American College of Rheumatology criteria for the classification of OA**

| | |
|---|---|
| **Hip (clinical and radiographic)** | |
| 1. | Hip pain for most days of the prior month |
| 2. | ESR =/< 20 mm/hr |
| 3. | Radiographic femoral and/or acetabular osteophytes |
| 4. | Radiographic joint space narrowing |
| (OA is present if features 1,2, and 3, or 1,2 and 4 or 1,3 and 4 are present) | |
| **Knee (clinical)** | |
| 1. | Knee pain for most days of the prior month |
| 2. | Crepitus on active joint motion |
| 3. | Morning stiffness =/< 30 mins in duration |
| 4. | Age =/> 38 yrs |
| 5. | Bony enlargement of the knee on examination |
| (OA present if 1,2,3 and 4, or 1,2 and 5 or 1, 4 and 5 present) | |
| **Hand (clinical)** | |
| 1. | Hand pain aching or stiffness for most days of the prior month |
| 2. | Hard tissue enlargement of =/>2 distal interphalangeal joints |
| 3. | Hard tissue enlargement of 2 of 10 other selected hand joints (proximal interpahalangeal and first carpometacarpal joints) |
| 4. | Swelling of =/< 2 metacarpophalangeal joints |
| 5. | Deformity of =/> 1 of 10 selected hand joints |
| (OA present if 1,2,3 and 4 or 1,3,4 and 5 present) | |

Note: These are not diagnostic criteria but they do document the main features of the condition which help distinguish it from other rheumatic diseases at each joint site.

What the above means is that the quality and amount of evidence available for particular treatments is not directly linked to its actual use. For example, all health professional groups recommend exercise for the treatment OA, but the amount of evidence available on its effectiveness is tiny compared to that for NSAIDs. This means that we do not know how effective exercise is for OA. However, a lack of research is not the same as saying that a treatment is not effective, it is just that we do not know if it is effective or not. A lack of a coherent research agenda for OA also means that there is only limited information on effectiveness of treatments at different stages of OA severity, for example, at what stage of disease severity is surgery most effective. This flaw in the research agenda now represents one of the significant problems for the establishment of a truly evidence based management strategy for OA. Unfortunately it seems unlikely that any coherent research agenda will emerge for OA, and the best hope is that those undertaking future studies will build into them the ability to investigate the question of how effectiveness changes with disease severity.

## Lay, Folk and Formal Management of OA

The actual of management for OA, like virtually all other conditions, is likely to rely on a mixture of lay, folk and formal medical information, interventions and management. It is important that health professionals are aware of the issues relating to these non-formal areas, as they are likely to have a significant impact on their own attempts to treat and manage, especially a chronic condition like OA.

The word 'lay' refers to something that is not endorsed with formal authority in a particular situation, for example a 'lay' preacher is someone who is not formally ordained within a religious organisation. In relation to healthcare this refers to areas where non-health professionals are involved in the healthcare of an individual, usually the individual themselves, friends, family and colleagues, and includes information provision, referral systems, and even treatment [24 25]. Research has found that in most situations patients use a variety of treatments that they have found themselves or have been recommended by other non-professionals [26]. Research also found that patients beliefs and information about a condition were heavily influenced by 'lay' beliefs and information rather than formal medical opinions [27 28]. Clearly this potentially has a major impact on management of a condition like OA. It is important that health professionals are aware of patients beliefs about their condition and are aware of all the treatments the patient is using for their condition, as these may impact on the success of the health professionals own management strategy.

The term 'folk' is used to describe practitioners, treatments and management that are not endorsed by the medical establishment (governing bodies) but which have their own formal belief system and for which a formal transaction (consultation) is often required by the patient. Folk treatments are often not based on the standard accepted view of science [29]. For example, homeopathy is based on the belief that disease should be treatment should be based on ingredients that produce similar symptoms to those of the disease, and that diluting a solution containing treatment actually increases its potency. The reason that it is important for health professionals to know about folk medicine is that research shows that a significant percentage of patients with OA use treatments that may be classified as folk [26 30]. Patients have a variety of reason for doing this – some out of a willingness to try anything that may help their condition, others out of desperation for an effective treatment, and others out of a clearly held belief that folk medicines are effective. Health professionals need to know if patients are using folk treatments as it may impact with their own treatments, especially if patients own beliefs about OA are influenced by folk interpretations of the condition.

The final area is formal medicine that covers those practitioners endorsed by the governing authorities as representing valid medical practices. This is the area within most formal research is undertaken, and therefore the focus of this review. Of course the distinction between groups is often blurred, for example, many formal medical practitioners use 'folk' medicines [29]. The main point is that patients belief and understanding will often be influenced by opinions from outside formal medical practice, and patients are likely use a variety of treatments not formally recommended for use by a health professionals. These issues will impact on a health professionals' attempts to manage a condition, so they must be aware of them.

What the above section shows is that formal medicine is only provides some of the information and interventions that a patient will use in the management of their condition. This is important for the health professional to know for a number of reasons. Firstly, it is important that the health professionals knows all treatments a patient is using in order to assess the impact of any additional treatments they may recommend. Secondly, it is important that health professionals assess that patients are using treatments correctly, and that the treatment is appropriate for the patient. For example, patients often use joint supports, but if these are not used correctly then they can do more harm than good. Thirdly, the health professional will often have to work with patients who have different beliefs of the disease and treatment based on lay and folk information, it therefore important that they understand the patient beliefs and is able to work with them rather than ignoring them –this is especially true for OA where most treatment is delivered via self-management [31 32].

# Patient Self-management

A key theme with the treatment of most chronic disease is the high degree to which patients are expected to self-manage their condition [33 34 35 36 37]. The reason for this is not any lack of commitment on the part of health professionals, but that the practicality of treatment means that patients have to undertake most of it unsupervised. In the case of OA, as will be shown, a variety of treatments are used with a varying degree of self-management needed, but for non-surgical patients it will be themselves or a carer will undertake the majority of treatment they receive. It is therefore obvious that in order for patients to self-manage they have to be educated in order to be able to do this effectively. This education can range from basic advice on how to take treatments to more in-depth education on how to change life-styles and cope with OA. However, as will also be outlined later, self-management does not mean that patients do not require continued support and help with their treatment, so there will continue to be a need for professional input in the management process, and research shows it is this issue that is at the heart of patients ability to self-manage.

In recent years the issue of patient empowerment has been raised as a means to improving disease management in general, and patient self-management in particular. The argument is that if patients become more empowered within the healthcare process, a position they have not traditionally enjoyed, that they will be able to get the services they want in the form they want, and so will be more satisfied and compliant, which in turn will lead to improved outcomes. This issue is examined in more depth below.

## Patient Empowerment

Patient empowerment is a popular term used in healthcare these days, but is almost never defined. The dictionary definition of empowerment means: giving something or someone power that they did not previously have. Patient empowerment relates to a wide range of issues from the empowerment of patient groups in the control of health services to empowerment of individual patients in the relationship they have with health professionals. Here we are interest in the latter of these. The traditional structure of the health professional-patient relationship has been one of health professionals dominance or paternalism, this being due to their control of knowledge and resources that the patient will need. The patient therefore has traditional been in a subordinate and even submissive role to the health professional – being expected to comply with the doctors orders without question. This model emerged when the majority of diseases treated in health systems where acute and when society was far more hierarchical than it is now. However, it is argued that this model is no longer applicably in modern society and leads to low satisfaction, compliance and poor outcome, especially in chronic diseases. And research has shown that compliance with treatment is a major issue with chronic conditions, with patients not following health professionals orders [31 38], but that patients have valid reasons for not complying [31]. The reason that the paternalistic model seems to fail, particularly in chronic disease, is that the needs of the patients are not taken into account, and the patient is not involved in decision-making. It is argued this is where patient empowerment will help improve disease management.

Patient empowerment means that the patient is given a greater role in the management decisions for their condition. They, after all, are the people administering most of the treatment and living long-term with the results of compliance and non-compliance. The health professional and patient work as a team designing a treatment regime that is both effective and that the patient feels able to comply with. The health professional brings their expertise with treatment, and the patient brings their expertise with coping and living with the condition. The advantage of this concept is that the planned and actual outcomes of long-term treatment are likely to closer than if the health professional dictates orders. Of course, with empowerment comes responsibility for the patient. Health professionals must make sure that the patient wants to take the responsibility for decision-making, as many patients prefer to listen to the expert rather than making decisions themselves. The patient empowerment/ shared-decision making model is almost universally accepted in healthcare – but it is still important that health professionals are aware that when dealing with non-surgical OA that patient empowerment is essential to long-term compliance.

**Table 3. Summary of Available Treatments, Available Research and Efficacy/Effectiveness of Treatments**

| Intervention | Amount of research | Efficacy of intervention |
|---|---|---|
| Education | Low | Low |
| Exercise | Moderate | Moderate |
| Nutrient Supplements, including glucosamine, chondroitin | Moderate | Low |
| Physical supports | Low | Low |
| Simple analgesics - acetaminophen | Moderate | Moderate – short term |
| Systemic non-steroidal anti-inflammatory drugs, including coxibs | High | Moderate – short term |
| Tramadol and opiod analgesics | Low | Moderate – short term |
| Topical agents, including capsaicin and NSAID creams and gels | Low | Low – short term |
| Intra-articular injections, including steroids and hyaluronan | Moderate | Moderate |
| Arthroscopic surgery | Moderate | Unpredictable – possible placebo effect |
| Other surgery, including osteotomy | Low | Moderate |
| Joint replacement surgery | High | High |
| Alternative and complementary interventions | Low | Low |

Amount of evidence: low = <15 Large primary studies; Moderate = <25 large primary studies; High 26> large primary studies

Efficacy: Low = little impact on symptoms for majority of patients, moderate = good impact on symptoms for majority of patients, high = excellent impact on symptoms for majority of patients

# Treatment of Osteoarthritis

A number of treatments are available for use on osteoarthritis. These are often used in combination with one another, but unfortunately there is no research evidence on the effectiveness of different management strategies or at what stage of OA severity it is most effective to use a particular treatment. In this section the effectiveness of most commonly used treatments for OA are summarised (Table 3).

## Primary Prevention of OA

Primary prevention is the term used to describe preventing a disease from occurring in the first place, and is mainly related to the modification of risk factors associated with the development of a condition (table 1). There is a reasonable amount of epidemiological research on OA showing the main risk factors associated with the disease, these being: age, weight, gender, repetitive joint use and joint injury. Other factors that have been suggested are based on ethnic and genetic markers, but research remains limited and often contradictory [39 40 41 42 43 44]. Of the factors outlined, weight and joint use are the only modifiable factors (though impact of HRT on OA levels in women has been examined there are potential risks with using this treatment that may outweigh protection it affords [45]). Research estimates that between 25 and 30% of knee OA is preventable via reducing obesity, and 25 to 30% is preventable via avoiding repetitive activities [46]. Therefore health professionals should routinely be recommending weight lose to obese patients - and should add OA to the list of disease linked with obesity. Advice on joint use is slightly harder to target, but people presenting to health professionals with repetitive work or sports injuries should be advised of the potential risks.

It is clear that primary prevention is largely based on patient life-style changes over long periods of time, and that such interventions will be delivered via public health education. The problem with this life-style advice is that the impact of OA is unlikely to be seen for many years, so people may discount the risk and so ignore the advice. For example, despite the on-going anti-smoking campaign numbers of smokers in many developed countries are actually rising. It is also unlikely that major funding would be available for such campaigns given the very limited funding for disease prevention, and the low priority given to OA as a condition compared to heart disease or cancer associated with obesity and smoking.

## Secondary Prevention

Secondary prevention relates to slowing or stopping disease progress once it has started. Central to this issue has been improving our understanding of the actual disease mechanisms involved in OA, and a large amount of research effort has gone into this area over recent years. The aim has been to discover a pharmacological intervention that interferes with the disease mechanisms, and such Disease Modifying Drugs (DMOADs) are the 'Holy Grail' of OA research. Unfortunately, although a number of agents are being tested none have yet been conclusively shown to modify the disease process [47 48 49 50] . Recently much interest has been given to the potentially disease modifying effects of glucosamine, with two RCTs showing a significant reduction in joint space narrowing [51 52]. However, the results of these RCT results have yet to be independently confirmed.

## Tertiary Prevention and Symptom Management

Given that primary prevention seems only likely to have a limited impact, and effective secondary prevention is currently not available, it seems that there will continue to be a need for more active treatment to slow disease progress and tackle disease symptoms. Below the treatment options available to health professionals are outlined along with the available information on their effectiveness.

## Education

The patients themselves, through self-management, control the utilisation of most non-surgical interventions. This means that information provision and education are particularly important in relation to non-surgical management of OA. Patients should always be told what is wrong, what treatments are available to help them, and the advantages or disadvantages of each, in language that they can understand.

However, within osteoarthritis research the term education has been extended to more life management issues, encompassing interventions involving behavioural change, environmental adaptation, psychological support and social support. The main reason for being included under the education heading is that they all involve a major educational element compared to the actual level of physical treatment. A number of patient education programmes have been developed over the years, probably the best known being the Arthritis Self-Management Programme (ASMP) from the USA (http://patienteducation.stanford.edu/programs/asmp.html) [37]. The ASMP uses a holistic to the self-management of arthritis, not only examining the actual treatment but also incorporating issues like communicating with friends and family about arthritis.

Unfortunately the evidence of the effectiveness of formal education programs shows only small effect sizes. Meta-analyses are available on educational interventions. The earliest found effect sizes associated with education were not significant for pain (WMD 0.16, 95% CI -0.69 to +1.02) or disability (WMD 0, 95% CI -0.61 to +0.61). The next showed only a small non-significant effect size of pain (-0.10, 95% CI -0.19 to 0.01). The most recent review of 17 studies found an effect size for pain of 0.12 (95% CI 0.00, 0.024) and for disability of 0.07 (95% CI 0.00, 0.15) [53 54 55]. Even the most recent RCTs show mixed results [56 57].

However, the aim of most educational interventions is not to reduce absolute pain or disability levels (as was tested by the meta-analysis), but reduce disease impact by changing behaviour, improving compliance with other treatment, or improving psychological well-being. Therefore, beneficial effects of education may relate more to a decrease in perceived psycho-social consequences of OA and improved compliance with other treatments, than to absolute pain reduction. Nevertheless, given the limited effectiveness demonstrated by research evidence for formal educational programmes the use of such interventions cannot currently be recommended. This does not mean that education should be abandoned, just that the currently available programmes may not be effective and need further development [37 58]. And patients will continue to require general education on the use of treatments from health professionals.

### *Behavioural and Environmental Coping Strategies*

The aims of behavioural and environmental coping strategies are to reduce the symptoms of OA, and the impact that they have on an individual's life. Examples include diet, weight loss, exercise, and adaptations to the home or the workplace [59 60]. These changes are strongly linked with education of the patient to enable them to make such changes to behaviour and environment. Referral to an occupational therapist is recommended to facilitate these approaches, particularly if home or workplace adaptations appear to be of special importance to the individual. Evidence of the effectiveness of this type of behavioural change on OA is almost non-existent, but epidemiological data show that repetitive joint use is a causal risk factors in OA. As was shown above more formal education programs appear to show little impact on symptoms.

### *Psychological and Social Support*

OA often causes major psychological and social problems: enforced changes in life roles, and anxiety about the future are frequent complaints. Depression is common, and an important determinant of pain severity and disability. The aim of psychological and social support is to relieve the impact of OA, and is highly dependent on the individual patient and their disease severity [60 61 62]. Psychological support ranges from family networks to formalised psychologist led interventions aimed at reducing symptoms of anxiety or depression. Similarly, social support can range from family networks to formal social service interventions. As with most treatment referral to specialists such as psychologists and social workers may be necessary when disease impact is severe.

Although social and psychological impacts of disease can be seen as secondary to those of the physical impact, it is important in chronic disease that these issues are properly addressed. There is very little evidence available on the effectiveness of these interventions in OA. This means no definitive recommendation can be made on the use of these interventions with OA. However, health professionals managing OA should not ignore the social and psychological impacts of chronic disease.

## Exercise

Exercise is one of the most frequently recommended treatments for OA of the hip or knee. It can be divided into two main types: local to treat specific joints (usually exercises to improve muscle strength and range of movement), and general activity training (such as aerobic exercises). With both types the aim is to reduce pain and disability. Muscle strengthening can reduce the load on joints and improve stability, aerobic exercises increase general fitness, and may aid beneficial weight loss [63].

A number of systematic reviews and RCTs are available on exercise treatments for osteoarthritis [64 65 66 67 68 69 70 71 72 73]. More recently RCTs tend to be larger and higher quality than earlier RCTs, and these more recent RCTs have all found small to moderate effects sizes from exercise. A recent meta-analysis which includes most of the more recent large RCTs found a pooled treatment effect size for exercise of: -0.46, 95% CI -0.62 to -0.31, however there was a great deal of heterogeneity with these results: Q=23.9 , P=0.002, which probably reflects the variation in interventions used (which range from simple advice to walk more, to complex packages of supervised physical therapy) [54]. This finding was confirmed by another meta-analysis of 16 trials of exercise for hip and knee OA which found an effect size on pain of –0.46 95% CI –0.57, -0.35 [74].

One of the most interesting findings of these more recent RCTs was that long-term effectiveness of exercise declined (decrease in effect size per month of follow-up 0.02, 95% CI 0.00 to 0.03, p=0.01) and concluded that this was due to poor patient compliance than decline in treatment effectiveness [71]. The authors recommended that patients receive 'boosters' in order for them to maintain the long-term benefits of exercise. Therefore, one of the main issues that has to be addressed by health professionals is how to maintain patient compliance with exercise. Patients often find it difficult to exercise due to the pain caused by their joints, and they often believe that exercise will worsen their condition rather than improve it. It is therefore necessary for health professionals to encourage patient to continue with exercise, in spite of the pain, and to education patients about the benefits of exercise on their OA. Another RCT demonstrated that the cost-effectiveness of exercise interventions may be greatly improved by group exercise sessions, which were shown to be at least as effective as individual sessions in one trial [72]. A recent review comparing one-to-one, group and home exercise programmes found standard mean differences (SMD) for pain of 0.52(0.32, 0.72), 0.47 (0.34, 0.60), 0.28(0.16, 0.40) against placebo respectively, and for function 0.32 (0.12, 0.52), 0.39 (0.25, 0.52), 0.27(0.16, 0.38) against placebo respectively. What this suggests is that group therapy is the most effective format for the delivery of exercise for OA [75].

As with the previous options the heterogeneity of interventions and lack of any standardised treatment regime means recommendation of specific exercises is not possible. However, referral to physiotherapists may be a cost-effective option if they are providing group treatment sessions. Overall what the evidence shows is that moderate exercise, in the form of aerobic and muscle strengthening, is an effective treatment for OA and should be routinely recommended by health professionals.

## Physical Aids and Supports

Aids used in the management of OA include joint braces, shoe wedges/insoles, walking aids, and taping of joints. The use of these can be traced back hundreds, if not thousand of years. However, there are only a small number of RCTs available on the most popular forms of physical aids – shoe in-soles and joint braces [76 77 78]. Overall the results of research on physical supports shows they are effective, however due to the limits of size and quality recommendations on the use of supports cannot be made until much larger scale RCTs have been undertaken. However, as has been stated, people have been reporting benefits from the use of canes and applying devices to their joints for centuries, and the evidence from individual trials shows significant improvements in pain and function from some interventions, including knee braces, wedged shoe insoles and canes [1]. The major advantage of physical aids is that treatment is reversible and non-invasive. However, a major concern with physical aids is ensuring that the patient uses them correctly, as improperly used equipment can cause damage if used over prolonged periods. This was found in one RCT where 13% of participants using a brace reported adverse effects [76]. It is therefore important that when recommendations on the use of this type of product are made it is followed-up with education on use of these products. Unfortunately a large number of products are freely available to patients. It is therefore important that health professionals pre-empt problems and ensure that patients are informed about the negative, as well as the positive aspects of this type of treatment. However, as with so many treatments for OA, the lack of evidence means it is unknown if such treatment are of any benefit or not.

## Dietary Supplements

Dietary supplements are commonly prescribed by health professionals and used as self-medication by patients. A number of supplements are available and these are used both individually and in combination. The amount of evidence available on their effectiveness has improved dramatically over recent years.

### *Glucosamine and Chondroitin*

Glucosamine and chondroitin are dietary supplements ('nutriceuticals'), used alone or in combination, that may reduce the symptoms of OA, and possibly retard the progression of the condition [79 80 81]. A number of systematic reviews and RCTs are available examining the effective of these agents. These reviews report small to moderate treatment effects sizes. One review reported a pooled effect size for 7 RCTs for glucosamine *v* placebo of 1.40, 95% CI 0.65 to 2.14) [81]. The same review reported that the safety profile of glucosamine in the 16 RCTs was excellent [71]. Out of the nearly 1000 people randomised to glucosamine treatment in the RCTs, 14 were withdrawn because of toxicity (comparative figures not provided) but it found insufficient evidence on long term tolerance. A more recent meta-analysis found a pooled effect size on pain for glucosamine versus placebo of: -0.18, 95% CI –0.28 to –0.09 and for chondroitin versus placebo pooled effect size: -0.78, 95% CI –1.00 to –0.54 [54]. However, research has also shown the heterogeneity of products sold as glucosamine, with a range of 59 to 138% of content stated on labels [82]. This may have a major impact on the effectiveness of the product experienced by individuals, though it is unknown if this issue has impacted on research where it is hoped more stringent controls would be in place. Many of the reviews have highlighted the potential of commercial bias affecting the research results.

Longer-term studies have highlighted potential protective properties of glucosamine (secondary prevention), specifically as reducing the rate of joint space narrowing in OA patients. Issues have been raised about these results, but if they can be repeated in other long-term studies then a potential effective and safe preventive treatment for OA may have emerged [51 52]. Major public health issues arise if the long-term protective effects of glucosamine are proven to be correct. Questions such as: when should people start taking glucosamine? And, should certain high-risk groups be targeted?

Given the excellent safety profiles and that both are inexpensive there is no reason for people not to use them if they find them effective even though this may be a placebo effect. However, at present evidence suggests that short-term use of glucosamine at best provides small benefits for patients.

### *Ginger, Avocado and Soybean Extracts*

Plant extracts are increasingly being investigated as potential safe and effective treatments for osteoarthritis. Evidence remains limited on these agents. Only one short-term large-scale trial including 261 patients compared ginger extract with placebo. It found a small to moderate benefit after 6 weeks (effect size 0.31, 95% CI 0.56-0.06). Four large-scale trials [83 84 85 86] found a combination of avocado and soybean extracts to have a moderate benefit for pain relief (pooled effect size –0.43, 95%-CI –0.74 to –0.13 [54]), but heterogeneity in these results means that they have to be treated with caution.

Dietary supplements offer the patient potential benefits with seemingly few side-effects. Therefore there seems no reason to discourage patients from using them if they find them effective, especially for pain control. However, no formal endorsement can be made, as there is currently not enough evidence to do so.

## Pharmacological Pain Relief

### *Acetaminophen*

Evidence evaluating its effectiveness of acetaminophen is surprisingly scarce. Three systematic reviews were identified which include use of acetaminophen on osteoarthritis. The first (search date 1994, 3 RCTs) evaluating simple analgesics in osteoarthritis of the hip [87], the second (search date 1994) evaluating simple analgesics in osteoarthritis of the knee [88], and the third evaluating acetaminophen against placebo and NSAIDs [89]2003). The reviews found limited evidence that simple analgesics were effective in controlling pain associated with osteoarthritis compared with placebo.

More studies are available of acetaminophen versus NSAIDS. The three systematic reviews mentioned above cover this comparison [87 88 89] and several additional RCTs are available. The systematic reviews found no evidence for the superiority of NSAIDs over simple analgesics. Subsequent RCT evidence further supports this conclusion, with only one study finding NSAIDs to be significantly better than acetaminophen. The conclusion of one n-of-1 trial probably reflects the reality of the situation – some patient do better on acetaminophen and some do better on NSAIDs, until the individual patients compares their effectiveness it is unknown which is preferable [90].

Given its relatively satisfactory long-term safety profile and accepted short-term analgesic effect [91], it seems prudent to recommend it as the initial form of pharmaceutical pain-relief for OA. And this is the conclusion made by most available guidelines [92,93].

### NSAIDs

There are hundreds of trials on NSAIDs; they report effective pain relief in OA, but that long-term use is likely to result in gastrointestinal or other complications. There is no evidence that any one NSAID is superior to another [1]. Similarly, there is no evidence to help indicate which patients should be treated with an NSAID rather than an analgesic. Two systematic reviews are available, one for the hip (search date 1996) and one for the knee (search date 1996). Both reviews found that NSAIDs provided good pain relief, but that long-term use was associated with GI side-effects. Neither review found sufficient evidence to recommend one NSAID compared to another. A recent meta-analysis found only a small benefit of NSAIDs compared with acetaminophen (effect size 0.28, 95%CI 0.48-0.08), while n-of-1 trials and surveys suggest that a proportion of patients will respond better to either approach [87 94]. Use of NSAIDs should be considered when simple analgesics are failing to provide adequate pain relief, and where there are no contra-indications to their use (existing GI problems). Simple analgesics and NSAIDs can be used in conjunction with one another.

A concern raised about NSAID trials is that the exclusion criteria applied due to concerns about subject safety mean that results are not representative of the actual population and so their practical usefulness is reduced [95]. This inclusivity debate raises some basic ethical issues in relation to medical research, and goes far wider than just NSAIDs.

### Coxibs

Coxibs (COX-2 selective inhibitors) represent the new generation of NSAIDs. They are meant to provide similar pain relief to non-selective NSAIDs, but with reduced GI side-effects. The COX-2 selectivity of these agents is on a scale rather than a binary difference, so, in theory, the more selective an agent the lower the GI adverse events [96]. Randomised trial evidence suggests that coxibs are indeed as effective as traditional NSAIDs [97 98 99 100 101 102 103 104]. However, recent re-analyses have questioned the claims of improved safety of these expensive drugs [105 106]: the moderately COX-2 selective celcoxib may not have improved GI safety, while the highly selective rofecoxib may lead to an increase in cardiovascular adverse events [107]. These problems may be dose related, and dose reduction might improve long-term safety. However, this hypothesis remains to be tested in adequately powered, long-term trials. Use of COX-2s should only be used where simple analgesics have failed; there are contra-indications for use of non-selective NSAIDs.

It is clear that there is still some way to go in the debate about the use of COX-2s, and that this will hamper recommendations on the use of them for the foreseeable future.

## Opiates

Interest in the use of opiates, such as tramadol and codeine, for pain management in OA has been increasing. A number of RCTs are now available showing that tramadol is an effective analgesic, comparable to NSAIDs, and no reported serious adverse events or treatment abuse was reported [108 109 110].

The use of opiates for pain control in chronic disease is controversial. Therefore caution is recommended in their use, and alternatives such as acetaminophen and NSAIDs should be considered before opiates.

## Other Pharmaceutical Interventions

Diacerhein is slow-acting drug for osteoarthritis (SADOAs). Evidence is limited, but results from two recent large scale trials indicate that diacerhein has only a small benefit (pooled effect size –0.18, 95%-CI –0.34 to – 0.01), even though it may have some beneficial effects on disease progression [111]).

## Topical Agents

Topical agents, most of which contain NSAIDs or capsaicin, are seen as a safer option for pain control in OA than oral pharmaceuticals. The amount of evidence available on these agents is minimal compared to oral pain relief, and this probably reflects a generally sceptical view on the theoretical basis for topical agents of this type. A review conducted on the effect of topical NSAIDs compared to placebo in OA found a relative risk (RR) for relief from pain of 2.0 (95%-CI 1.5-2.7) [112]. However, it seems likely that the large effect sizes found in smaller trials had a disproportionate impact on the analysis. This notion is supported by a subsequent large-scale trials [113 114], which failed to detect a significant difference between a topical NSAID and placebo. However, work is continuing on this form of intervention for NSAIDs using newer vehicle gels, as it offers such an attractive methods of treatment [115].

Capsaicin-containing products may have rather different effects, and have been found to have some efficacy in predominantly small trials [116]. A subsequent large-scale trial, however, found only a small benefit (effect size –0.25, 95%-CI –0.69 to 0.19) [117].

Recommendations on use of topical NSAIDs cannot be made, as the evidence is still not strong enough to make any clear conclusions. However, given the excellent safety profile of topical agents their use should not be prevented if found to be effective, and the main issue is cost of such treatments, but the benefit of formal prescription of such products is debateable.

## Injections

Intra-articular injections of agents are popular amongst health professionals, as a method for directly applying treatment to the problem site but without the need for surgery

### *Glucocorticoids*

One systematic review [118] and two subsequent RCT are available on this treatment [119]. The systematic review found that intra-articular injection of glucocorticoids into the knee (1 trial used 4 injections, the rest used single injections) provided a little additional pain relief compared with placebo (not defined). The subsequent RCT [119] found a short-term benefit (1- 4 wks) of the steroid injection compared with placebo (saline) for both pain and for a functional index [119]. The second recently published trial suggested that long-term injections were not associated with detrimental effects on joint space, it did not provide evidence for a beneficial long-term effect of steroids on pain either, with an effect size of 0.12 after two years (95%-CI –0.36 to 0.60) [120]. However, given the relatively small effect size shown for this intervention its use cannot be recommended.

### *Hyaluronan*

Hyaluronic acid (HA) is a naturally occurring polysaccharide. As the viscous component of synovial fluid, it acts as a lubricant and shock absorber [121]. The standard treatment regimen is 3-5 injections over the course of a few weeks, and courses may be repeated every 6-12 months. One meta-analysis, one systematic review [118] and several RCTs were identified [122 123 124 125]. The review found slightly greater benefit with the injections versus placebo at 1-6 months after treatment. However, RCTs published since then have reported mixed results but with the balance in favour of the use of injections. A recent meta-analysis found a pooled effect size for pain of: -0.48, 95% CI –0.72 to –0.23 [54]. This represents a moderate treatment effect, so making injections one of the more effective treatments for OA. However, as with all pharmacological interventions, the effects of injections are not permanent, and there are also few studies on the repeated long-term use of injections in patients.

## Arthroscopic Surgery for Knee Joint OA

Arthroscopic surgery is a very popular form of surgery for OA of the knee and is seen as useful for patients not yet suitable for total joint replacement, particularly younger patients. Surgery involves either the wash-out the joint to remove fragments of material that may be causing problems and/or the repair and removal of abnormalities of the bone or cartilage.

Several RCTs and observational studies have claimed that these procedures are effective [126 127 128 129 130 131 132]. However, in a recent trial, Moseley et al, compared arthroscopic lavage and arthroscopic débridement with sham surgery and found a trend towards increased pain in both active groups with an effect size of 0.28 (95%-CI –0.07 to 0.64) for lavage and 0.13 (95%-CI –0.23 to 0.49). The 95%-CIs excluded any clinically meaningful benefit of arthroscopic interventions [133]. The results of this RCT may explain the findings of earlier non-placebo controlled RCTs and observational studies [128,130 131] that highlighted unpredictability of results for arthroscopic surgery, which may have been due to a placebo effect. Of course, further trials are needed these findings, but if true have major financial and ethical implications – could the money be put to better use; and is it ethical to provide a treatment that is no better than placebo, even though it produces a large and long-term placebo effect? What this trial also highlights is the need for RCT evidence about treatment efficacy and effectiveness for all treatments.

## Osteotomy

Osteotomy is a surgical intervention that involves the removal of a wedge of bone tibia in order to bring the joint alignment to within normal ranges. Four RCTs of osteotomy versus other surgical treatments [134 135 136 137]. These showed that osteotomy was as effective as TJR in selected groups.

## Total Joint Replacement

Total joint replacement (TJR) represents the most invasive treatment available for osteoarthritis. It involves major surgery and a long period of rehabilitation for patients. Patients are selected based on age (usually older than 55), disease severity (pain not controlled by other treatments), and contra-indications to surgery (weight, co-morbidities). Although joint replacement has not been subjected to randomised trials compared to sham treatment or no intervention, it is clear from the large volume of observational data that it is an effective and cost-effective intervention for severe OA of the hip or knee joint [138 139 140], and there a number of large surgical registries that monitor the progress of patients [141 142 143].

However, problems remain, including morbidity, and the fact that some 10% of those operated on appear to obtain relatively little benefit [144 145 146]. The main issue with the use of TJR is the selection of people for surgery. There is no evidence available to help aid prospective selection of people for surgery, not even case-control studies, so it is entirely left to the surgeon's own decision, based on the personal experience and results of observational studies. The major problem with observational studies is that all patients have been selected for surgery rather than being randomly allocated to surgery and are not compared with other matched non-surgical groups, so it is unknown who benefits most from surgery and when surgery is most beneficial for particular groups of people. It is therefore essential that at the very least case-control studies be undertaken to examine which patients should be selected for surgery.

Overall joint replacement surgery represents the most effective intervention for moderate to severe OA. It is therefore important that health professionals are able to appropriately refer patients for surgery and that capacity is in place for surgery to be delivered.

# Complementary and Alternative Therapies

Complementary and alternative therapies are widely used by people with OA. Evidence on the effectiveness of these interventions is very limited [147]. Acupuncture, is the only modality with a reasonable level of research evidence to support its use: two systematic reviews of acupuncture found evidence of effectiveness on pain and but not on function when compared to sham treatment [148 149]. Other complementary therapies include: homeopathy, herbal remedies (such as Willow Bark), and massage. Glucosamine is often categorised as a CAM therapy, but due to the level of interest in dietary supplements these have been afforded their own section. Evidence on effectiveness is very limited and what evidence is available points to a placebo effect in most cases. However, if the treatment is safe, easily reversible and most importantly the patient derives benefit from it's use then health professionals should not dissuade patients from using such products in conjunction with more conventional therapies. Given the limited evidence on CAM therapies the formal recommendation on their use cannot be made, and prescription of such therapies without further evidence is debateable. However, as was shown earlier, a significant percentage of patients with OA use CAM treatments [30 150]. This means that health professionals cannot ignore or dismiss these treatments, but instead will have to learn to work with these therapies.

# Summary of Treatments

The above section shows the range of available treatments for OA and the range of reported effectiveness from each intervention. Table 3 and figure 2 provide a summary of treatments and management options for OA. However, a number of factors will impact the effectiveness of a treatment, including: patient compliance, health professional technical skill and knowledge, and timing of treatment. All will have an impact on the outcome of a treatment.

Another issue with the evidence available on effectiveness is the lack of it for many of the available options (table 3). It is impossible to make recommendations on the use of treatment where no evidence is available on its effectiveness; the obvious example here is individual types of exercise. Having said this there does appear to be a core number of treatments that are effective and should be provided by health services, and figure 2 outlines a theoretical outline for how treatment for OA would proceed. The management of OA should be concentrated on a gradual intensification of treatment depending on disease severity and impact that is present to the health professional. As will be outlined below the actual application of treatments requires a number of elements to be in place to ensure the successful management of OA. Health professionals should not recommend those treatments outlined above where evidence suggest little effectiveness (not where evidence was not available), but they should not prevent patients from accessing these treatments if this is what they want.

Another major issue facing the use of evidence in the treatment of OA is the lack of data on how treatment effectiveness varies with disease severity, both physical and overall. This presents a major barrier to the successful management of OA, as it is unknown at what severity each treatment is most effective, when they should be introduced and when, or if, treatment should be stopped. Addressing this issue requires studies sizes to increase considerable in order to the required statistical power to be obtained and for such sub-group analysis to be outlined in study designs.

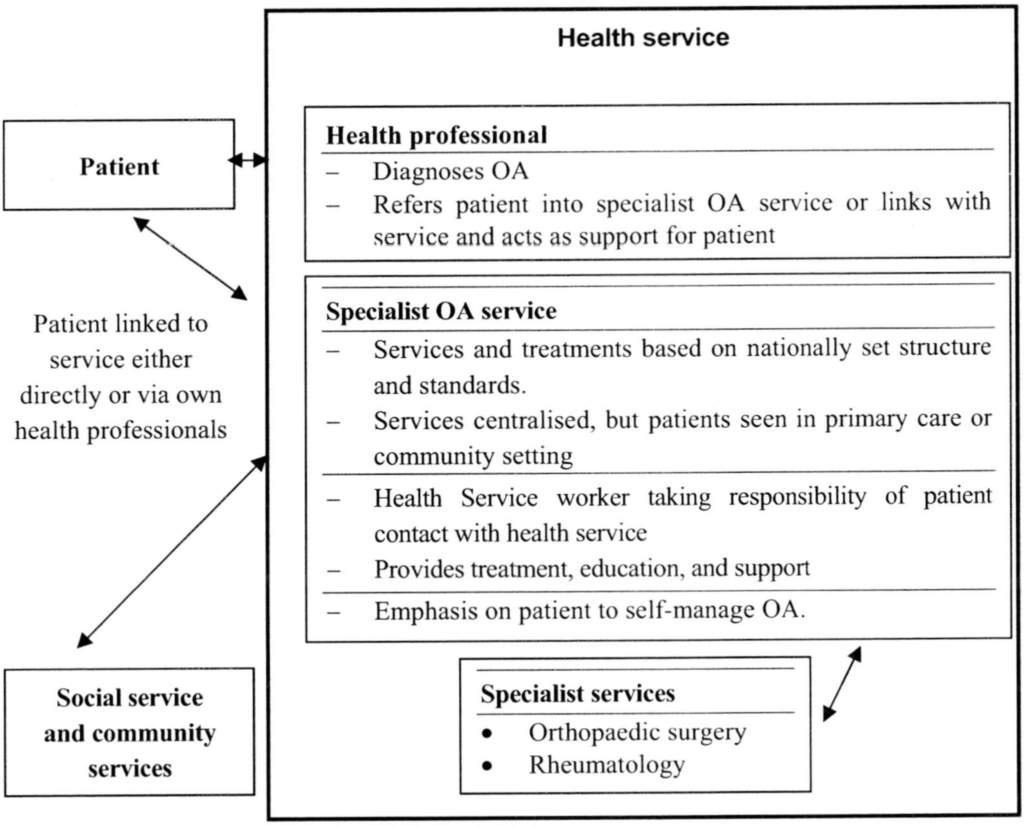


Figure 2. A suggested service structure for OA.

# Services for OA

It is relatively straightforward to provide a summary of advances in available treatment for osteoarthritis. However, the practical use of such articles is often questionably as they provide no insight into the true complexity of dealing with a condition like osteoarthritis.

Treatments reviews only concentrate on the efficacy and effectiveness of treatment, leaving the actual application and organisation of treatment to the individual health professional or organisation. Such an approach is justified given the limited remit of treatment reviews, however, it overlooks the importance that delivery of services has, especially with chronic diseases like OA where treatment may be required over many years. It is therefore important, with a disease like OA, to examine service delivery issues. Health professionals may not see it as their role to develop services, but the fact is that they play a key role in the development of all services, so must therefore be aware of the issues involved.

In order to provide a high quality service a series of resources need to be in place, and it is these that will determine the quality of service that is provided. While there is little available evidence specifically on the development of services for OA, there is a vast amount of general research on service development and structure that can be used [151 152]. The main resources that influence a service are: treatments – an intervention is available to give to patients, staffing – staff are available to provide treatments and support services, knowledge – staff have the necessary knowledge to apply treatments, working relationship – communication and cop-operation between staff and between staff and patients, equipment & facilities – physical infrastructure needed for service, motivation – staff want to provide service, service organisation & planning – a structure has been put in place for the deliver of a service, finance – money is available for service provision, and power – those in position of power endorse provision of service. The aim of any service is to organise resources to provide the highest quality possible. A number of definitions are available of how to measure quality are available, and more or less cover the same items [153 154]. One of the most commonly used is that outlined by the Joint Commission on the Accreditation of Healthcare Organisations (JCAHO). This defines six factors central to service quality: efficacy – research shows that treatment provide benefit, effectiveness – research shows that treatment provided benefit in normal healthcare setting, efficiency – services are cost-effective, and organised to maximise resources, appropriateness – that patients get the treatment they need when they need it, access – that people have easy administrative and physical access to services, and continuity – that services are provide in a reliable and responsive manner.

However, recent qualitative research undertaken by the author shows that in the case of OA a number of issues relating to resources mean that currently high quality services for OA are not available [155 156]. The themes outlined below are based on the results of 42 one-to-one interviews undertaken with patients, health professionals, and mangers involved with the management of OA in the United Kingdom.

- *Few efficacious treatments* – There is a generally held view, backed by research evidence, that the only 'cure' is joint replacement surgery, and that other treatments are only likely to provide moderate short-term benefits due to low efficacious or poor effectiveness. This is a fundamental issue in the provision of any service, especially for a chronic condition where treatment is required over long periods.

- *High prevalence* – As the figures outlined above show, OA has very high prevalence. This is viewed as a major burden on health services, especially as no efficacious treatments are available, except surgery, meaning that long-term management is required. Many health professionals and managers are concerned that any service for OA would be swamped as staffing and facilities would not be available to cope with demand.
- *Perceived low impact of OA* – Osteoarthritis is viewed as a low impact condition due to being slow to progress and non-fatal, especially when compared to other conditions such as cancer or rheumatoid arthritis. For this reason managers and health professionals in resource limited services give priority to services for condition where treatment is more effective or disease impact is seen as greater.
- *Limited motivation to manage OA amongst health professionals* – Many health professionals groups often see the management of OA as a 'heart sink' condition. This is due to the lack of efficacious treatment and the requirement for long-term management, naturally this makes health professionals reluctant to take on the management of OA. Research shows that health professionals are unwilling to provide the long-term support that many patients want. Research also shows that this situation is reversed in orthopaedic surgery where an effective treatment is available. Here OA patients account for 80% of elective workload, and surgeons are enthusiastic to take on the management of suitable patients.

Low motivation also has an impact on the quality of referrals, with many health professionals inappropriately referring patients to colleagues, especially surgeons, in order to off-load a group of patient they feel they cannot help and do not want to manage. The result is that patients are often moved around a health system looking for a health professional willing to help, but responsibility usually remains with primary care physicians.

- *Large number of health professionals treating OA* – A large number of groups help with the treatment of OA: primary care physicians, specialist-nurses, rheumatologists, physiotherapists, occupational therapists, and orthopaedic surgeons. The large number of groups treating OA means that the likelihood of inappropriate referral is increased as patients are moved around the system.
- *Financial resources limited health services* – Basic to any health service is a limit on available financial resources. The actual ceiling of available resources varies between countries, so some are able to provide a wider range of services than others, but in all cases the factors outlined above combine to mean that OA is given a low priority compared to other conditions. The result is that only in orthopaedic surgery are significant resources committed for the treatment of OA.
- *Power and control of services and resources* – Important to any service is that those in charge of resources are committed to the establishment of the service, otherwise the necessary resources will not be available, and so the service will not be able to introduced. The limited motivation amongst health professionals

and managers for managing OA means that there is no attempt to provide comprehensive services. So while patients with OA, especially non-surgical patients, may want a more comprehensive service because they have little power in the provision of most services they do not get want they want. This situation is only reversed in situations of private healthcare where the patient directly pays for services so can demand what they want, but even in these situation no service has been formally planned or organised.

All the above factors contribute to OA being given a low priority for service provision. It is only when patients enter orthopaedic service that OA become a higher priority, mainly due to the effectiveness of surgical interventions, which has a 'knock on' effect on all other factors. Unfortunately only a minority of people with OA will receive surgery, and a large percentage of those sent for surgery are inappropriately referred. Therefore there is a need for more work on service provision for non-surgical services.

## What would a Service for OA Look Like?

The limited evidence of dedicated services for osteoarthritis means making recommendations of service structure based on evidence difficult. However the evidence from qualitative research that does exist clearly shows that existence of a service structure is better than its absence, and work from Germany shows that integrated rheumatology services are successful [157].

This section on services for OA is based on the assumption that resources, in the form of staff, finance, equipment, facilities, and time, are made available to create such a service. If resources were not made available then it would be impossible to provide a service, as it could not be introduced alongside existing services.

A suggested structure for an OA service is outlined in figure 2. The initial point of contact can be via any health professional that the patient consults. The health professional has to make an initial diagnosis of OA, but then has the option to take on the support role for the patient or refer the patient on to a dedicated case manager within the OA service. If the health professional decides to continue with management then they must have they must have the undertaken the appropriate training. The patient too must decide who they want to act as support for the management of their condition. Whoever is the point of contact for the patient will link into a clearly defined service structure. The OA service provides the equipment, facilities, time, staff over a prolonged period of time and at the local level that the patient requires. Thus, the patient is provided with appropriate treatment, monitoring and support. When and if patients require help that the case manager cannot provide then they are able to access the appropriate professional – orthopaedic surgery.

This relatively simple service structure appears to mirrors that which already exist in most healthcare settings, and this is true. However, the service has a significant number of advantages over existing services structure for OA.

- Firstly, the main emphasis of the service is supporting patient self-management, rather than continually providing treatment. One of the key elements for patient self-management is that a support structure is put in place for the patient to access when they are self-managing. Expecting the patient to self-manage with only *ad-hoc* support is only likely to lead to poor outcomes. The support structure would take the form of an open access case-worker(s) who could provide treatment and advice when the patient is facing problems, and, if necessary, referral to more specialist care.
- Secondly, the service would be independent of the individual practitioner. The service structure would ensure the reliability and responsiveness without being dependent on the motivation of a particular health professional. Support can be provided via telephone or at outreach clinics based in primary care settings where patients would have access to case workers (most likely trained physiotherapists or extended role nurses), and, perhaps, more specialised health professionals.
- Thirdly, one of the key figures in the service structure that has been outlined is the case manager. Case managers have been successfully used in other areas of healthcare [158 159]. The advantages of using a case manger against a physician are that the physicians time is freed to concentrate on individuals where their expertise is likely to produce benefits, and the case-manager can give more time to the individual patient than it is likely that the physician could. The case manager can be trained in the treatment, service provision and support for self-management.
- Fourthly, the service acts as a focal point for referral and filtering of all OA patients. Most of the present issues with services for OA relate to the lack of service for non-surgical cases. What this service provides is a service for these patients, while appropriately referring patients on to more specialist care, such as surgery.
- Fifthly, service would be for all OA patients (surgical and non-surgical), where as, at present, only limited support services are available for non-surgical patients.
- Sixthly, the service would use a 'hub and spokes' design. What this would mean is that the service would be centrally administered, but provided at a local level. This would allow the standard of the service to be monitored, and, more importantly, it would allow health professionals to maintain professional links rather than being isolated in community based services.

It could be argued that the provision of a dedicated service for OA, as outlined above, would be a waste of resource and so inefficient. This could be true, but that assumes the choice is between providing no service or providing a service, however this is not the case. People with OA will seek treatment and will require assistance no matter what the circumstances. What the service shown here does is formalise the current informal arrangement for service organisation for OA, which will hopefully lead to quality improvements without requiring disproportionate resource increases.

## Conclusion

The evidence presented above provides a picture of the current situation relating to the management of osteoarthritis. It is clear that OA is a large and growing issue for health services that will have to be addressed. The research evidence on treatment efficacy and effectiveness shows that moderate effect sizes are possible with non-surgical interventions, and large effect sizes are possible with surgical interventions, however the amount of evidence available on many options is small so making any recommendations on use difficult.

While research continues on developing more effective treatments, and perhaps even cures for OA, the area that presently appears to require the most attention is the actual organisation and implementation of treatment. The current reality is that no service or pathway for OA is available, and health professionals have to rely on their on knowledge and resources to provide suitable management to patients. Although there is no evidence on services provision for OA, it is likely that the lack of any service structure will impact on patient outcome due to inappropriate referral, inappropriate treatment, staff motivation and delays in proper treatment. The service structure outlined in this chapter shows one possible service structure that will address many of the service quality issue raised by health professionals, patients and managers. However, this structure has not been tested, so it is unknown what impact it would have on service quality.

Successful management of OA is possible, even using non-surgical interventions, but requires a great deal of effort from both health professionals and patients over a long period of time. If either group do not take an active role in management then it is unlikely to be beneficial. Introduction of more formalised service structures for the management of OA would seem to offer a way of improving the quality of service provided, and so increasing the likelihood of successful management of OA.

## References

[1] Scott D, Smith C, Lohmander S, Chard JA. Osteoarthritis. In: Godlee F, ed. *Clinical Evidence*. London: BMJ, 2003.

[2] Chard JA, Dieppe PA. The case for nonpharmacologic therapy of osteoarthritis. *Current Rheumatology Reports* 2001;*3*:251-257.

[3] Creamer P, Hochberg MC. Why does osteoarthritis of the knee hurt - sometimes? *British Journal of Rheumatology* 1997;*36*:726-728.

[4] Petersson IF. Occurence of osteoarthritis of the peripheral joints in European populations. *Annals of the Rheumatic Diseases* 1996;*55*:659-664.

[5] Felson DT. Epidemiology of hip and knee osteoartritis. *Epidemiological Review* 1988;*10*:1-28.

[6] Dieppe PA, Cushnaghan J, Tucker M, Browning S, Shepstone L. The Bristol 'OA500 study': progression and impact of the disease after 8 years. *Osteoarthritis and Cartilage* 2000;*8*:63-68.

[7] Petersson IF. Occurence of osteoarthritis of the peripheral joints in European populations. *Ann Rheum Dis* 1996;*55*:659-664.

[8] Gaffney K, Ledingham J, Perry JD. Intra-articular triamcinolone hexacetonide in knee osteoarthritis: Factors influencing the clinical response. *Ann Rheum Dis* 1995;*54*:379-381.

[9] Pavelka JK, Sedlackova M, Gatterova J, Becvar R, Pavelka SK. Glycosaminoglycan polysulfuric acid (GAGPS) in osteoarthritis of the knee. *Osteoarthritis & Cartilage* 1995;*3*:15-23.

[10] Brooks P. Impact of osteoarthritis on individuals and society: how much disability? Social consequences and health economic implications. *Current Opinion in Rheumatology* 2003;*14*:573-577.

[11] Dieppe PA, Chard JA, Faulkner A, Lohmander S. Osteoarthritis. In: Godlee F, ed. *Clinical Evidence*. London: BMJ Publications, 2000;437-447.

[12] Hosie G, Dickson J. *Managing osteoarthritis in primary care*. London: Blackwell Science, 2000.

[13] Yelin E. The economics of osteoarthrits. In: Anonymous1997.

[14] Yelin E. The earnings, income, and assets of persons aged 51-61 with and without musculoskeletal conditions. *J Rheumatol* 1997;*24*:2024-2030.

[15] Murray CJL, Lopez AD. *The global burden of disease: A comprehensive assessment of mortality and disabilty from diseases, injuries, and risk factors in 1990 and projected to 2002.* Geneva: World Health Organisation, 1996.

[16] Altman R, Alarcon G, Appelrouth D, et al. The American-College-of-Rheumatology Criteria for the Classification and Reporting of Osteoarthritis of the Hip. *Arthritis and Rheumatism* 1991;*34*:505-514.

[17] Altman R, Alarcon G, Appelrouth D, et al. The American-College-of-Rheumatology Criteria for the Classification and Reporting of Osteoarthritis of the Hand. *Arthritis and Rheumatism* 1990;*33*:1601-1610.

[18] Altman RD, Block DA, Brandt KD, et al. Osteoarthritis - Definitions And Criteria. *Annals of the Rheumatic Diseases* 1990;*49*:201.

[19] Altman RD, Bloch DA, Bole GG, et al. Development Of Clinical-Criteria For Osteoarthritis. *J Rheumatol* 1987;*14*:3-6.

[20] Altman R, Asch E, Bloch D, Et Al. Development Of Criteria For The Classification And Reporting Of Osteoarthritis - Classification Of Osteoarthritis Of The Knee. *Arthritis and Rheumatism* 1986;*29*:1039-1049.

[21] Bellamy N, Buchanan WW, Goldsmith CH, Campbell J, Stitt LW. Validation study of WOMAC: a health status instrument for measuring clinically important patient relevant

outcomes to antirheumatic drug therapy in patients with osteorthritis of the hip or knee. *J.Rheumatol.* 1988;*15*:1833-1840.

[22] Chard JA, Tallon D, Dieppe PA. Epidemiology of research into interventions for the treatment of osteoarthritis of the knee joint. *Ann.Rheum.Dis.* 2000;*59*:414-418.

[23] Pendleton A, Arden N, Dougados M, et al. EULAR recommendations for the management of knee osteoarthritis: report of a task force of the standing committee for international clinical studies including therapeutic trials (ESCISIT). *Ann Rheum Dis* 2000;*59*:936-944.

[24] Calnan M. *Health and Ilness: the lay persepctive.* London: Tavistock, 1987.

[25] Williams SJ, Calnan M. *Modern medicine :lay perspectives and experiences.* London: UCL Press, 1996.

[26] Ramos-Remus C, Gutierrez-Urena S, Davis P. Epidemiology of complementary and alternative practices in rheumatology. *Rheumatic Disease Clinics of North America* 1999;*25*:789-+.

[27] Donovan J. Patient education and the consultation: the importance of lay beliefs. *Ann Rheum.Dis* 1991;*50 Suppl 3*:418-421.

[28] Donovan JL, Blake DR, Fleming WG. The patient is not a blank sheet: lay beliefs and their relevance to patient education. *Br J Rheumatol.* 1989;*28*:58-61.

[29] Mann J. *Murder, magic and medicine.* Oxford: Oxford University Press, 1992.

[30] Rao JK, Mihaliak K, Kroenke K, Bradley J, Tierney WM, Weinberger M. Use of complementary therapies for arthritis among patients of rheumatologists. *Annals of Internal Medicine* 1999;*131*:409-416.

[31] Donovan JL, Blake DR. Patient non-compliance: Deviance or reasoned decision-making? *Social Science and Medicine* 1992;*34*:507-513.

[32] Ramos-Remus C, Gutierrez-Urena S, Davis P. Epidemiology of complementary and alternative practices in rheumatology. *Rheumatic Disease Clinics of North America* 1999;*25*:789-+.

[33] Barlow JH, Williams B, Wright CC. Improving arthritis self-management among older adults: 'Just what the doctor didn't order'. *British Journal of Health Psychology* 1997;*2*:175-186.

[34] Beaven DW, Helm A, Stafford JA, Hunter AD. Patient self-sufficiency: Re-organisation of a diabetes clinic. *N Z Med J* 1978;*88*:253-256.

[35] Edelman P, Guihan M, BudimenMak. Arthritis self-management: Patient and physician knowledge/attitudes/behavior. *Arthritis and Rheumatism* 1997;*40*:AND.

[36] Edworthy SM. How important is patient self-management? *Best Practice & Research in Clinical Rheumatology* 2000;*14*:705-714.

[37] Fries JF, Lorig K, Holman HR. Patient self-management in arthritis? Yes! *Journal of Rheuamatology* 2003;*30*:

[38] Campbell R, Evans M, Tucker M, Quilty B, Dieppe P, Donovan JL. Why don't patients do their exercises? Understanding non- compliance with physiotherapy in patients with osteoarthritis of the knee. *J Epidemiol Community Health* 2001;*55*:132-138.

[39] Manek NJ, HART D, Spector TD, MacGregor AJ. The association of body mass index and osteoarthritis of the knee joint: an examination of genetic and environmental influences. *Arthritis Rheum.* 2003;*48*:1024-1029.

[40] Lievense AM, Bierma-Zeinstra SM, Verhagen AP, van Baar ME, Verhaar JA, Koes BW. Influence of obesity on the development of osteoarthritis of the hip: a systematic review. *Rheumatology (Oxford)* 2002;*41*:1155-1162.

[41] Hunter DJ, March L, Sambrook PN. Knee osteoarthritis: the influence of environmental factors. *Clin Exp Rheumatol.* 2002;*20*:93-100.

[42] Sowers M. Epidemiology of risk factors for osteoarthritis: systemic factors. *Curr Opin.Rheumatol.* 2001;*13*:447-451.

[43] Cooper C, Inskip H, Croft P, et al. Individual risk factors for hip osteoarthritis: obesity, hip injury, and physical activity. *Am J Epidemiol* 1998;*147*:516-522.

[44] Felson DT, Zhang Y, Hannan MT, et al. Risk factors for incident radiographic knee osteoarthritis in the elderly: the Framingham Study. *Arthritis Rheum.* 1997;*40*:728-733.

[45] Reginster JY, Kvasz A, Bruyere O, Henrotin Y. Is there any rationale for prescribing hormone replacement therapy (HRT) to prevent or to treat osteoarthritis? *Osteoarthritis and Cartilage* 2003;*11*:87-91.

[46] Felson DT. Preventing knee and hip osteoarthritis. *Bull.Rheum.Dis* 1998;*47*:1-4.

[47] Pelletier JP. Long-term treatment with diacerein has a structure/disease modifying effect on hip osteoarthritis. *Clin Exp Rheumatol.* 2003;*21*:152-154.

[48] Ayral X, Mackillop N, Genant HK, et al. Arthroscopic evaluation of potential structure-modifying drug in osteoarthritis of the knee. A multicenter, randomized, double-blind comparison of tenidap sodium vs piroxicam. *Osteoarthritis Cartilage* 2003;*11*:198-207.

[49] Bruyere O, Honore A, Ethgen O, et al. Correlation between radiographic severity of knee osteoarthritis and future disease progression. Results from a 3-year prospective, placebo-controlled study evaluating the effect of glucosamine sulfate. *Osteoarthritis Cartilage* 2003;*11*:1-5.

[50] Beary JF, III. Joint structure modification in osteoarthritis: development of SMOAD drugs. *Curr Rheumatol.Rep* 2001;*3*:506-512.

[51] Pavelka K, Gatterova J, Oletarova M, Machacek S, Giacovelli G, Rovati LC. Glucosamine sulfate decreases progression of knee osteoarthritis in a long-term randomized, placebo-controlled independent, confirmatory trial. *Arthritis and Rheumatism* 2000;*43*:1908.

[52] Reginster JY, Deroisy R, Rovati LC, et al. Long-term effects of glucosamine sulphate on osteoarthritis progression: a randomised, placebo-controlled clinical trial. *Lancet* 2001;*357*:251-256.

[53] Superio-Cabuslay E, Ward MM, Lorig KR. Patient education interventions in osteoarthritis and rheumatoid arthritis: a meta-analytic comparison with nonsteroidal antiinflammatory drug treatment. *Arthritis Care & Research* 1996;*9*:292-301.

[54] Dieppe P, Chard JA, Juni P. *The Management of Osteoarthritis*. 2003;(UnPub)

[55] Warsi A, LaValley MP, Wang PS, Avorn J, Solomon DH. Arthritis self-management education programs: a meta-analyisi of the effect on pain and disability. *Arthritis & Rheumatism* 2003;*48*:2207-2213.

[56] Solomon DH, Warsi A, Brown-Stevenson T, et al. Does self-management education benefit all populations with arthritis? A randomized controlled trial in a primary care physician network. *J Rheumatol* 2002;*29*:362-368.

[57] Osborne RH, Lorig K, McColl GJ. Does self-management lead to sustainable change? A two-year follow-up of 452 Australians. *Osteoarthritis & Cartilage* 2003;s118(Abstract)

[58] Solomon DH, Lee TH. Patient self-management in arthritis? Yes, more research! *Journal of Rheuamatology* 2003;*30*:

[59] Clark BM. Physical and occupational therapy in the management of arthritis. *Canadian Medical Association Journal* 2003;*163*:999-1005.

[60] Gignac MA, Cott C, Badley EM. Adaptation to chronic illness and disability and its relationship to perceptions of independence and dependence. *Journal of Gerontology* 2003;*55*:362-372.

[61] Salaffi F, Cavalieri F, Nolli M, Ferraccioli G. Analysis of disability in knee osteoarthritis. Relationship with age and psychological variables but not with radiographic score. *J Rheumatol* 1991;*18*:1581-1586.

[62] van Baar ME, Dekker J, Lemmens JAM, Oostendorp RAB, Bijlsma JWJ. Pain and disability in patients with osteoarthritis of hip or knee: the relationship with articular, kinesiological, and psychological characteristics. *J Rheumatol* 1998;*25*:125-133.

[63] Minor MA. Exercise in the treatment of osteoarthritis. *Rheumatic Diseases Clinics of North America* 1999;*25*:397-415.

[64] Fransen M, McConnell S, Bell M. Therapeutic exercise for people with osteoarthritis of the hip or knee. A systematic review. *J Rheumatol* 2002;*29*:1737-1745.

[65] van Baar ME, Assendelft WJJ, Dekker, Oostendorp RAB, Bijlsma JWJ. Effectiveness of exercise therapy in patients with osteoarthritis of the hip or knee: a systematic review of randomized clinical trials. *Arthritis & Rheumatism* 1999;*42*:1361-1369.

[66] Kovar PA, Allegrante JP, MacKenzie CR, Gutin B, Charlson ME. Supervised Fitness Walking In Patients With Osteoarthritis Of The Knee - A Randomized, Controlled Trial. *Annals of Internal Medicine* 1992;*116*:529-534.

[67] Ettinger WH, Jr., Burns R, Messier SP, et al. A randomized trial comparing aerobic exercise and resistance exercise with a health education program in older adults with knee osteoarthritis. The Fitness Arthritis and Seniors Trial (FAST). *JAMA* 1997;*277*:25-31.

[68] O'Reilly SC, Muir KR, Doherty M. Effectiveness of home exercise on pain and disability from osteoarthritis of the knee: a randomised controlled trial. *Annals of the Rheumatic Diseases* 1999;*58*:15-19.

[69] Peloquin L, Bravo G, Gauthier P, Lacombe G, Billiard JS. Effects of a cross-training exercise program in persons with osteoarthritis of the knee a randomized controlled trial. *Jcr-Journal of Clinical Rheumatology* 1999;*5*:126-136.

[70] Petrella RJ, Bartha C. Home based exercise therapy for older patients with knee osteoarthritis: a randomized clinical trial. *J Rheumatol* 2000;*27*:2215-2221.

[71] van Baar ME, Dekker J, Oostendorp RAB, Voorn TB, Bijlsma JWJ. Effectiveness of exercise in patients with osteoarthritis of hip or knee: nine months' follow up. *Annals of the Rheumatic Diseases* 2001;*60*:1123-1130.

[72] Fransen M, Crosbie J, Edmonds J. Physical therapy is effective for patients with osteoarthritis of the knee: a randomized controlled clinical trial. *J Rheumatol* 2001;*28*:156-164.

[73] Thomas KS, Muir KR, Doherty M, Jones AC, O'Reilly SC, Bassey EJ. Home based exercise programme for knee pain and knee osteoarthritis: randomised controlled trial. *BMJ* 2002;*325*:752.

[74] Fransen M, Crosbie J, Edmonds J. Physical therapy is effective for patients with osteoarthritis of the knee: a randomized controlled clinical trial. *J Rheumatol* 2001;*28*:156-164.

[75] Fransen M, McConnell S, Bell M. Meta-analysis of exercise for knee OA: differential effectiveness of one-to-one treatments, exercise classes and home programs. *Osteoarthritis & Cartilage* 2003;s4(Abstract)

[76] Kirkley A, Webster-Bogaert S, Litchfield R, et al. The effect of bracing on varus gonarthrosis. *Journal of Bone & Joint Surgery (am)* 1999;*81A*:539-548.

[77] Cushnaghan JM. Taping The Patella Medially - A New Treatment For Osteoarthritis Of The Knee-Joint. *British Medical Journal* 1994;*308*:753-755.

[78] Toda Y, Segal N, Kato A, Yamamoto S, Irie M. Effect of a novel insole on the subtalar joint of patients with medial compartment osteoarthritis of the knee. *J Rheumatol* 2001;*28*:2705-2710.

[79] McAlindon TE, LaValley MP, Felson DT. Efficacy of glucosamine and chondroitin for treatment of osteoarthritis. *JAMA* 2000;*284*:1241.

[80] Chard J, Dieppe P. Glucosamine for osteoarthritis: magic, hype, or confusion?. It's probably safe-but there's no good evidence that it works. *BMJ* 2001;*322*:1439-1440.

[81] Towheed TE, Anastassiades TP, Shea B, Houpt J, Welch V, Hochberg MC. Glucosamine therapy for treating osteoarthritis. *Cochrane.Database.Syst.Rev.* 2001;CD002946.

[82] Russell AS, Aghazadeh-Habashi A, Jamali F. Active ingredient consistency of commercially available glucosamine silfate products. *Journal of Rheuamatology* 2002;*29*:2407-2409.

[83] Blotman F, Maheu E, Wulwik A, Caspard H, Lopez A. Efficacy and safety of avocado/soybean unsaponifiables in the treatment of symptomatic osteoarthritis of the knee and hip - A prospective, multicenter, three-month, randomized, double- blind, placebo-controlled trial. *Revue du Rhumatisme* 1997;*64*:825-834.

[84] Maheu E, Mazieres B, Valat JP, et al. Symptomatic efficacy of avocado/soybean unsaponifiables in the treatment of osteoarthritis of the knee and hip - A prospective, randomized, double-blind, placebo-controlled, multicenter clinical trial with a six-month treatment period and a two-month followup demonstrating a persistent effect. *Arthritis and Rheumatism* 1998;*41*:81-91.

[85] Appelboom T, Schuermans J, Verbruggen G, Henrotin Y, Reginster JY. Symptoms modifying effect of avocado/soybean unsaponifiables (ASU) in knee osteoarthritis. A double blind, prospective, placebo-controlled study. *Scandinavian Journal of Rheumatology* 2001;*30*:242-247.

[86] Lequesne M, Maheu E, Cadet C, Dreiser RL. Structural effect of avocado/soybean unsaponifiables on joint space loss in osteoarthritis of the hip. *Arthritis & Rheumatism-Arthritis Care & Research* 2002;*47*:50-58.

[87] Towheed, T., Shea, B., Wells, G., and Hochberg, M. *Analgesia and non-aspirin, non-steriodal anti-inflammatory drugs for osteoarthritis of the hip*. 2000.

[88] Towheed TE, Hochberg MC. A systematic review of randomized controlled trials of pharmacological therapy in osteoarthritis of the knee, with an emphasis on trial methodology. *Seminars in Arthritis & Rheumatism* 1997;*26*:755-770.

[89] Zhang W, Jones A, Doherty M. Does paracetamol work fro osteoarthritis? - A meta-analysis of randomised controlled trials. *Osteoarthritis & Cartilage* 2003;s41(Abstract)

[90] March L, Irwig L, Schwarz J, Simpson J, Chick C, Brooks P. n of 1 trials comparing non-steroidal anti-inflammatory drug with paracetamol in osteoarthritis. *British Medical Journal* 1993;*309*:1041-1046.

[91] Courtney P, Doherty M. Key questions concerning paracetamol and NSAIDs for osteoarthritis. *Annals of the Rheumatic Diseases* 2002;*61*:767-773.

[92] Jordan KM, Arden NK, Doherty M, et al. *EULAR Recommendations 2003: An evidence based medicine approach to the management of knee osteoarthritis*. 2003;(UnPub)

[93] American college of rheumatology. Recommendations for the medical management of osteoarthritis of the hip and knee. *Arthritis & Rheumatism* 2000;*43*:1905-1915.

[94] March L, Irwig L, Schwarz J, Simpson J, Chock C, Brooks P. n Of 1 trials comparing a non-steroidal anti-inflammatory drug with paracetamol in osteoarthritis. *BMJ* 1994;*309*:1041-1045.

[95] Dieppe PA, Bartlett CJ, Davey P, Morrant C, MacDonald T. NSAID trials in OA lack approriate inclusivity. *Osteoarthritis & Cartilage* 2003;s78(Abstract)

[96] Anonymous. Selective COX-2 inhibitors: are they safer NSAIDs? *Therapeutics Initiative* 2002;

[97] Ehrich EW, Schnitzer TJ, McIlwain H, et al. Effect of specific COX-2 inhibition in osteoarthritis of the knee: A 6 week double blind, placebo controlled pilot study of rofecoxib. *J Rheumatol* 1999;*26*:2438-2447.

[98] McKenna F, Weaver A, Fiechtner JJ, Bello AE, Fort JG. COX-2 specific inhibitors in the management of osteoarthritis of the knee: A placebo-controlled, randomized, double-blind study. *Journal of Clinical Rheumatology* 2001;*7*:151-159.

[99] Acevedo E, Castaneda O, Ugaz M, et al. Tolerability profiles of rofecoxib (Vioxx (R)) and Arthrotoc (R) - A comparison of six weeks treatment in patients with osteoarthritis. *Scandinavian Journal of Rheumatology* 2001;*30*:19-24.

[100] Bensen WG, Fiechtner JJ, McMillen JI, et al. Treatment of osteoarthritis with celecoxib, a cyclooxygenase-2 inhibitor: A randomized controlled trial. *Mayo Clinic Proceedings* 1999;*74*:1095-1105.

[101] Bensen WG, Zhao SZ, Burke TA, et al. Upper gastrointestinal tolerability of celecoxib, a COX-2 specific inhibitor, compared to naproxen and placebo. *J Rheumatol* 2000;*27*:1876-1883.

[102] Cannon GW, Caldwell JR, Holt P, et al. Rofecoxib, a specific inhibitor of cyclooxygenase 2, with clinical efficacy comparable with that of diclofenac sodium - Results of a one-year, randomized, clinical trial in patients with osteoarthritis of the knee and hip. *Arthritis and Rheumatism* 2000;*43*:978-987.

[103] Goldstein JL, Correa P, Zhao WW, et al. Reduced incidence of gastroduodenal ulcers with celecoxib, a novel cyclooxygenase-2 inhibitor, compared to naproxen in patients with arthritis. *American Journal of Gastroenterology* 2001;*96*:1019-1027.

[104] Silverstein FE, Faich G, Goldstein JL, et al. Gastrointestinal toxicity with celecoxib vs nonsteroidal anti- inflammatory drugs for osteoarthritis and rheumatoid arthritis - The CLASS study: A randomized controlled trial. *Jama-Journal of the American Medical Association* 2000;*284*:1247-1255.

[105] 105. Juni P, Rutjes AW, Dieppe PA. Are selective COX 2 inhibitors superior to traditional non steroidal anti-inflammatory drugs? *BMJ* 2002;*324*:1287-1288.

[106] Jüni P, Dieppe P, Egger M. Risk of Myocardial Infarction Associated With Selective COX-2 Inhibitors: Questions Remain. *Arch Intern Med* 2002;*162*:2639-2642.

[107] Mukherjee D, Nissen SE, Topol EJ. Risk of cardiovascular events associated with selective COX-2 inhibitors. *Jama-Journal of the American Medical Association* 2001;*286*:954-959.

[108] Jensen EM, Ginsberg F. Tramadol versus dextropropoxyphene in the treatment of osteoarthritis: A short term double-blind study. *Drug Investigation* 1994;*8*:211-218.

[109] Bird HA, Hill J, Stratford ME, Fenn GC, Wright V. A double-blind cross-over study comparing the analgesic efficacy of tramadol with pentazocine in patients with osteoarthritis. *Journal of Drug Development & Clinical Practice* 1995;*7*:181-188.

[110] Fleischmann RM, Caldwell JR, Roth SH, Tesser JRP, Olson W, Kamin M. Tramadol for the treatment of joint pain associated with osteoarthritis: A randomized, double-blind, placebo-controlled trial. *Current Therapeutic Research, Clinical & Experimental* 2001;*62*:113-128.

[111] Marcolongo R, Fioravanti A, Adami S. Efficacy and tolerability of diacerhein in the treatment of osteoarthritis. *Current Therapeutic Research, Clinical & Experimental* 1988;*43*:878-887.

[112] Moore RA, Tramèr MR, Carroll D, Wiffen PJ, McQuay HJ. Quantitive systematic review of topically applied non-steroidal anti-inflammatory drugs. *BMJ* 1998;*316*:333-338.

[113] Grace D, Rogers J, Skeith K, Anderson K. Topical diclofenac versus placebo: a double blind, randomized clinical trial in patients with osteoarthritis of the knee. *J Rheumatol* 1999;*26*:2659-2663.

[114] Ottillinger B, Gomor B, Michel BA, Pavelka K, Beck W, Elsasser U. Efficacy and safety of eltenac gel in the treatment of knee osteoarthritis. *Osteoarthritis Cartilage* 2001;*9*:273-280.

[115] Rother M, Mazgareanu S, Cevc G. Placebo controlled efficacy of IDEA-033 - Results of two clinical studies in patients with osteoarhritis of the knee. *Osteoarthritis & Cartilage* 2003;s79(Abstract)

[116] Zhang WY, Li Wan Po A. The effectiveness of topically applied capsaicin. A meta-analysis. *European Journal of Clinical Pharmacology* 1994;*46*:517-522.

[117] McCleane G. The analgesic efficacy of topical capsaicin is enhanced by glyceryl trinitrate in painful osteoarthritis: a randomized, double blind, placebo controlled study. *European Journal of Pain* 2000;*4*:355-360.

[118] Kirwan JRR. Intra-articular therapy in osteoarthritis. *Baillieres Clinical Rheumatology* 1997;*11*:769-794.

[119] Ravaud P, Moulinier L, Giraudeau B, et al. Effects of joint lavage and steroid injection in patients with osteoarthritis of the knee - Results of a multicenter, randomized, controlled trial. *Arthritis and Rheumatism* 1999;*42*:475-482.

[120] Raynauld JP, Buckland-Wright C, Ward R, et al. Safety and efficacy of long-term intraarticular steroid injections in osteoarthritis of the knee - A randomized, double-blind, placebo-controlled trial. *Arthritis and Rheumatism* 2003;*48*:370-377.

[121] Brandt KD, Smith GN, Jr., Simon LS. Intraarticular injection of hyaluronan as treatment for knee osteoarthritis: what is the evidence? *Arthritis Rheum* 2000;*43*:1192-1203.

[122] Altman RD, Moskowitz RW. Intraarticular sodium hyaluronate (Hyalgan (R)) in the treatment of patients with osteoarthritis of the knee: A randomized clinical trial. *J Rheumatol* 1998;*25*:2203-2212.

[123] Hochberg MC. Role of intra-articular hyaluronic acid preparations in medical management of osteoarthritis of the knee. *Seminars in Arthritis and Rheumatism* 2000;*30*:2-10.

[124] Petrella RJ, DiSilvestro MD, Hildebrand C. Effects of hyaluronate sodium on pain and physical functioning in osteoarthritis of the knee - A randomized, double-blind, placebo-controlled clinical trial. *Archives of Internal Medicine* 2002;*162*:292-298.

[125] Karlsson J, Sjogren LS, Lohmander LS. Comparison of two hyaluronan drugs and placebo in patients with knee osteoarthritis. A controlled, randomized, double-blind, parallel-design multicentre study. *Rheumatology* 2002;*41*:1240-1248.

[126] Gross DE, Brenner Sl, Estormes I, Gross ML. The arthroscopic treatment of degenerative joint disease in the knee. *Journal of Orthopedics* 1991;*14*:1317.

[127] Livesley PJD. Arthroscopic lavage of osteoarthritic knees. *Journal of Bone and Joint Surgery* 1991; *73-B*:922-926.

[128] McLaren AC, Blokker CP, Fowler PJ, Roth JN, Rock MG. Arthroscopic debridement of the knee for osteoarthrosis see comments. *Canadian Journal of Surgery* 1991;*34*:595-598.

[129] Ike RW, Arnold WJ, Rothschild EW, Shaw HL. Tidal irrigation versus conservative medical management in patients with osteoarthritis of the knee: A prospective randomized study. *J Rheumatol* 1992;*19*:772-779.

[130] Chang RW, Falconer J, Stulberg S, Arnold WJ, Manheim LM, Dyer AR. A randomized, controlled trial of arthroscopic surgery versus closed-needle joint lavage for patients with osteoarthritis of the knee. *Arthritis & Rheumatism* 1993;*36*:289-295.

[131] Mceldowney A. Open-Knee Magnuson Debridement As Conservative Treatment For Degenerative Osteoarthritis Of The Knee. *Journal of Arthroplasty* 1995;*10*:805-809.

[132] Ravaud P, Moulinier L, Giraudeau B, et al. Effects of joint lavage and steroid injection in patients with osteoarthritis of the knee - Results of a multicenter, randomized, controlled trial. *Arthritis and Rheumatism* 1999;*42*:475-482.

[133] Moseley JB, O'Malley K, Petersen NJ, et al. A controlled trial of arthroscopic surgery for osteoarthritis of the knee. *N Engl J Med* 2002;*347*:81-88.

[134] Stukenborg-Colsman C, Wirth CJ, Lazovic D, Wefer A. High tibial osteotomy versus unicompartmental joint replacement in unicompartmental knee joint osteoarthritis: 7-10-year follow-up prospective randomised study. *Knee* 2001;*8*:187-194.

[135] Broughton NS, Newman JH, Baily RAJ. Unicompartmental replacement and high tibial osteotomy for osteoarthritis of the knee. A comparative study after 5-10 years follow up. *Journal of Bone & Joint Surgery* 1986;*68-B*:447-452.

[136] Magyar G, Ahl TL, Vibe P, Toksvig-Larsen S, Lindstrand A. Open-wedge osteotomy by hemicallotasis or the closed-wedge technique for osteoarthritis of the knee - A randomised study of 50 operations. *Journal of Bone and Joint Surgery-British Volume* 1999;*81B*:444-448.

[137] Korovessis P, Katsoudas G, Salonikides P, Stamatakis M, Baikousis A. Medium- and long-term results of high tibial osteotomy for varus gonarthrosis in an agricultural population. *Orthopedics* 1999;*22*:729-735.

[138] Callahan CD. Patient outcomes following uni-compartmentla or bi-compartmental knee arthroplasty: a meta analysis. *Journal of Arthroplasty* 1995;*10*:141-150.

[139] Callahan CM, Drake BG, Heck DA, Dittus RS. Patient outcomes following tricompartmental total knee replacement: A meta-analysis. *Journal of the American Medical Association* 1994;*271*:1349-1357.

[140] Hajat S, Fitzpatrick R, Morris R, et al. Doea waiting for total hip replacement matter? prospective cohort study. *J Health Serv Res Pol* 2002;*7*:19-25.

[141] Norwegian Arthroplasty Registry *Report 2002: hip and knee prostheses*. Bergen: Haukeland University Hospital, 2002.

[142] Knutson K, Lewold S, Robertsson O, Lidgren L. The Swedish knee arthroplasty register. A nation-wide study of 30,003 knees 1976-1992. *Acta Orthopaedica Scandinavica* 1994;*65*:375-386.

[143] Swedish Knee Arthroplasty Register *Annual Report 2002*. Lund: 2003.

[144] Fortin PR, Penrod JR, Clarke AE, et al. Timing of total joint replacement affects clinical outcomes among patients with osteoarthritis of the hip or knee. *Arthritis Rheum*. 2002;*46*:3327-3330.

[145] Murray DW, Britton AR, Bulstrode CJK. Loss to follow-up matters. *Journal of Bone and Joint Surgery-British Volume* 1997;*79B*:254-257.

[146] Ashworth, M. A., Brule, C., Day, A., Harrison, M., Hopman, W., and Rudan, J. *The development of an orthopedic waiting list algorithm for elective total hip and total knee replacement surgery*. Canadian Health Services Research Foundation, 2002.

[147] Ernst E. Complementary and alternative medicine in rheumatology. *Best Practice & Research in Clinical Rheumatology* 2000;*14*:731-749.

[148] Ezzo J, Hadhazy V, Birch S, et al. Acupuncture for osteoarthritis of the knee - A systematic review. *Arthritis and Rheumatism* 2001;*44*:819-825.

[149] Ernst E. Acupuncture as a symptomatic treatment of osteoarthritis - A systematic review. *Scandinavian Journal of Rheumatology* 1997;*26*:444-447.

[150] Ramos-Remus C, Gutierrez-Urena S, Davis P. Epidemiology of complementary and alternative practices in rheumatology. *Rheumatic Disease Clinics of North America* 1999;*25* :789-800.

[151] Ovretveit J. Quality evaluation and indicator comparison in health care. *International Journal of Health Planning and Management* 2001;*16*:229-241.

[152] Donabedian A. The quality of care - How can it be assessed? *JAMA* 1988;*260*:1743-1748.

[153] Maxwell Rj. Quality Assessment In Health. *Br Med J* 1984;*288*:1470-1472.

[154] http://www.jcaho.org

[155] Tallon D, Chard JA, Dieppe PA. Exploring the priorities of patients with osteoarthritis of the knee. *Arthritis Care & Research* 2000;*13*:312-319.

[156] Chard JA, Dickson J, Tallon D, Dieppe PA. A comparison of the views of rheumatologists, general practitioners and patients on the treatment of osteoarthritis. *Rheumatology* 2002;*41*:1208-1210.

[157] Specker C, Richter J, Take A, Sangha O, Schneider M. RheumaNet - A novel Internet-based rheumatology information network in Germany. *British Journal of Rheumatology* 1998;*37*:1015-1019.

[158] Middleton J. The effect of case management on glycemic control in patients with type 2 diabetes. *Case Manager*. 2003;*14*:43-47.

[159] Thompson E, Dixon J, Duveneck S, et al. Creating solutions: A case management model for the 21st century. *Case Manager.* 2002;*13*:63-67.
[160] Dieppe PA, Chard JA, Juni P. *The management of osteoarthritis*. 2003;(UnPub)

## Acknowledgements

Many thanks to Prof Paul Dieppe and Dr Peter Juni for their advice on this chapter.

In: Arthritis Research: Treatment and Management
Editor: F. Columbus, pp. 185-226
ISBN 1-59033-984-3


*Chapter VIII*

# Etiology, Pathophysiology, Diagnosis and Conservative Management of Degenerative Joint Disease

***Slavica Jandric****

Institute for Rehabilitation "Dr Miroslav Zotovic", 78 000 Banja Luka, Republika Srpska, Bosnia and Herzegovina

## Abstract

### Etiology of Degenerative Joint Disease

Degenerative joint disease which results in deterioration of joint structure and function is the most common cause of long-term disability and has significant economic impact. It affects people in all geographic locations. There is a strong association between joint degeneration and age. Etiology of degenerative joint disease is still not clearly understood and there is no specific management for this group of diseases. Various pathological conditions cause damage of the articular cartilage and lead to clinically and radiographically recognized impairment of the patients. Biomechanical, metabolic, genetic factors, inflammation and other risk factors contribute to the development of osteoarthrosis.

---

* Address of the author: Prof. Slavica Jandric, MD, PhD, Marka Kraljevica 20, 51 000 Banjaluka, RS, Bosnia and Herzegovina, Phone +38751 461 770, fax +38751 301 533, E- mail: slavicajandric@yahoo.com

## Pathophysiology of Degenerative Joint Disease

Osteoarthrosis is characterized by progressive erosion of articular cartilage and bony overgrowth at the joint margins. Cartilage integrity requires a balance between synthesis and degradation of matrix components. Chondocytes react to various mechanical and chemical stresses and try to stabilize and restore the tissue. Failures in stabilizing and restoring the tissue lead to the phase of cartilage degeneration that may be irreversible. For better understanding of conservative management of degenerative joint diseases it is important to know the influence of pathophysiology mechanisms in development of degenerative joint diseases. There is a great variability in the rate of progression of the erosive processes in articular cartilage in the clinical, radiographic signs and the course of the disease. This is in relation with many factors, as well as with management and response to the therapy.

## Diagnosis of Degenerative Joint Disease

OA is characterized by pain, stiffness, swelling, deformity, loss of mobility and it diminishes the quality of life. Three radiographic markers of OA include narrowed joint space, increased density of subchondral bone and osteophytes. Criteria for the diagnosis and classification of symptomatic OA based on clinical and radiographic signs for the most frequently involved joints. The diagnosis of OA is usually based on the history and physical findings. Radiographic changes confirm the diagnosis. Other imaging studies including bone scans, computed tomography (CT) and magnetic resonance imaging (MRI), may help in evaluating OA, but they are rarely necessary for establishing the diagnosis. Improved methods of cartilage imaging, including MRI, combined with biochemical markers of OA (levels of cartilage proteoglycan, collagen fragments in synovial fluid, serum or urine), may help for detecting subtle changes in the joint tissue in the early stages of OA.

## Treatment of Degenerative Joint Disease

Treatment should vary according to the severity of disease and patient's expectations and the level of activity. Pain management in OA should start with education, psychological support, physical therapy, exercise therapy and environmental measures. Many non-pharmacological, conventional and nonconventional treatments and techniques can be used for the management of osteoarthrosis. These can reduce drug consumption and toxicity or even delay the need for joint replacement surgery. Physiotherapy and exercises are very important for maintaining muscle strength, joint stability and mobility, but should be closely monitored for optimal efficacy.

Analgesics, nonsteroidal anti-inflammatory drugs (NSAIDs) and intraarticular corticosteroids are current pharmacologic treatments for OA. The so-called "simple" analgesics (Paracetamol) are often recommended as first-choice agents for pain relief in

OA as a less toxic yet potent alternative to NSAIDs. NSAIDs have become a routine treatment for pain and stiffness due to OA. This class of medication offers a potential advantage because they suppress any inflammation as well. But clinical studies have not shown NSAIDs to have a clear advantage over analgesic drugs. New NSAIDs are still under development. There is evidence that symptomatic slow acting drugs may relieve pain and improve disease severity of OA, but more studies using standardized methodology are required.

***Keywords:*** osteoarthrosis + etiology + physiopathology + diagnosis + therapy + rehabilitation

# Introduction

Degenerative joint diseases are designated as osteoarthrosis (OA) and describe both osteoarthrosis and intervertebral disc degeneration.

Synonyms for this disease such as "osteoarthritis" reflect the varied etiology of the disease. Term "osteoarthritis" is often used and it is preserve in Anglo-Saxon literature, but many prefer the term osteoarthrosis. This term emphasizes the distinction from primary inflammatory joint disease.

OA is the most frequent and the oldest of the joint diseases of humanity. Degenerative changes of articular cartilage and joint structures have been noted in the fossils of vertebrates and man, the remains of prehistoric times. Their trails are also found in philogenesis of reptiles.

Results of common researches of rheumatologists from "Saint Mary's Hospital" and Institute for archeology in London indicate that the sure signs of OA occur in 168 from 3788 examined skeletons which originate before 15$^{th}$ century [1].

The first description of OA was given by Hippocrates. He described it as "an arthritis which seizes great joints but which does not actually go beyond these". William Heberden (1806.) described only the nodes of the distal interphalangeal joints and did not link these nodes with OA at other sites. Detailed and clinically accurate description of OA was given by Haygarth in 1805. Spender defined OA in 1876. but definitive clinical and radiological differentiation from rheumatoid arthritis was published in 1907. by AE Garrod [2]. OA was not widely accepted as a distinct rheumatic disease until the paper of Cecil and Archer in 1926.

Degenerative joint diseases are the clinical manifestation of degenerative joint changes [3]. It may be defined in pathological terms as a degenerative condition affecting the axial skeleton and peripheral diarthrodial joints. Degeneration of articular cartilage, reactive changes in synovial tissue with low grade inflammation and remodeling of the subchondral bone with increased density and osteophytes are characteristic changes of the disease. The terms with the most functional determinants designate OA as a disease which lead to static and dynamic unbalance because of degenerative changes of joint and adjacent anatomical structures and some other factors.

For better understanding of pathophysiology and methodology of management of degenerative joint disease, we should remind ourselves of certain features of a healthy mature synovial joint, before considering the changes that occur in OA.

# Biology and Biomechanic Principles of Synovial Joints

The upright posture and bipedal gait of man present unique problems in biomechanical terms. Muscular contractions, transmitted through ligaments and tendons, act upon bone to effect movements that are facilitated by the joints. Synovial joints (diarthroses) are one of two fundamental joint types. There are both cavity and free movements. In some joints articular geometry obviously contributes to stability.

## Types of Joints

Synovial joints vary in size, number of articulating surfaces, shape, range of motion, and type of motion. Joints that permit movement in one plane only are uniaxial. When movement is allowed in two mutually perpendicular axes the joint is called biaxial. The most mobile synovial joints are multiaxial. The hip and the shoulder joints are ball-and-socket (spheroidal) joints that move in multiple planes. They permit flexion/extension, abduction/adduction and rotation. These joints depend largely on muscles stability.

## Articular Cartilage

Load-bearing and movement at synovial joints are facilitated by the juxtaposition of two or more surfaces covered, sometimes incompletely, by hyaline (glass-like) cartilage.

Articular cartilage has a lamellar organization and consists of four successive zones and forms bearing surfaces that have low-friction gliding properties and ability to distribute loads applied to synovial joints, minimizing stresses on subchondral bone. Normal articular cartilage has a unique elasticity and compressibility conferred by its molecular constituents.

Articular cartilage contains only one cell type (the chondrocyte), an extracellular matrix and no nerve cell processes or blood vessels. Chondrocytes synthesize collagen and hydrophilic proteoglycans which interact with collagen fibrils to form hydrated macromolecular matrix of articular cartilage. Chondrocytes depend on diffusion of nutrients and metabolites through the matrix, yet they maintain a level of metabolic activity similar to that of some cells in vascularized tissues.

Following the completion of skeletal growth, chondrocytes rarely divide. They degrade and synthesize matrix macromolecules with proteoglycan aggregate. Cartilage integrity requires a balance between synthesis and degradation of matrix components. The cytokines with catabolic and anabolic effects appear to have important roles in maintaining balance between catabolic and anabolic activities (interleukin (IL-1), insulin-like growth factor I (IGF-I), transforming growth factor beta (TGF-ß). Chemokines are a novel class of small cytokines and have a wide range of effects both inside and outside of the immune system. Their actions are mediated by a family of 7-transmembrane G-protein-coupled receptors [4].

Chondrocytes attach themselves to the matrix macromolecular framework that occupied by a hydrated proteoglycan gel. The water contributes 60% to 70% of the wet weight of cartilage matrix. Proteoglycans consist of a protein core filament and one or more glycosaminoglycan chains that contain chondroitin sulfate, keratan sulfate and dermatan sulfate. Negatively charged glycosaminoglycan side chains attract positively charged ions or water molecules increasing matrix volume.

There is a unique hydraulic permeability system. Glycosaminoglycan chains are closer to each other and forcing water out of the molecular domain following compression. The process is reversible and the molecules are reexpanded when the load is removed.

This hydraulic permeability serves not only to protect the underlying bone from injury, but also provides nutritiens for the chondrocytes and their own synthetic activities.

Collagen forms a fibrillar meshwork that provides tensile strength, form and stiffness. 90% to 95% of total cartilage collagen consists of type II collagen. Interactions between these elements and collagen fibril network give cartilage its stiffness and resilience. Collagen meshwork limits the expansion of the molecule and matrix volume. Disruption of the collagen network allows the proteoglycans to expand, thereby increasing the water concentration and decreasing the proteoglycan concentration.

### *Cartilage Repair*

When holes are drilled experimentally into hyaline cartilage, a defect persists unless the hole extends through the calcified cartilage into the vascular bone. Under these circumstances, the defect is repaired by a new formation of fibrocartilage. The main collagen in such defects is initially type I but becomes to a greater extent, yet never completely, type II [5].

### *Blood Vessels and Cartilage*

Normally, hyaline cartilage does not undergo vascularisation. Their resistance to vascular invasion is due to the presence of diffusible anti invasion factor(s), substances that inhibit capillary endothelial cell growth. The factors display activity against a variety of proteinases, including collagenases and proteoglycan-degrading enzymes and play an important part in protecting articular cartilage from the adverse inflammatory responses.

By contrast, synovium in particular form, contains and liberates angiogenesis factors that in the artificial circumstances causes an extensive loss of proteoglycan and of collagen with fibroblastic transformation of the chondrocytes [6].

### *Synovium and Synovial Fluid*

The synovium consists essentially of a discontinuous intimal lining layer of cells, synoviocytes and subjacent adipose of fibrous tissue. The collagens are of type I and III.

Two types of synovial cells (A and B) have been identified. Cells may produce hyaluronic acid for the synovial fluid and have phagocytic capability, and B cells synthesize proteins including enzymes. Hyaluronic acid, the main constituent of joint fluid, found in articular cartilage and participates in the boundary lubrication of cartilage. The synovial fluid consists of a plasma ultra filtrate plus materials added by the synovial tissues.

### *Joint Capsules and Ligaments*

Joint capsules form fibrous tissue cuffs that enclose synovial joints while ligaments consist of distinct fibrous tissue cords or bands. Both restrict abnormal joint motion and contain nerves that may sense joint motion and displacement.

Neuromuscular control of joint movement is mediated on the afferent side by sensory receptors in ligaments, joint capsule and extra capsular structures. The nerve fibers probably function as pain receptors, vasomotor efferent and mechanoreceptors sensitive to stretch or distortion. The mechanoreceptors may sense loads applied to ligaments and capsules and may have a role in initiating protective reflexes that oppose potentially damaging joint movements.

Menisci are interposed between articular cartilage surfaces. They increase joint stability, bear load, absorb shock and help lubricate the joint.

### *Joint Muscles*

Most of the stresses generated across the joints can be absorbed by muscle contraction. Failure of joint and muscular mechanisms in load distribution can increase stresses on cartilage and subchondral and metaphyseal bone, thereby contributing to joint degeneration.

### *Synovial Joint Biomechanics*

For different daily activities, the role of mechanical factors that provided stability during motion, joint lubrication and load distribution across joint and their action on synovial joint are very important.

The rapid, painless movement is necessary for daily activities, recreation and work. This movement is the result from the action of muscles across synovial joints. For apparently simple activities, a controlled efficient movement of more than 20 synovial joints is required, and for playing basketball, more than 100 synovial joints.

### *Biomechanical Homeostasis of the Normal Joint*

The applied stress to chondro-osseous unit of the synovial joint affects the articular cartilage and subchondral bone and if it exceeds its strength, mechanical failure occurs. However, the chondroosseous unit also possesses biologic properties that can respond to the applied stress. Remodeling occurs in accordance with Wolf's law for bone and Heuter-Volkmann's principle for articular cartilage (the amount of matrix in the articular cartilage is proportional to the stress distributed on it) [7]. There is a static and dynamic balance between applied stress and reaction of the chondro-osseous unit to the applied stress mechanically and biologically. As long as the applied stress remains within normal limits, mechanical and biologic changes are reversible.

Synovial joints share the same basic structure that provided: stability during motion, joint lubrication that allows the low-friction gliding of cartilage surfaces and load distribution across joints.

Dynamic joint stability is necessary for providing efficient, controlled movement. Within the normal range of movement, stability is maintained by musculoligamentous tension. Loss of dynamic joint stability not only compromises function but also leads to joint degeneration in many instances.

Static joint stability depends primarily on joint shape and the restraint of abnormal or excessive motion provided by ligaments and joint capsules.

Lubrication mechanisms have an important role in maintaining of joint biomechanical homeostasis. Many details of the joint lubrication systems remain unknown, but at least two mechanisms have been identified: boundary layer lubrication and hydrodynamic lubrication. In boundary lubrication the frictional force is a function of the properties of the opposing surfaces and of properties of the lubricant other than its viscosity. In hydrodynamic lubrication, lubrication under pressure, the shape and relative motion of the sliding surfaces cause the formation of a fluid film having sufficient pressure to separate the surfaces.

Load distribution is an important factor in contributing to joint degeneration. The elastic behavior of articular cartilage, menisci and subchondral and metaphyseal bone helps distribute compressive stresses applied to joints. This mechanism would quickly fail if the muscles did not absorb most of the compressive stresses generated across the joints.

# Pathology and Pathogenesis

## Pathology

### *Cartilage Changes*

The efficiency of biomechanical system is profoundly impaired by the progressive attrition of OA. Fibrillation, softening and ulceration of cartilage are the most important structural changes. Localized fibrillation is the earliest visible sign of OA. The lesions appear first in the load-bearing areas. As the cartilage fissures grow deeper, the superficial tips of the fibrillated cartilage tear, releasing free fragments into the joint space and decreasing the cartilage thickness, so that the progressive loss of articular cartilage leaves only exposed bone. During the course of OA, there is thinning and loss of cartilage, but paradoxically there is often thickening of cartilage in the early stages. Many of the mechanisms responsible for progressive loss of cartilage in degenerative joint disease remain unknown, but the process can be divided into three overlapping phases: cartilage damage, chondrocyte response and decline of the chondrocyte response. In the first phase, either before or during the appearance of fibrillation, the matrix macromolecular framework is disrupted or the water content increases. Chondrocytes detect tissue damage and respond to variety of mechanical and chemical stresses, possibly as a result of changes in osmolarity or charge density or strain applied through cell membrane-bound matrix molecules. They release mediators that stimulate a tissue response. Nitric oxide probably has a role in this response and can induce production of IL-1, which stimulates the expression of metalloproteases that degrade the matrix macromolecules. Proteoglycan content decreases as a result of degradation by stromelysin, a metalloprotease and other enzymes.

The destructive process is accompanied by efforts to repair with synthesis of matrix components, particularly proteoglycans. Chondrocytes have a limited capacity for proliferation, but clusters of newly generated cells may be found in OA cartilage. This repair response counters the catabolic effects of the proteases and may stabilize or, in some instances, even restore the tissue. Failure to stabilize or restore the tissue leads to the third phase of cartilage degeneration, a decline in the chondrocytes response that may be irreversible.

Denuded areas may be filled in with fibrocartilage with inferior mechanical properties.

### *Bone Changes*

Bone changes play a clinical and biomechanical role in OA. Recent work suggests that, very early in the OA process, biological and morphological disturbances occur at the subchondral bone and may have a role in the modulation of articular cartilage metabolism.

When fibrillation has progressed to the deep layers of the cartilage there is usually radiological evidence of remodeling of the subchondral and metaphyseal bone. Alteration of the subchondral bone include increased subchondral bone density, formation of cyst-like bone cavities and the appearance of regenerating cartilage within and on the subchondral bone surface. Increased bone density is a result of formation of new layers of bone on existing trabeculae. Loss of trabecular bone leads to formation of subchondral bone cysts.

Marginal growth of osteophytes may change the configuration of the joint and reduce its motion. Osteophytes may appear early, even before cartilage thickness and be radiographically diminished of "joint space". They may have a protective role with regard to articular cartilage to provide an enlarged surface at the joint margins thus increasing the area available to absorb mechanical forces. Presence or absence of a definite osteophyte is the most sensitive and specific indicator of OA of the knee.

At the end stage of the disease, the articular cartilage is completely lost. Alteration in the shape of a joint reflects bone rather than cartilaginous change. It occurs in response to mechanical forces and vascularisation of the calcification front. Increased femoral intramedullary pressure and altered osseous circulation have been demonstrated in OA of the hip by impaired venous drainage and nocturnal pain (bone engorgement syndrome).

The bone remodeling combined with the loss of articular cartilage changes the shape of the joint and can lead to limb shortening, deformity and instability.

### *Synovium Changes*

The inner layer of the joint capsule may be normal, inflamed or fibroses. In patients with coxarthrosis and gonarthrosis some degree of synovial inflammatory cell infiltration was found. When present, the synovitis in OA is usually mild and changes closely resemble those found in patients with "posttraumatic synovitis". Recent studies have demonstrated that there is a strong correlation between synovial inflammation and OA progression as well as an association with strong risk factors [8]. Serum hyaluronic acid seems to be a predictor of disease progression in OA of the knee [9].

## Pathogenesis

Maintaining the tissue requires a balance between catabolic and anabolic activities in articular cartilage.

### *Cartilage Degradation*

Progression of OA changes is a function of the degree of imbalance between degradation and repair, in this metabolically active tissue. Synthesis rates of matrix components increase in OA, but fail to keep pace with the losses. Chondrocyte activation may be related to cytokines, particularly interleukin1 (IL-1) that usually produces monocyte/macrophage cells of the synovial tissue. Perhaps interleukin-6 (IL6) and tumor necrosis factor alpha (TNF-$\alpha$) also have a role in OA. IL-1 has multiple actions on the chondrocyte: synthesis of matrix components is reduced, production of degradative enzymes is increased and proliferation of chondrocytes is inhibited.

Chondrocyte-derived metalloproteinase's, particularly stromelysin and collagenases are the most important enzymes that degrade the matrix macromolecules. The degradation of type IX and XI collagens and other molecules may destabilize the type II collagen fibril meshwork. There are qualitative changes in proteoglycan content. Proteolysis results in smaller molecules and replacement molecules may have altered composition and aggregation properties. As a result of a damaged collagen network, a net loss of proteoglycan occurs [10].

Accelerated cartilage degradation may occur as a result of hereditary enzyme deficiency (ochronosis).

### *Cartilage Repair*

Insulin-like growth factor 1 (IGF-1), fibroblast growth factor and transforming growth factor may affect the anabolic process in cartilage. Growth factors may increase proteoglycan synthesis and inhibit the catabolic effects of IL-1. Diseased chondrocytes have a diminished response to the growth factor.

## *Mechanisms of Joint Destruction in Osteoarthrosis*

### The Role of Aging

The development of primary joint degeneration is strongly associated with age although this relationship remains unclear. 60% to 90% of persons, older than 65 years have an evidence for OA, while this percentage in age category from 15 to 44 less than of 5%, and in age group from 45 to 64 is 25% to 30% [11].

Involutive processes of the articular cartilage do not develop clinical symptoms. OA is not simply due to wear and ageing of articular cartilage but involves some other pathophysiological mechanisms.

Biochemical study of cartilage shows that minor changes do occur during adult life. These normal changes are different from those found in the fibrillated cartilage of OA and they include: a fall in water content with no change in cartilage thickness, a rise in total glucosaminoglycan content due to an increase in keratan sulphate, a rise in the protein to hyaluronic acid ratio and the keratan sulphate to chondroitin sulphate ratio. The proteoglycans of macroscopically healthy but aging cartilage remain capable of aggregation.

Although the cause of OA is often unknown, recent findings suggest that inevitable consequence of aging is fact of life and there may be ways to slow the progression of OA.

### The Role of the Mechanical Factors

Regular activity is important for maintaining joint function. Cyclic loading of cartilage stimulates matrix synthesis, whereas prolonged static loading or the absence of loading and motion leads to joint degeneration.Regular moderate activity does not appear to cause or accelerate OA in normal joints.

However, some types of repetitive joint use-such as repetitive lifting or carrying heavy objects, awkward work posture, vibration and continuously repeated movements –apparently do hasten the development of OA. It is considered that overloading of the joint is the initial and the main factor of later OA changes. The people in some professions (farmers, metal workers, miners) may be at greater factor for early onset of joint degeneration because their occupations expose them to repetitive and intense joint loading.

Participation in sports that repeatedly expose joints to high levels of impact and/or torsion loading also increases the risk of joint degeneration [12,13]. Disturbances of joint or muscle innervations, and inadequate muscle strength or endurance also cause degenerative joint changes. In these conditions, the loads on the joints are greater than those of normal daily activities and that may lead to further increase of the risk from disease.

Prospective following up lasting several years shows that patients with rupture cruciate ligament of the knee and damaged meniscus, have severe increasing of proteoglycans in synovial fluid immediately after trauma. The increased values of proteoglycans in the synovial fluid with maintenance of symptoms indicate of remodeling in the cartilage. These conditions may later lead into the development of OA and proteoglycans may have role of a marker. They increase expression and activity of stromelysin in the cartilage and synovial membrane in various models of arthropathy on the animals [14].

## Metabolic and Genetic Factors

There is great variability in the rate of progression of the erosive process in articular cartilage. The traditional view in which mechanical factors are assigned a central role must now be modified [15].

In accordance to new knowledge, metabolic events in cartilage are more often of prime importance in relation to mechanical factors. OA may be viewed as an insufficiency of the joint that can be due either to abnormal physical stresses on normal cartilage or normal stress on abnormal cartilage. Progression is a function of the degree of imbalance between degradation and repair in this metabolically active tissue. Degradation of matrix components increases in OA because of acting hondrocyte-derived metalloproteinase's, particularly stromelysin and collagenase. Synthesis rates increase but fail to keep pace with the losses of matrix components. There also are qualitative changes in proteoglycan content (smaller molecules, altered composition and aggregation properties).

There was an interesting research of osseal molecular density in patients with OA of the hip and osteoporosis [16 ]. It show that osteoarthritis of the hip is negative risk factor for compressive fracture of the spine. It seems that there is a genetic factor in primary generalized OA (Kellgren, Lawrence, and Bier) and association between cartilage-specific gene and primary OA. A pattern of heredity for Heberden's nodes involves an autosomal dominant gene in women and recessive gene in men. Non-nodal OA in contrast of nodal generalized OA appears to have polygenic modes of inheritance.

Dequeker reported that patients with postmenopausal osteoporosis and these with OA are anthropometrically different population [16].

There is knowledge about possible genetic factors that are responsible for anomalies of cartilage matrix or some growth factors which lead to disturbing of balance between proteases and antiproteases. An abnormal collagen network resulting from a mutation in the gene for type II procollagen leads to premature generalized articular cartilage failure [18].

The study that explored the therapeutic effect of interleukin-1 receptor antagonist (IL-1Ra), administered by gene transfer, on the progression of osteoarthritic (OA) lesions in an experimental dog model.showed that a local increase in IL-1Ra production in OA knee joints by intraarticular injection of transduced synovial cells can reduce the progression of experimentally induced lesions [17].

## The Role of Inflammation in Osteoarthrosis

Pathologic changes in OA are different from pathologic inflammatory changes in arthritis. This knowledge is based on clinical, biological and anatomic dates. The most attractive recent findings are the data pointing to an association between inflammation and disease appearance and progression. There are several studies in which the levels of biomarkers such as cartilage oligoprotein, hyaluronic acid, or C reactive protein were measured in patients with OA.

Recently researches have shown an increase of rate of serum CRP in patients with OA of the knee and acute effusion. Highly sensitive dosage settings may be used to prove the biologic markers of inflammation which point out an early degradation of joint [6, 11].

Joint laxity may be more important than excessive use as a cause of synovitis in young adults. Some subsets of osteoarthrosis are characterized by more synovial inflammation, both clinically and pathologically. Erosive osteoarthritis of the interphalangeal joints of the fingers is associated with greater destruction than the usual no inflammatory variety [19].

Although a primary etiological role for inflammation has been suggested in ordinary OA, it is more likely to be a secondary phenomenon induced by cartilage debris or crystals [20].

Chondrocytes are responsible for metabolism of proteoglycans. They produce many enzymes: proteases and antiproteases. Cytokines (IL-1 and TNF alpha) produced by activated chondrocytes. These enzymes can found in synovial fluid at the time of acute effusion in OA [11]. During the time of acute OA, chondrocytes can secrete of lipid proinflammatory mediators, especially prostaglandin E2. This activity is due to increased synthesis of phospholypasis A2 and cycloooxigenasis and participation of nitric oxide (NO), through NO synthetasis from chondrocytes.

Recent studies have demonstrated that chondrocytes co-express chemokines and their receptors, and that the interaction of chemokines with their receptors results in the release of cartilage matrix-degrading proteinases, and affect proteoglycan metabolism in chondrocytes.

The C-C chemokines and their receptors CCR-2 and CCR-5 were found to be expressed in normal and OA chondrocytes. However, regulation of chemokine expression by IL-1beta and TNF alpha differed between normal and OA chondrocytes [4].

This differential expression of chemokines and their receptors suggests that the cytokine-triggered chemokine system may play a key role in the cartilage degradation of OA, possibly acting in an autocrine/paracrine manner.

There are a number of ways by which the production or activity of cytokines could be reduced. The action of cytokines can be reduced at the cell membrane level by decreasing the membrane receptor level or by the use of receptor antagonists or soluble receptors. The action of the cytokine can also be reduced by blocking the intracellular signalling pathways.

Of the catabolic pathways activated by inflammation, synthesis of nitric oxide (NO) is an interesting one in the context of OA. NO may induce chondrocyte death by apoptosis. It may also stimulate the synthesis and activities of matrix metalloproteinases (MMP), and reduce the anabolism of cartilage by inhibiting the synthesis of the major matrix components, collagen and proteoglycan. Moreover, NO is capable of increasing the activity of COX-2 and consequently appears to be responsible for an increase in the signs and symptoms of the disease. Reducing its excess production may not only reduce the symptoms but also reduce the progression of the disease [8].

Many of hypotheses have been proposed for explanation of mechanism activation of chondrocytes. The first hypothesis states that products of degradation of cartilage matrix lead to releasing of various proinflammatory mediators. The second hypothesis proposes that cartilage only participates in the activation of the chondrocytes through recently proved mechanoreceptors, placed on the surfaces of the chondrocytes. It is shown that intermittent, mild and modest pressure stimulates matrix synthesis, while abnormally increased pressure diminishes the production of matrix. This is may have the importance in prescribing a dose of loading in the patients with OA.

Despite these newly investigations and evidences about the role of inflammation in OA, we could say that inflammation of the synovium is gentle and variable characteristic in OA. It is generally believed that clinical signs of an active disease suggest the likelihood of rapid progression of the disease. Moreover, there are a number of pathways linked to inflammation that represent the most interesting therapeutic targets.

## Origins of the Pain and Disability

The determinants of pain and disability in OA are complex. The articular cartilage has no nerve supply, but the joint capsule, supporting ligaments and periosteum are innervated. In the synovium, nerve fibres are found in close apposition to blood vessels. A complex neural system monitors joint position and movement separately.

Symptomatic change in OA perhaps reflects decreasing thresholds and enlarging receptive fields. With the induction of experimental OA the small-diameter fibres are active even without mechanical stimulation and also become sensitive to motion. Stimulation small-diameter unmyelinated nerve fibres experimentally or after tissue injury may result in transmission of impulses to the spinal cord, thalamus and eventually reach cerebral cortex. The dorsal horn neurons become more sensitive to further stimuli [21].

Neuropeptides are small peptides synthesized in the dorsal root ganglia. The greatest impact on pain perception has substance P. In addition to inducing vasodilatation and vascular permeability, it has effects on the inflammatory cascade.

Activation of opioid receptors inhibits both neuronal stimulation and neuropeptide release [22]. The endogenous opioid peptides such as ß-endorphin and met-encephalin play a role in modulating pain.

Pain has an articular or periarticular source other than articular cartilage. However, the perception of pain and its severity is a central phenomenon. This includes life style, psychosocial factors, family support, job satisfaction, muscle weakness and comorbities. Nocturnal pain may be related to stimulation of unmyelinated fibres in subchondral bone by increased intra-osseous pressure. The pain and disability and their severity often correlate poorly with the degree of anatomical change. The role of inflammation is uncertain in most cases.

An appreciation of the contributions of various pathogenetic factors may be useful in recommending therapies, designed to ameliorate pain postpone disability and retard the degenerative process.

# Clinical Aspects of Osteoarthrosis

## Prevalence of Osteoarthrosis

Degenerative joint diseases are the most common medical problems and cause of disability in middle-aged and older people in most populations. The disease can lead to insufficiency of the joint. This condition of the joints is analogous to cardiac or renal failure.

The disease affects people of all ethnic groups and all geographical locations. Researchers estimate that 24.3 million Americans ages 35 to 65 suffer from some degree of OA [23].

The exact prevalence has been difficult to establish. There is difficulty in defining the condition under study. If radiological criteria alone are used to detect OA then a high prevalence figure will emerge. If clinical criteria are added then the prevalence figure is lower.

OA changes were radiologically found in more than 80% of subjects over age 55 whereas clinical manifestation had only 15 to 20%. Cobb found that only 30% of persons with radiological OA had symptoms in the diseased joint. Lawrence found radiological prevalence of OA of the distal interphalangeal joints of the hands in 56% of males, yet only 9% had symptomatic. In weight-bearing joints the correlation between radiological and symptoms findings is closer but never very strong [24].

Localization of asymptomatic OA radiographic changes are 30% hands, 21% feet, 3% knees/hips in general population, and symptomatic OA have all adults in 4% men and 9% women. Persons over 60 years have symptomatic OA in 17% men and 30% women.A strong association exists between joint degeneration and age. The prevalence and incidence of OA increase with age, and is especially high among people with over 50 years of age. There is evidence that 90% of people with over 75 years of age have evidence of OA [25], and that 60% of persons with over 35 years have clinical manifestation of the disease. In Lawrence's study in 1966. the prevalence of radiologically defined OA increased with age.

The disease is more common in women. Epidemiological works of Kellgren and Lawrence showed that 87% women and 83% men have OA radiological changes in one or more joints. The primary differences in incidence between males and females are related to the sites affected by OA. The most common sites affected in females are distal interphalangeal joints (DIP). Males suffer from OA before 45 years, possibly because of higher incidence of posttraumatic OA. After 45 years, females suffer more frequently from OA and tend to have more severe disease than men do.

No significant correlation exists between incidence of osteoarthritis and the race, with the exception of decreased incidence among the Chinese. Local factors do appear to modify the prevalence of OA of certain joints, e.g. OA of the hip is less common in the Southern Chinese than in Caucasian populations [26].

The incidence of OA of the hip is much high among the Caucasian populations than among the other races [27-30]. It is relatively more in the Japan. It is unknown whether the difference is reflected in genetic predisposition in the Caucasian in the development of OA of the hip, or factors such as disease of the hip in childhood, deformity of the hip, anthropological differences or type daily activities are responsible for differences [26].

Identification of genetic factors and environmental factors may help to clarify of etiology and prevention of OA.

# Classification of Osteoarthrosis

The classification and diagnosis of OA is difficult in everyday practice because of different forms of the disease and heterogeneity in localization, presenting symptoms and final outcome. Degenerative joint disease has been categorized in many ways. Diagnostic and classification guidelines for OA based on clinical and radiographic signs for the most frequently involved joints have been developed by American College of Rheumatology (ACR).

As a clinical entity, OA can be divided into primary and secondary forms. Clinicians may classify it by the number of joints involved into monoarticular, oligoarticular and polyarticular types.

## Primary Osteoarthrosis

Etiology of primary (idiopathic) OA is still not clearly understood. Despite the fact that the etiology is not clear, there are many common characteristics of the disease.

It is considered that genetic and hormonal factors can play a very important role, such as in the development of Haberden's nodes and primary generalized OA.

The role of genetic factor suggests different prevalence of OA on some joints in different geographical regions. In Greenland OA of the knee is more common amongst women on the west coast than amongst those on the east coast. The diagnostic criteria used in the race studies of the geographic prevalence of OA were not uniform and the explanation for the differences in the prevalence is speculative.

Recent findings suggest a role of immunologic mechanisms [31]. Certain unrecognizable anatomical abnormalities of joint anatomy or function may also play a role in development of primary OA.

The dates show that the other factors such as obesity, regular and occupational activity have a role in the etiology of OA, but there is no evidence that any of them have a crucial role in development of the disease. Association between obesity and joint degeneration is not completely clear. It suggests positive correlation between obesity and OA of different localizations such as the knee (weight-bearing joint), and also non-weight-bearing joints such as the sternoclavicular and distal interphalangeal joints. Other radiological studies have not shown any excess of OA in joint of an overweight study group as well as animal work [32-33]. Recent study of 1021 males and females ranging in age from 23 to 94 years and requiring surgery for end-stage hip joint OA were analyzed to find the prevalence of high body weights at the time of surgery. 68% of the patients surveyed were recorded as overweight and 53.3% of patients aged 30-39 years nearly reached the lower limit defined for obesity [34].

### *Clinical Subgroups of Primary Osteoarthrosis*

Generalized OA and Heberden's nodes are a subgroup of OA that occurs mostly in female patients with mean age of 52 years. 20% gave a family history of similar joint diseases, suggesting a hereditary influence in its development. This disease has the characteristic pattern of joint involvement, presentation and course. The joints affected most often are: distal interphalangeal joints, carpometacarpal joints, knee, spine, proximal interphalangeal joints and hips.

*Erosive OA* is a subgroup of OA and characteristically seen in postmenopausal women. This OA present occasionally such an acute painful inflammatory arthritis of the distal interphalangeal and proximal interphalangeal joints of the hand. Affected joints may be red, warm and swollen. Joint deformity and ankylosis may occur. Radiologically changes may show loss of joint space, subchondral sclerosis, osteophytes and bony erosion. Histology findings show non-specific inflammatory features.

*Ankylosing hyperostosis (Forestier's disease).* The disease is characterized by florid form of OA of the spine and by large marginal osteophyte formation. The new bone is laid down on the localization aspect of the dorsal vertebrae across the front of the vertebral disc. Bony spur formation is usually more marked on the right side of the spine. Spinal ankylosis has occurred. Sacroiliac joints are normal and disc spaces are often well preserved. The tendency to florid ossification is seen at cervical, lumbar spine, calcaneum. Despite these findings, patient is often asymptomatic. Bony ankylosis in OA may also occur in erosive OA.

The exact prevalence of primary and secondary OA has been difficult to establish. There is no clear accepted limit between primary and secondary OA but according to present knowledge, the majority of cases of OA fall into primary category. In the case of the hip joint, for example predisposing abnormalities underlies the later development of OA changes in a significant number of cases. Murray has suggested that majority of patients have primary OA of the hip and that 65% of them can be shown to have a pre-existing anatomical abnormality of the joint.

## Secondary Osteoarthrosis

Secondary OA are diseases which develop after the influence of some known etiological factor on the joint causing damage to articular cartilage: inflammatory joint diseases (infectious arthritis, psoriatic arthritis, Reiter's syndrome, ankylosing spondylitis), , metabolic and endocrine diseases (crystal deposition disease, haemochromatosis, ochronosis, Wilson's disease, bleeding disorders, acromegaly), dysplastic and hereditary conditions (congenital hip dysplasia, epiphyseal dysplasia, chondrodysplasia, Perthes' disease, joint hypermobility, and bone disorders (osteonecrosis, osteochondritis, Paget's disease of bone), traumatic lesions (acute injury, fractures, meniscus tears, repetitive microtraumas), overuse of the joints (work-load, chronic occupational overuse, sports overuse, neuropathic arthropathy-Charcot joint). The interval between injury and ensuing OA varies from a months after fracture to 10 to 15 years (after meniscectomy).

Many researches of association between occupations and OA have shown that chronic trauma can predispose development of OA. There are evidences that repetitive and intense of loads impact greater than those of normal daily activities in some profession may predispose development of clinical and radiological OA changes. Hadler has shown in 1981.that OA is more severe and common in the joints which are more used.

Participation in sports may increase the risk of joint degeneration [13,35 ]. Recent research has shown that former soccer players have significant higher prevalence of OA of the hip [12].

Various metabolic processes that damage articular cartilage may lead to joint degeneration. OA of acromegaly is similar to primary OA. In this condition in which a pituitary tumor causes excessive growth factor generation, results in a generalized over proliferation of chondrocytes and overproduction of cartilage matrix.

Haemochromatosis, the disease of iron metabolism can resemble primary OA. Congenital or developmental abnormalities can predispose appearance of OA. The importance of incongruity of the articular surface (because of morphologic deviations from normal shape of articulating surfaces) in development of OA of the hip has proved in many clinical and experimental researches [36-37]. In 20-50% of cases of OA, predisposing factors are congenital hip dysplasia, Legg-Perthes disease and slipped femoral epiphysis.

# Diagnostic Evaluation

OA is one of the most frequent causes of the pain and physical disability of the adult persons. This is a slow progressive, evolutive disease.

## Clinical Manifestation

Clinical conditions are characterized by gradual development of the joint pain, stiffness, decreased of movement, functional disturbance, and depend of the localization and of the evolutive stage of the disease. There are mentions that muscle strength and psychosocial factors the main and decisive factor of the pain and disability [38-39].

The presence of the degenerative processes on the joints and their clinical manifestation in the interaction and combination of the different mechanisms, have as results also changes on the adjacent joint structures. As epiphenomena of the diseased joint and adjacent connective tissue structures, occur muscle weak, fatigue, atrophy and dysfunction [40]. Decreased of range of motion, the pain and deformities, instabilities [41], reduction of functional performances [42-43] , as well as muscle strength [41, 42, 44] in the patients with OA, occur in different degree. The increased magnitude of gluteus medius activation in the group with OA is the evidence of a muscular dysfunction associated with hip disease. This has implications for the progressive nature of the disease and for its conservative management [45].

### *History*

Careful patient history involves questioning the patient about the following: the time of occurrence of initial symptoms and signs, the circumstances in which first symptoms and signs appeared previous infection, underlying diseases, the pattern of pain and stiffness and the incidence of OA in the family.

In addition to documenting joint symptoms and their impact on patient's daily activities and lifestyle, the physician should evaluate the patient's general health as well as medical history injuries, medications, alcohol consumption and other illnesses that may complicate the treatment of the joint disease.

### *Physical Examination*

One of the most important tasks of physical examination is to elicit the pain the patient is complaining of and to determine its source. Patients often describe the activity-associated pain that is poorly localized and typically begins immediately or shortly after the patients begins to use the joint and may persist for hours after the activity is stopped.

Most patients also notice joint stiffness, particularly in the morning or after prolonged inactivity.

The second important part of the physical examination is evaluation of swelling and deformity. "Hard swelling" or "hard nodes" around the joint are characteristic of OA (Heberden's nodes, Bouchard's nodes, and nodes around medial and lateral tibiofemoral compartments of the knee joint). The nodes are palpable much earlier than they can be recognized on x-rays. At this stage they are visible on bone scintigrams as hot spots.

Soft tissue swelling may also be a feature of OA. Palpable joint effusion is often present in PIP, DIP and knee joint. Palpation of crepitus may occasionally be of importance. Coarse cracking felt with movement may be due to severe damage of the cartilage. One or two cracks felt over the knee can be a sign of a loose body or meniscus tear.

Examination of joint function may have diagnostic value. Physical examination starts with inspection. Examination includes assessment of the range of motion, muscle strength, circumferences of the joint, circumferences and length of the extremity. In diagnostic terms it may consist of series of functional tests and also of different special tests.

When joint degeneration progresses, patients may notice the loss of motion and feel crepitus, catching and grinding sensations in the joint with active motion. For example in OA of the hip initially internal rotation and abduction are restricted.

Abnormal passive movements are common, especially in the knee and finger joints of OA patients and are due to laxity of capsule and ligaments.

In some patients with advanced degenerative disease, muscle spasms develop and contribute to contractures.

Since muscle atrophy occurs with longstanding severe disease, the circumference of the involved limb should be measured and compared with the opposite limb. The assessment of the muscle strength becomes in a great extent useful component for diagnostic and therapy, in practice as research framework.

## Localization and Characteristic Osteoarthrosis

It is described particular clinical forms of OA: OA of the knee, OA of the hand OA of the hip joints, Osteoarthrosis of the spine.Although OA affects every synovial joints, the knee, hip, distal interphalangeal joints, the first metacarpophalangeal joint and the cervical and lumbar apophyseal joints of the spine are affected more often.

Agreement and modified combination of clinical, laboratory and radiological variables make criteria for diagnosis of symptomatic OA [46 ] (Table1, 2,3).

### *Osteoarthrosis of the Knee (Gonarthrosis)*

OA of the knee can be usually seen as the part of the clinical pictures of the generalized OA. The osteoarthritic knee is frequently the site of deposition of crystals of calcium pyrophosphate dihydrate. In contrast to usually chronic course of disease, the crystals, if released into the joint space, will cause episodes of acute synovitis.

As is the case with other weight-bearing joints, OA of the knee is likely to present with symptoms in the contrast to OA of the small joints of the hands. OA can affect the three main compartments of the knee joint differently. The medial tibiofemoral compartment is the most frequently involved (75%). The coexistence of medial tibiofemoral and patellofemoral OA is the most frequent combination. The different compartments are susceptible to different risk factors: obesity, knee injury and meniscetomy for tibiofemoral OA, and post-traumatic states, subluxation of the patella and valgus deformity of the knee for patellofemoral OA.

**Table 1. Classification criteria for OA of the knee**

| Clinical | | Clinical, laboratory and radiographic | |
|---|---|---|---|
| 1. Knee pain (on most days of previous month) | | 1. Knee pain (on most days of previous month) | |
| 2. Crepitus | | 2. Osteophyte | |
| 3. Morning stiffness<30min | | 3. Synovial fluid typical of OA | |
| 4.Age>38 years | | 4. Age>40years | |
| 5. Bony enlargement | | 5. Morning stiffness<30min | |
| | | 6. Crepitus | |
| Criteria fulfilled if: | 1,2,3& 4 | Criteria fulfilled if: | 1&2 |
| | 1,2&5 | | 1,3,5&6 |
| | 1,4&5 | | 1,4,5&6 |

OA causes pain with motion, stiffness after inactivity and limitation of motion. Physical examination may show enlarged knee, either as a result of synovial effusion, or as a consequence of bony overgrowth due to marginal osteophyte formation. The joint margins are often tender on palpation. The movement of the knee, particularly in the patellofemoral joint, produces crepitus. The varus or valgus deformity will be accompanied by instability of the joint. Progressive wasting of the quadriceps and the lack of muscular support for the joint may further impair the patient's mobility, causing functional impairment.

### *Osteoarthrosis of the Hand*

This presentation of OA is usually the part of the clinical pattern of generalized OA. Some patients develop classic signs of joint distribution: the distal interphalangeal joints (Heberden's nodes) and Bouchard nodes over the proximal interphalangeal joints (PIP). DIP joints are affected in about 70% of cases, the first metacarpophalangeal joints in 60% and all other joints of the hand in less than 30%.

**Table 2. Classification Criteria for OA of the Hand**

| ***Clinical*** | |
|---|---|
| 1. Hand pain, aching or stiffness (on most days of previous month) | |
| 2. Hard tissue enlargement>2 of 10 hand joints* | |
| 3. Metacarpophalangeal swelling <2 joints | |
| 4. Bony enlargement >2 or more distal interphalangeal joints | |
| 5. Deformity > 1 of 10 hand joints* | |
| ***Criteria fulfilled if:*** | 1,2,3&4 |
| | 1,2,3&5 |

* Second and third distal interphalangeal, second and third proximal interphalangeal, and first carpometacarpal in both hands.

The changes often develop slowly and without symptoms over many years. Occasionally the onset is sudden, painful and associated with signs of inflammation such as redness, swelling and cyst formation. Inflammation may cause the nodes to be tender, but they later become asymptomatic. Section through interphalangeal joint shows irregular, hyperplastic bony nodules at articular margins of phalanx. Though movement may be restricted they have surprisingly little effect on hand function. Interphalangeal joint OA is strongly associated with obesity and medial tibiofemoral OA. It is thought that repetitive loading and excessive use may influence the development of Heberden's nodes.

### *Osteoarthrosis of the Hip (Coxarthrosis)*

OA of the hip has specific distribution sites: the superolateral subset is the commonest (60%), medial poll hip disease is less common and can cause protrusion acetabuli. The concentric type is rare but this form is more strongly linked with the generalized forms of the OA than the other two forms.

In the contrast OA of the knee there is a weaker association with obesity, hip injury and Heberden's nodes, but a marked association with occupational activity such as farming.

Degenerative changes of eccentric idiopathic (primary) OA had deteriorated rapidly. Hips with concentric idiopathic OA underwent total hip arthroplasty (THA) at 10 years and with eccentric OA at an average of 4 years, after symptoms onset [47].

**Table 3. Classification Criteria for OA of the Hip**

| *Clinical* | | ***Clinical, laboratory and radiographic*** | |
|---|---|---|---|
| 1.Hip pain (on most days of previous month) | | 1. Hip pain (on most days of previous month) | |
| 2. Internal rotation<15 | | 2. ESR<20mm/h | |
| 3. ESR<45mm/h | | 3. Radiographic osteophytes | |
| 4.Hip flexion<115 | | 4. Radiographic joint space narrowing | |
| 5.Internal rotation >15 | | | |
| 6. Morning stiffness<60min | | | |
| 7. Age>50years | | | |
| 8. Pain on internal rotation | | | |
| ***Criteria fulfilled if:*** | 1,2&3 | ***Criteria fulfilled if:*** | 1,2&3 |
| | 1,2&4 | | 1,2&4 |
| | 1,5,6,7&8 | | 1,3&4 |

OA of the hip may develop slowly and cause a pain that is felt on the outer aspect of the hip or in the groin area, the inner thigh, buttocks or knee and painful antalgic gait. Stiffness on rising and after inactivity is also characteristic symptoms.

Restriction of movement may not be noticed by the patient initially, as flexion of the joint tends to preserved. Internal rotation and extension movements are usually the first to be restricted and later abduction and flexion are compromised. Patients characteristically hold the affected limb externally rotated and the hip flexed and adducted. Some patients with longstanding hip disease develop a Trendelenberg gait because of their hip adduction deformity and associated abductor muscle weakness. There is weakness of the other hip muscle also. With progression of the disease limitation of joint motion makes sitting down and rising very difficult and limb shortening may occur due to proximal subluxation of femoral head. The final stage is the phase of definite disability with severe pain, very restricted movements and greater functional disturbances.

*Osteoarthrosis of the Spine*

The spine is the most frequently affected by OA. It is often accompanied by OA at other sites. In regard to spine the term is used to encompass degeneration of both the fibrocartilaginous disc and the diarthrodial apophyseal joints. As the intervertebral disc degeneration and the disc space narrows, osteophytes develop along the margins of the vertebrae. Degenerative changes occur also in the apophyseal joints and posterolaterally around neural foramina.

The OA changes are usually most severe at the apices of the lordotic segments of the spine. Pain and stiffness as well as discomfort and in some patient's neurological symptoms are the characteristic symptoms of OA of the spine. The pain and neurological symptoms with referred radicular pain and paraesthesiae may be the result of osteophytes pressing on the spinal cord or narrowing intervertebral foramina, degenerative disc protrusion or apophyseal joint subluxation.

Cervical spine involvement may lead to neurological problems and compromise blood flow through the vertebral arteries, causing dizziness, visual problems, headaches, nausea, ataxia and vertigo. Referred pain and paraesthesiae are most common in the C5, C6 and C7 dermatomes of the arms and may be associated with alteration of sensation, power and reflexes in the affected limbs. Occasionally entrapment of the lowest cervical and upper thoracic nerve roots may give rise to chest wall pain which can be mistaken for ischemic cardiac pain.

OA of the lumbar spine is a common cause of low back pain. Radicular pain, paraesthesiae and neurological symptoms are most common in the L4, L5 and S1 dermatomes. Osteophyte formation within the spinal canal may also compress the blood supply to the spinal cord, causing a spinal claudication syndrome. Most common of these is claudication of the cauda equina in which the patient complain of pain and paraesthesia in the legs which are related to exercise and the neurological deficit may be apparent only after exercise.

# Diagnostic Techniques

The diagnosis of OA is usually based on the history and physical findings but laboratory tests, radiography and other imaging studies may help in evaluating OA.

## Radiography

X-rays may provide useful confirmatory evidence of the condition. Three radiographic markers of joint degeneration often occur together: narrowed joint space, increased density of subchondral bone and osteophytes. In some joints only one or two of radiographic markers may be visible on standard radiographs. The earliest change on X-ray in OA is joint space narrowing. This is usually accompanied by bony sclerosis around the joint margins. With advancement of disease, marginal osteophytes and subchondral bone cysts will develop. Finally in end stage disease, gross bony deformity will be evident.

Calcification within the articular soft tissues is an extremely common finding in OA. It may take the form of chondrocalcinosis with characteristic sites for crystal deposits in the knee, wrist and symphysis pubis. In advanced disease are commonly seen non-linear deposits of calcium crystals in periarticular soft tissues. The loose bodies are usually within the synovial tissues.

For weight-bearing joints, x-ray films should always be taken in a weight-bearing position. Careful and reproducible positioning is essential for imaging both the tibiofemoral and the patellofemoral compartments of the knee.

## Other Imaging Studies

Other imaging studies may have value in selected cases.

Bone scintigraphy is a sensitive measure of bone activity and may show the level of activity in OA during the course of the disease. In situation when radiography may not show pathological alteration scintigrams performed and may provide diagnostic clues, showing accumulation of the nuclide around DIP joints.

Ultrasound is theoretically useful in measuring the width of cartilage, but this procedure has not yet been standardized. Ultrasound is largely used for detection of effusion in the hip joint, for Bakers cyst and for diagnosing ligamentous and/or tendinous tears.

CT demonstrates subtle changes in joint congruity, alignment, thickening of subchondral bone and loss of joint space.

MRI provides visualization some localized osteochondral abnormalities, changes in the soft tissues, ligamentous, meniscal abnormalities. It can provide very early differential diagnosis of avascular necrosis of the femoral head and swelling and cyst formation of the apophyseal joints of the spine. Recent advances in this technology have led to significant improvement in spatial resolution and contrast, enabling researchers to evaluate anatomical damage of all these joint structures across sagittal, coronal, and axial planes. MRI system makes a highly reliable quantification of cartilage volume possible. Recently, the quantitative assessment of knee cartilage volume has become possible. Such technology will be critical for the analysis of disease progression over time.

## Laboratory Tests

The blood count, erythrocyte sedimentation rate and bone biochemistry are normal. Synovial fluid in advanced disease will contain fragments of the degenerating articular surface. When calcium crystals are released into the joint space a vigorous inflammatory response is provoked. These tests may help exclude other causes of joint pain.

### Biochemical Markers

Sensitive and specific biochemical markers of OA may help for early diagnosis and objective monitoring of course of the disease. Markers under investigation include cartilage components (keratan sulfat epitopes which indicate catabolic activity and occur primarily after joint trauma; different types chondroitin sulfate epitopes, type II collagen propeptide–C, cartilage oligometric matrix protein, seem to be sensitive markers of cartilage anabolic activity), bone derived markers (pyridinoline and deoxypyridinoline-indicate catabolic action and osteocalcin and alkaline phosphatase-increased anabolic processes in the subchondral bone), and markers of synovial proliferation (III collagen propeptides, serum hyaluronic acid). The importance of this markers in the following of the OA, for the estimate of the activity of disease, the early diagnosis as well as the possibility of objective monitoring of both the natural course of the disease and the effect of therapy remains to assessment.

Diagnostic arthroscopy is rarely needed for the diagnosis of OA. Arthroscopy makes it possible to detect the earliest stages of articular cartilage degeneration and to identify other intraarticular problems.

Outcome measures can help us evaluate the functional status of the patients and they provide an objective tool for assessing the severity of impairment, functional disability and handicap at personal and community levels [48]. Health Assessment Questionnaire (HAQ), Arthritis Impact Measurement Scales (AIMS) and the MOS 36-Item Short Form Health Survey (SF-36) can be used for general outcome measures.

Specific outcome measures for OA have been developed: the Lequesne algofunctional index and the Western Ontario and McMaster Osteoarthritis Index (WOMAC), index for assessing the severity of OA of the knee and hip.

## Differential Diagnosis

When assessing a patient with joint pain the physician should consider other possible causes besides OA. Deformities caused by diseases other than OA may show very similar clinical signs and symptoms. These types of deformities include the following: rheumatoid arthritis, spondyloarthropathies and distal type of psoriatic arthritis involving interphalangeal joints; infectious arthritis; crystal arthropathy, including gout and pseudogout; hypertrophic osteoarthropaty which might be mistaken for generalized OA affecting the fingers, traumatic joint injuries, bleeding disorders and villonodular synovitis. The physician should also consider the all possible causes of secondary joint degeneration before make a definite diagnosis of primary OA.

# Management of Osteoarthrosis

Treatment of OA should vary according to the severity of disease and patient's expectations and level of activity. Initiation of complex therapeutical program early in the course of the disease can make a significant difference in the patient's quality of life and may help to slow the progression of the disease.

ACR is recently defined the recommendations for the progressive and slowly progressive management of OA of the hip and knee [49]. As a step one in management of OA is recommendation of nonpharmacologic therapy. It is considered a pharmacologic therapy is most effective when combined with nonpharmacologic therapy so that optimal management of OA requires a combination of pharmacological and non-pharmacological treatment. Step three in management of OA is surgical management in combination of nonpharmacological treatment and with/without pharmacologic therapy.

Except the conventional techniques in management of the OA, alternative therapeutic remedies are also used: diseases modifying drugs, chondroprotective drugs and structural modification.

The different approaches as an attempt for modifying of the disease are used in the researches of the management of the OA: modification of the risk factors, the therapy with cartilage components, antiinflammatory and antiprotheases therapy, cytokines manipulation, genetic therapy and cartilage replacement.

## Nonpharmacological Treatment

The use of nonpharmacologic interventions in OA is essential for good management of the disease. Many treatment or techniques have been developed to combat pain in OA. This therapy including patient education, self-management programs, personalized social support directly or via telephone contact, programs for aerobic exercise, weight loss (if overweight is present), physical therapy involving exercises and occupational therapy involving joint protection and energy conservation. These numerous nonpharmacologic treatments can reduce consumption and toxicity or even delay the need for joint replacement surgery. The patient should start the treatment of OA with education, psychological support and environmental measures.

### *Education and Psychological Support*

OA is chronic and potentially disabling disease and in management of pain patients should be reassured that such pain is a reversible state and not associated with irreversible loss of ability. Forman et al. in a survey of 682 elderly people demonstrated that the OA is not a severe disease that necessarily leads to major disability, e.g. inability to walk [50]. It has shown that pain or disability in OA does not correlate with cartilage loss [51]. Education and psychological support is becoming more popular. Patient information concerning the evolution and severity of the disease is essential. Physicians and therapists should reassure patients that most people can continue to lead active lives and that simple measures of treatment can reduce symptoms and improve function. Education should focus on outlining activities that should be avoided and encouraging appropriate types of activities.

Psychological support is essential for elderly people suffering from chronic disabling disease. Lack of understanding by family members can be a great problem. Some patients may also need counseling in order to relieve anxiety or depression and develop more optimistic outlook.

Evaluation of the patient's environment and alterations in physical and social factors are important. These can improve function and reduce pain with patients with OA.

### *Exercise and Physiotherapy in Osteoarthrosis*

It is conceived that muscle strength is the key of the pain and disability in the OA of the patients [39, 52]. The loss of muscle strength and function around the arthrotic joint is evident. The muscle can atrophy to 30% for one week [53]; end with completely rest will have the loss of function 3% daily. The aim of the kinesitherapeutical treatment is the pain relief, prevention or reduction of the contractures, preserving and restitution of the range of motions, muscle strength, conservation and preserving of the energy [41]. This is intended to attain of the function with minimal cost of energy and to avoid the muscle fatigue that has increased due to joint dysfunction.

Exercise therapy is irreplaceable method for maintaining the muscle strength, stability and movement of the joint in OA. But, it should be emphasized that kinesitherapeutical programs must be lead correctly in order to be effective and avoid danger from worsening of the disease because of inadequate dosage and loading. Exercise therapy could involve training or exercises focused on the OA joint. Some specific exercises, e.g. quadriceps exercises in patients with knee OA can reduce disability and pain. Exercises therapy for OA involves warm-up and range of motion, muscle strengthening and stretching exercises.

The therapeutical program should be applied to respect the principles of the optimal stimulation. Functional excitements stimulate physiologic activity only if they are middle and moderate, until too strong harm. When exercises carried out within the limits of normal joint motion and comfort exercises seem beneficial for pain and disability. The stronger muscle contractions increase intraarticular pressure, and repetitive stronger contractions can become associated with cartilage destruction and increases of the pain.

Excessive force of the contraction can lead to further OA changes, increasing of the pain with negative effect on the muscle and functional performances. In patients with advanced degenerative changes and in end-stage of OA, as well as in these with evidence of joint effusion, isometric exercises are preferable. In general, isometric exercises are used more often than isotonic because they build muscle as effectively as the latter, but impose less stress on a joint, as less traumatic [41], it would achieve improvement in muscle mass with minimizing of the risk from worsening. Fisher and Chamberlain have shown that quadriceps exercises in patients with knee of OA can reduce disability and pain during various activities after only 1 month of physical therapy and in some cases, even allowed the complete withdrawal of analgesic drugs [55].

If exercises lead to increased pain rest should be ordered and further exercises must be performed only with medical monitoring. Therapeutical exercises with optimal dose decrease the pain and disability. Increased muscle strength can protect the joint with resorption of the stress.

### *Physiotherapy in Osteoarthrosis*

The use of *heat* or *cold* in the various forms to treat joint pain has long been advocated and popular treatment. Many methods for applying heat can be used, including paraffin baths, simple warm bath, infrared bakers and diathermy.

Heat may facilitate muscle relaxation and has been suggested that it has an analgesic effect. The analgesic effect of therapy is explained by the pain modulation with the stimulation of the heat receptors.

The sufficient subjective improvement felt by the patients with OA makes these techniques very important in clinical use. Warmth can comfort the painful joint involved with OA. Cold therapy is used in the management of particularly painful OA joints. It is shown that it can be a practical method for acute pain relief during severe attacks of OA. Superficial cooling decreases muscle spasm, and it has been demonstrated to decrease muscle spindle activity and to raise the threshold of pain.

In summary, the efficacy of specific superficial heating measures and cooling measures (ice pack, ice massage) in terms of relief of pain or reduction of inflammation in OA has not been fully established. No definitive study has investigated the efficacy of either heat or cold.

Decisions about the use of superficial heat or cold for pain relief are based on empirical observations that the pain of acute inflammatory and traumatic disorders is best relieved by cold compresses, whereas subacute to chronic inflammation is best relieved by superficial heat. The application of the moderate heat may be useful to precede each exercise session to relieve pain and diminish stiffness.

Application of surface heat is less effective than diathermy and ultrasonic treatments in the management of the OA of the hip, because the hip is deep within tissue.

*Thermal baths.* They are a very fashionable and attractive form of therapy for the patients with OA. However, there have been very few rigorous studies of the efficacy of thermal water in treating of OA. There are some reports of the positive effects of this technique on the pain relief. They tried to prove the efficacy of spa therapy. The results showed that two weeks' treatment with mineral baths and mud packs produced significant pain relief, which lasted for 6 months. But, only a small sample was investigated [55].

*Massage* is comfortable and desirable procedure of physical therapy and may be valuable for the soft tissue contracture around of OA joints and in relieving the muscle spasm. Massage may be useful in acute and chronic low back pain.

*Shortwaves, microwaves, interferential current, and ultrasound* deliver deep heat. Deep heat is useful in treating painful musculoskeletal disorders. It affects the viscoelastic properties of collagen and may enhance the efficacy of stretching.

*Shortwave diathermy* has an analgesic effect which makes up over so-called endogenous heat. This heat is created in the tissues by conversion of electric power in the thermal energy. The favorable effect is a result of their deep action. That is very important in region which is being treated such as hip because it has more high penetration than exogenous heat.

Close correlations were found to exist between magnitude of blood flow, length of treatment and therapeutic intensity. The medium level of energy application was considered to be a highly favorable approach in terms of intensity. Segmental high-frequency application likewise resulted in increased blood flow in both legs, though intensity values thus achieved were below results of locally delimited calf treatment.

*Interferential current* becomes endogenous in the treating area by interference of middle-frequent power from two independent circuits. They act analgesic and attribute effect on the vessel's blood and regeneration of the tissue. Lower frequency and shorter duration are used when disease activity is lower.

*Ultrasound therapy* is used in the therapy of the OA. The different therapeutical results of this form of therapy are reported in the literature. There are statements that therapeutical doses of ultrasound have analgesic, vasodilatatory, fibrinolytical, resorptive and spasmolitic effects. The mechanical action of the ultrasound consists of the change in the ultrasound pressure and acceleration of the tissue particles that vibrate. It is only proved that the ultrasound acting on the increasing of the elasticity of the soft tissue. This therapeutical effect would be useful in the therapy of muscle contractures and this is important in the therapy of the OA. It can be of the help for contractures of the knee. There are statements that more expressive effect of the ultrasound is when it is applied simultaneously with diadynamic current. ("Sonodynator"). With ultrasound a medication can also be applied (sonophoresis). Recent controlled study could not prove the analgesic effect of the ultrasound in the OA of the knee.

*Light therapy* and laser use are unconventional therapy techniques for some chronic pain conditions. The mechanism of the effect of laser use is not sufficiently known. It is mentioned that it has effect on decreasing of the acute and chronically muscle-skeletal pain, muscle spasms and neurogenical pain. The most of the studies of laser use for the relief of pain do not have suitable controls.

### Biomechanical Interventions

They correct the effects of the biomechanical factors on pathophysiology and progression of OA.

*Weight reduction* is a classic concept in OA of the hip and knee. The disease may be preventable in some instances by reducing risk factors associated with disease. Although, no study has shown that obesity directly causes the disease, it has been proven that obesity increases symptomatic OA. There are differences in the effects obesity as risk factor on knee OA compared with hip OA.

In the hip OA there is a weaker association with obesity. But, one recent study investigated 1021 males and females who were requiring surgery for end-stage hip joint OA to determine whether they were overweight or obese; a health risk is commonly associated with hip joint OA. A study has shown that overweight were recorded for 68% of the patients surveyed (the Body mass index-BMI > 30kg/m2), including younger adults. This study has also shown that patients whose BMIs are in the obese range may have increased risk of removal and reimplantation of their prosthesis [34]. For people with OA of the hip, knee, ankle, foot and possibly lumbar spine, weight loss may help decrease symptoms and slow disease progression. Weight loss should be prescribed for obese people with painful arthritis, but this goal is often difficult to reach because of the degree of inactivity imposed by the joint damage. The beneficial effects of weight loss presumably result from decreased joint loading.

### Supportive Aids and Appliances

The use of a wedged insole under static conditions of lower extremity leads to significant symptomatic improvement. Pain relief lasts significantly longer in the management of foot and ankle OA with wedged insole and orthotics, than with nonsteroidal drugs. Bandaging of the knee seems to provide symptomatic improvement in knee OA. Impact-absorbing shoes and shock absorbing heel pads provide a lot of relief for many people with lower limb and back OA. Walking sticks and walkers are necessary to maintain better functional status and prevent of exacerbation of pain in elderly people. Modifications of the home and work environment allow people with OA to perform common activities more easily. Raised seating and mounted grab bar make entering and exiting car easier. The orthosis or spinal brace is indicated for symptomatic back pain unresponsive to conservative measures. Orthosis may help rest inflamed tissue by immobilization and may reduce lordosis as well as unload the spine and reinforce abdominal muscles. But, activity and carefully prescribed abdominal muscle strengthening are to be encouraged to tolerance in an attempt to discontinue the use of the orthosis at the earliest possible time.

### *Nonconventional Therapies*

*Acupuncture* may have an analgesic effect that was shown in clinical practice. Acupuncture can also have an effect on reducing of analgesic drug consumption in patients with OA pain. But, to our present knowledge, there is no other valuable study investigating the efficacy of acupuncture in OA pain.

*Transucutaneous electrical nerve stimulation (TENS)* is effective in some conditions of neuropathic pain. Taylor et al. have reported that it can provide analgesia greater than the one that is obtained with placebo even after long term use [56]. Therapeutical effect of TENS is explanation by the gate control theory of pain. Essentially, TENS is designed to preferentially stimulate large-diameter cutaneous fibers in an effort to inhibit transmission of painful stimuli to the spinal cord.

It is supposed that secretion of the endogenous opioid peptides such as ß-endorphin and met-encephalin plays a role in modulating pain. These opioid peptides have been demonstrated in synovial lining cells, lymphocytes and macrophages. A few forms of the stimulation are used toward frequency, intensity and time of during of the procedure. The segmental application is preferable in patients with severe disease activity.

*Homeopathy.* Only placebo effect which is sometimes useful effect of homeopathy is proved by now.

*Osteopathy and chiropractics* are very fashionable methods. There have been attempts to apply them to OA, particularly in the knee joint. Typically, osteopathy is proposed in France and chiropractic is a classic approach in the US. They are on the range of the experiment for OA joints.

*Pulsed electromagnetic fields* have recently been used to treat OA. In patients with symptomatic osteoarthritis of the knee, pulsed electromagnetic fields (PMF) treatment can reduce impairment in activities of daily life and improve knee function [54]. Analgesics effect of the pulsed electromagnetic fields reported in majority of the studies [55]. In the conditions of the acute pain recommended parameters are lower frequencies, intensity and duration of the procedure.

Further research is required to improve the evidence base of nonpharmacologic interventions in and the overall management of OA.

## Pharmacological Treatment of Osteoarthrosis

For the successful pharmacological treatment of the OA it should be provided that a drug fulfills following expectation (prerequisites): to provide chondroprotective effect, to improve or at least to stop developed damage of the joint, to pain relief and to improve symptoms which negative influence on function.

Pharmacological treatment of the OA until today did not achieve the expected results. There is no specific medication which can be used to change the course of the disease and repair developed damage of the joint, but there is a range of medications that can relief the pain, accompanying synovitis, improve function and quality of life.

Pain and stiffness are dominant symptoms in developing OA. It is recommended that analgesics should be used for pain control in the patients with OA.

Analgesics are initial therapeutic approach for mild-to-moderate pain symptom control. Paracetamol, the oral analgesic, should be given first. Topical capsaicin or methyl salicylate cream should be considered in patients who do not respond to paracetamol or do not wish to take systemic therapy.

For moderate-to-severe pain and swollen joints, a prescription of nonsteroidal anti-inflammatory drug (NSAIDs) should be considered. The same goes with intraarticular injections of long acting steroids.

When initial therapy yields inadequate response an alternative options can be used. These include cyclooxygenase 2 (COX-2) specific inhibitors and Tramadol for patients with moderate-to-severe pain and who have contraindications to COX-2 specific inhibitors and NSAIDs.

Treatment and pharmacological agents should vary according to the severity of disease, of the involved joint, clinical findings and individual tolerability and response of the drug.

### *Analgesics*

One of the most important symptoms of the OA is the pain because of which the patients ask for medical help. "Simple" analgesics are often recommended as first-choice agents for pain relief in OA (paracetamol or other analgesics according to chose of the doctor).

In many investigations paracetamol has proved to be an effective medication for decreases of the pain in OA. It is more and more of interest for paracetamol, today. This medication is less toxic among OA pharmacological agents, but is still powerful alternative to NSAIDs. NSAIDs are used, although, more than paracetamol despite the fact that they cause more adverse effects than paracetamol. Comparison of the efficacy of the paracetamol in dose of 4g daily with Ibuprofen of 1200 mg and 2400 mg daily shows the same effect.

The effective dose of paracetamol is about 4g daily, although its suggested dose_is 1 to 3 g. Full dose of paracetamol may be useful also in combination with low doses of naproxen. The efficacy of the NSAIDs is first of all realized with analgesic and no anti-inflammatory features, but with more severe adverse effects. It is especially important for older people with significantly less functional reserve of liver and significant risk of bleeding from gastrointestinal tract. Relief of constant pain is usually best achieved with regular doses of analgesics. Adverse effects associated with paracetamol include rashes and hepatotoxicity. It may be contraindicated in patients with compromised renal or hepatic function. Paracetamol should be used cautiously in patients with existing liver disease and avoided in patients with chronic alcohol abuse.

Therefore, paracetamol has an important place in the management of OA, although further investigations are needed. The role of paracetamol in the control of pain in osteoarthritis is still in need of better definition.

### *Nonsteroidal Anti-inflammatory Drugs*

Nonsteroidal anti-inflammatory drugs (COX-1 or COX-2 inhibitors- Ibuprofen, Diclofenac etc., Meloxicam, Nimesulid) have become a routine treatment for pain and stiffness due to degenerative joint disease. The accelerated development of the pharmaceutical technology in the last decades the number of the NSAIDs is increasing in clinical practice.

This medication's name indicates the anti-inflammatory effect. They were first used for joining herb extracts which contained salicylates. For pain relief and decreasing of fever, Hippocrates suggests the use of the extract of willow bark. At the beginning of this century, a lot of medications were sintetized which had the same therapeutical effect. These medications were named by the drugs similar to aspirin. Because of obvious differences toward corticosteroids they were named nonsteroidal anti-inflammatory drugs. NSAIDs offer a potential advantage because they suppress any inflammation as well.

Anti-inflammatory effect is based on experimental evidence, but this has been less well documented in clinical practice, where analgesic effects dominate [57]. The mechanisms of their acting are still not completely clear. Inhibition of the synthesis of the proinflammatory mediators of the prostaglandin, which are at the end of the metabolic path of the arachidonic acid are the important factor of that action.

The enzyme cyclooxigenase (COX) acts on the arachidonic acid and leads to synthesis of the prostaglandin. This enzyme exists in the less of the two forms isoenzymes, so-called COX-1 and COX-2. It is attractive supposition that in essence, anti-inflammatory activity of the NSAIDs is the consequence of the inhibition COX-2, while adverse effects (gastric intolerance, impairment of the liver) are consequences of the inhibition of the constitutive enzyme COX-1, which have obvious physiologic (antitrombogenic, citoprotective) function.

Although inhibition of cyclo-oxygenase (COX) is common to all NSAID, it has been known for a long time that there is no close quantitative relationship between inhibition and analgesic or anti-inflammatory effect [58]. Inducible isoform COX-2 was found 1992. Its synthesis can start a number of proinflammatory stimuli which act on the cells.

Today is known that NSAIDs show the different selectivity toward COX-1 and COX-2, is inhibiting stronger or poor some enzymes. The most selective of NSAIDs toward COX-2 isoenzym, have the same antiinflammatory activity compared with standard NSAIDs, but much less impact on the physiologic production PG. It is reason of substantially better relation of the risk and benefit during their using.

Previous results of the use of selective COX-2 inhibitors are used to point out a conclusion that relation between COX-2/COX-1 of the inhibition would be crucial in the estimate of the therapeutically-safety profile of NSAIDs in the inflammatory rheumatic diseases. The new forms of NSAIDs (COX-2 specific inhibitors) are still developed [59].

While it has been hard to document relevant overall differences in efficacy between currently used NSAIDs evidence of real differences in toxicity is accumulating. Indomethacin has the most pronounced sedative effect, while hepatotoxicity is more commonly reported for diclofenac. Aseptic meningitis is rare but alarming adverse reaction reported with ibuprofen and sulindac. Cystitis is a complication peculiar to tiaprofenic acid and alveolitis may be induced by naproxen.

Clinical studies have not shown NSAIDs to have a clear advantage over analgesic drugs. In vitro and animal studies suggest that some NSAIDs may accelerate joint degeneration; other NSAIDs may help preserve articular cartilage. There is evidence that indomethacin accelerates degeneration of human hip joints.

When the patient has the severe pain, the drug should be administered in the full dosage during at least 10 to 14 days. The dose of the drug can be decreased when there is a pain relief. At this time, NSAIDs we can change with analgesics.

NSAIDs can have toxic effects, especially gastrointestinal bleeding that may occur in absence of symptoms. There is an overall relative risk of hospitalization for bleeding and perforation [60] of 3 to 4. Older women appear to be particularly vulnerable to this side effect. There is no "safe" NSAID in this respect, but evidence from several newer independent studies indicates that ibuprofen and diclofenac are the safest among a number of NSAID. These drugs can also cause rashes and hypersensitivity reactions adversely affect kidney, liver and bone marrow function, impair platelet aggregation, prolonging bleeding time. In the term to prevention of adverse side effects it is used means which protect of mucous of the digestive tract. It has been shown that treatment with Misoprostol, a stabilized prostaglandin E, reduces the risk of ulcer development without reducing the therapeutic effect of diclofenac. [61]

### *Intraarticular Glucocorticoids*

Glucocorticoids inhibit the synthesis of interleukin-1ß and tumor necrosis factor-α in cultures of OA synovial tissue and may exert a favorable influence on tissue destruction. Indications for intraarticular glucocorticoids are inflammatory episodes with joint effusion or permanent pain. Arthrocentesis as such may have lasting symptom-relieving effects. Controlled trials show that the improvement is not longer than a few weeks. Published data on the use of intra-articular corticosteroids for OA have shown short term (up to four weeks) improvement in signs and symptoms compared with placebo.

Complications of corticosteroid injection include infection and cutaneous atrophy; repeated injections may also accelerate joint degeneration.

One recent study have demonstrated that long-term treatment of knee OA with repeated steroid injections appears to be clinically effective for the relief of symptoms of the disease. No deleterious effects of the long-term administration of intraarticular steroids on the anatomical structure of the knee were noted [62].

There has been speculation that intra-articular corticosteroid administration may have a disease modifying effect in OA. However, a recent structural outcome study in humans did not validate such a hypothesis [7].

### *Opioids*

Tramadol is synthetic opioid which is effective after oral, rectal or parenteral administration. It is may be effective in symptomatic treatment of OA although published results are limited. Symptom improvement was reported by 70% after tramadol and 50% after dextropropoxyphene [63]. Another unpublished study show that pain relief after 1 and 4 weeks was similar with tramadol 50 to 100mg 3 times daily and diclofenac 25 to 50 mg.Tramadol was associated with more frequent adverse reactions (nausea, constipation, drowsiness). Tramadol may be useful in the symptomatic treatment of OA in patients who do not tolerate or respond to paracetamol or NSAIDs, but the frequent occurrence of adverse reactions seems to limit its usefulness in the reported dosage.

### *Transcutaneous Therapies*

Topical liniments, gels, and creams, with contents like salicylates, camphor, local anesthetics and various vasodilating and skin-penetrating components, have been and are still being used to treat musculoskeletal pains. The efficacy of such self-medication has little support from controlled studies. Diclofenac applied percutaneosly was better than placebo. Capsaicin also resulted in significant pain relief compared with placebo vehicle after local application. It is a potent rubefacient that causes depletion of substance P.

In the management of the OA alternative pharmacologic remedy are uses, also: symptomatic slow acting drugs and chondroprotective agents.

### *Symptomatic Slow Acting Drugs for Osteoarthrosis*

Hyaluronic acid, diacerein, chondroitin sulphate, glucosamine sulphate and S-adenosil metionin may possess structure modification properties but more studies using standardized methodology are required.

#### Hyaluronan

(Arzal, Hyalgan), designated hyaluronic acid has attracted considerable interest as a physiological therapeutic agent. Hyaluronic acid polymers have been found to be useful as viscosupplements for the treatment of OA in a number of clinical studies. In experimental canine OA, intra-articular injections of hyaluronan had beneficial effects [64]. Hyaluronan can relieve knee pain and improved disease severity more than placebo [65].

#### Diacerein

It is an interesting drug without effects on cyclo-oxygenase or lipooxygenase but effective in animal models of OA and with interleukin-1-inhibiting effects.

It has good effect on the simptomatology in OA and positive effect on the integrity of extracelular matrix of the cartilage [66]. One research on 288 patients with OA of the hip has shown that combination of the therapy of the diacerein and tenoxicam has a priority over monotherapy only by Diacerein. The onset of action was rapid with tenoxicam but occurred after 6 weeks with diacerein.

So, complementary management is proposed in the initial phase of OA which is especially painful. Tolerability of oral administrated Diacerein is good. Mild diarrhea was seen in 37% of patients receiving diacerein [67]. The color change of urine in the red or brown is without pathologic importance. It is because of excretion of the drug metabolites. Gastric tolerability is better than for NSAIDs. This drug will have to prove its usefulness alone or in combination in further trials.

#### Chondroitin Sulfate

*Chondroitin sulfate* has shown itself better than placebo and is well tolerated. It has slow effect and symptomatic effect after 1 to 2 months and maintains effect of two months after the end of the therapy. Some of the patients are not good reaction on the therapy. They don't show clinical and subjective improvement or it is completely a little.

### Glycosamin Sulphate

It is found that the drug is moderately effective orally and intramuscularly administrated in short-term studies. The mechanisms of acting are unclear. The effect on the pain in the OA happens later, after 30 days, and remains 2 months after break of the therapy. The new experimental research have shown positive effect glycosamine hydrochloride on repairing processes on the model of the posttraumatic arthrosis in articulare cartilage [68].

Recently there is a great deal of interest and investigation for potential therapeutic properties of *S-adenosil metionin* (SAMe). SAMe is a biological compound that is found in virtually every living cell of the human body. It is a metabolite of the amino acid methionine, a key element in methylation and critical component in cartilage production [69].

It has shown that it stimulates the proliferation of the hondrocytes in experimental OA. of the rabbit. SAMe was investigated by researchers in the treatment of age–related diseases such as OA. Numerous research studies have found that raising the level of SAMe in the body reduces the age-related biological processes. A study tested the effectiveness of SAMe in 108 patients with OA of the knee, hip and spine during the 24-month study has shown improvement of clinical symptoms after two weeks. In only 20% of the patient, minor, non-specific side effects such as nausea occurred [70].

### *Chondroprotective Agents*

The idea of chondroprotection is attractive and is exciting in the sense of being able to preserve cartilage from deteriorating in the course of OA Chondroprotection has never been documented in human disease and it may not exist. It has been discussed whether certain NSAIDs as well as some drugs used for intraarticular injection could prevent cartilage damage. Using of glycosaminoglycan and cartilage preparation did not show significant therapeutically effects.

Two preparations that were used for decades in some countries, Rumalon®, a glycosaminoglycan peptide complex extracted from bovine cartilage and Arteparon® a glycosaminoglycan polysulfate with heparinoid actions have both been withdrawn because of the occurrence of unusual cases of fatal adverse reactions [71].

The pharmacotherapy of OA is at present mainly symptomatic and past claims of disease modification and chondroprotection remain unproven. The goal of preventing or delaying, or even improving, tissue damage in OA will remain high on the list of priorities of investigators. One line of investigation is the search for means of stimulating matrix synthesis or of inhibiting its degradation.

## Comment

It is now widely accepted that OA is the most frequent of joint diseases and represents a heterogeneous pattern (group of overlapping pathological conditions), causing damage of the articular cartilage and periarticular structures, with clinically and radiographically impairment of the joint and disability of the patient. OA is a major health problem, the most common cause of chronic disabilities for working and self-care among middle-aged and older people and has significant social and economic impact.

Many studies about the impact of these diseases on the quality of life, have shown that the high degree of impairment of physical and social function have impact on the work efficiency, decreased employment opportunities and decreased standard of living of the patients.

Physician visits, diagnostic studies, medications, physical therapy, surgery and no medical costs are large burden on individuals and healthcare systems. The enormous economic consequences of this common disease are evident in the fact that OA is responsible for the loss 4.7 million days from work per year in the United Kingdom [25].

OA has been divided into two main categories. In primary OA initiating event despite many anatomic, biochemical, immunological, biomechanical, genetic, pathophysiologic and clinical studies is still not clearly defined. Secondary OA may be due to many different factors.

The most attractive recent findings are the data pointing to an association between inflammation and disease appearance and progression. IL1ß and other proinflammatory cytokines or inflammatory factors, are probably responsible for the signs and symptoms of inflammation present in patients with OA. A clearer understanding of the pathophysiology of this disease has facilitated the development of new approaches for treatments aimed at specifically and effectively retarding disease progress.

Further studies will lead to a better understanding of the osteoarthritic process.

Slow progress of the joint pain, stiffness, limitation of movement, swelling, development of joint deformity and joint instability, especially of hip and knee, can lead to functional impairment and diminishes the quality of life. The main radiological characteristic of these conditions are joint space narrowing (thinning of articular cartilage), bony sclerosis with subchondral cysts and marginal osteophytes.

Other imaging methods (ultrasound, CT, MRI) and laboratory studies may have diagnostic value in some cases. Although anatomical changes in the cartilage can be seen, quantification of these changes remains difficult. Recently, the quantitative assessment of knee cartilage volume has become possible using MRI.

Methods for detecting and monitoring subtle changes in cartilage metabolism are needed to identify the joint changes that precede loss of articular cartilage. Detection of the earliest signs of OA may allow physicians to intervene in preventing progression of the disease or reverse the course of the disease.

There is no specific management but we have wide diapason of abilities for symptomatic treatment of OA. General goals of the management are: restorative goal, maintenance goal and preventive goal. Specific goals include: relief of pain, maintenance of strength and range of motion, preservation of energy and supportive measures. Optimal management of OA is dependent on many variables including the patient's age, weight, amount of disability and desired activity level, the stage of the OA process, the state of the science of treatment modalities available and ability of the physician.

Guidelines for management of OA have been developed by the American College of Rheumatology. These guidelines include three steps in management: nonpharmacological, pharmacological approaches and preventive surgery. Pain management in OA should start with education, psychological support exercises, physiotherapy and environmental measures. Interventions that may prevent progression include lifestyle and activity modifications, weight loss, correction of mechanical abnormalities in joints, exercise programs etc. These treatments can reduce drug consumption and toxicity as well as reduce joint deformity, to build up muscle power to support damaged joints and protect joint alignment.

Analgesics are an important part of the treatment. When an inflammation is a significant source of pain, anti-inflammatory drugs are helpful. Opioids are used in combination with paracetamol when pain is not controlled with NSAIDs or in patients intolerant to NSAIDs.

Some controlled studies seem to demonstrate an analgesic superiority of the non steroidal anti-inflammatory drugs versus paracetamol, but NSAIDs can have more severe adverse effects than paracetamol. Some studies suggest the potential structural effect of so called slow-acting symptom modifying drugs. Among the local treatments, the interest of the viscosupplementation seems well established.

New forms of pharmacological and nonpharmacological treatment of OA are still under development. Disease modification and chondroprotection are interesting fields for future research.

Further work is also needed, to define the clinical efficacy of these medications. Researches are implanting artificial matrices, growth factors, and transplanted chondrocytes or mesenchymal stem cells into cartilage defects to stimulate of a new articular surface. However, this approach has not yet been shown to be effective in osteoarthritic joints.

In the light of several recent international guidelines, it seems necessary to optimise in the individual patient the best possible combination of nonpharmacological and pharmacological therapeutic modalities. The place and the modalities of use of the slow-acting symptom modifying drugs remain to be determined more precisely [72].

Therefore, the early detection and management of OA are important. In the early stage of the disease there is a great potential for preventing the progression of OA.

# Lists of Abbreviations

| | |
|---|---|
| ACR | American College of Rheumatology |
| AIMS | Arthritis Impact Measurement Scales |
| COX-1 and COX-2 | Cyclooxygenase -1 and Cyclooxygenase-2 |
| CRP | C-reactive protein |
| CT | Computed tomography |
| DIP joints | Distal interphalangeal joints |

| | |
|---|---|
| ESR | Erythrocyte sedimentation rate |
| HAQ | Health Assessment Questionnaire |
| IGF-I | Insulin-like growth factor I |
| IL-1 | Interleukin-1 |
| IL-6 | Interleukin-6 |
| MMP | Matrix metalloproteinases |
| MRI | Magnetic resonance imaging |
| NO | Nitric oxide |
| NSAID | Nonsteroidal anti-inflammatory drug |
| OA | Osteoarthrosis |
| PGE2 | Prostaglandin E2 |
| PIP joints | Proximal interphalangeal joints |
| PMF | Pulsed magnetic field therapy |
| SAMe | S-adenosil metionin |
| SF-36 | MOS 36-Item Short Form Health Survey |
| TENS | Transucutaneous electrical nerve stimulation |
| TGF-ß | Transforming growth factor beta |
| THA | Total hip arthroplasty |
| TNF-α | Tumor necrosis factor-alpha |
| WOMAC | Western Ontario and McMaster Osteoarthritis Index |

## References

[1] Waldron HA. Osteoarthritis of the hands in early populations. *Br J Rheumatol.* 1996; 35:1292-1298.

[2] Hart DJ, Spector TD. Radiographic criteria for epidemiologic studies of osteoarthritis. *J.Rheumatol.* 1995; 22 suppl 43: 46-48.

[3] Dürrigl Th. Degenerative joint disease. In: *Konecni J*, ed. *Clinical rheumatology*. Belgrade-Zagreb: PA: Medical book, Inc; 1984: 493-499.

[4] Yuan GH, Masuko-Hongo K, Sakata M, et al. The role of C-C chemokines and their receptors in osteoarthritis. *Arthritis Rheum.* 2001; 44:1056-1070.

[5] Furukawa T, Eyre DR, Koide S, Glimcher MJ. Biochemical studies on repair cartilage resurfacing experimental defects in the rabbit knee. *Journal of Bone and Joint Surgery.*1980; 62:79-89.

[6] Jubb RW. Breakdown of articular cartilage by vascular tissue. *Journal of Pathology.*1982; 136:333-343.

[7] Freeman MAR. Adult Articular Cartilage. *Tunbridge Wells: Pitman Medical Publishing Co*; 1973.

[8] Pelletier JP, Martel-Pelletier J.Therapeutic targets in osteoarthritis: from today to tomorrow with new imaging technology. Annals of the Rheumatic Diseases. 2003; 62:79.

[9] Sharif M, George E, Stepstone L, et al. Serum hyaluronic acid predicts disease progression on osteoarthritis of the knee. *Arthritis Rheum*. 1995;38:760-767.

[10] Rizkalla G, Reiner A, Bogoch E, et al. Studies of the articular cartilage proteoglycan aggrecan in health and osteoarthritis. *J Clin Invest.*1992; 90:2268-2277.

[11] Buckwalter JA, Martin J. Degenerative Joint Disease. *Clinical Symposia.*1995; 47:2-3.

[12] Shepard GJ, Banks AJ, Ryan WG. Ex-professional association footballers have an increased prevalence of osteoarthritis of the hip compared with age matched controls despite not having sustained notable hip injuries.*Br J Sports Med.* 2003; 37:80-81.

[13] Spector TD, Harris PA, Hart DJ, et al. Risk of osteoarthritis associated with long-term weight-bearing sports: a radiologic survey of the hips and knees in female ex-athletes and population controls. *Arthritis-Rheum.* 1996; 39:988-995.

[14] Stankovic A. Etiopathogenesis of osteoarthrosis. *Balneoclimatologia.* 1998; Suppl.1: 9-15.

[15] Pinals RS. Mechanism of Joint Destruction, Pain and Disability in Osteoarthritis. *Drugs.* 1996; 52 Suppl 3:14-20.

[16] Lethbridge -Cejku M, Tobin JD, Scott WJR, et al. Axial and hip bone mineral density and radiographic changes of osteoarthritis of the knee: data from the Baltimore longitudinal study of aging. *J Rheumatol.* 1996; 23: 1943-1947.

[17] Jimenez SA, Dharmavaram RM. Genetic aspects of familial osteoarthritis. *Ann Rheum Dis.* 1994; 53: 789-797.

[18] Pelletier JP, Caron JP, Evans C, et al. In vivo suppression of early experimental osteoarthritis by interleukin-1 receptor antagonist using gene therapy. *Arthritis Rheum.* 1997; 40:1012-1019.

[19] Belhorn LR, Hess EV. Erosive osteoarthritis. *Semin Arthritis Rheum.* 1993; 22:298-306.

[20] Pattrick M, Hamilton E, Wilson R. et al. Radiographic changes of osteoarthritis, symptoms and synovial fluid particles in 300 knees. *Ann Rheum Dis.* 1993; 52: 97-103.

[21] Grigg P. Schaible H, Schmidt RF. Mechanical sensitivity of group III and IV afferents from posterior articular nerve in normal and inflamed cat knee. *J Neurophysiol* 1986; 55: 635-643.

[22] Stein C. The control of pain in peripheral tissue by opioids. *N Eng J Med.* 1995; 332:1685-1690.

[23] Singh G, et al. Prevalence of cardiovascular disease risk factors among U.S. adults with self-reported osteoarthritis: data from the Third National Health and Nutrition Examination Survey. *Am J Manag Care.* 2002; 8: S383-391.

[24] Doyle D. Clinical aspects of osteoarthrosis. In: Scott JT, ed. *Copeman's Textbook of the Rheumatic Diseases*.6th ed. Edinburgh, London, Melbourne and New York: Churchill Livingstone, Inc; 1986: 846-873.

[25] Hinton R et al. Osteoarthritis: diagnosis and therapeutic considerations. *Am Fam Physician*. 2002; 65: 841-848.

[26] Hoaglund FT, Yau AC, Wong WL. Osteoarthritis of the hip and other joints in southern Chinese in Hong Kong. *J Bone Joint Surg*. 1973; 55A: 545-557.

[27] Byers PD, Hoaglund FT, Purewal GS, et al. Articular cartilage changes in Caucasian and Asian hip joints. *Ann Rheum Dis* .1974; 33:157-161.

[28] Mukhopadhaya B, Barooah B. Osteoarthritis of the hip in Indians: An anatomical and clinical study. *Indian J Orthop*. 1967; 1:55-62.

[29] Solomon L, Beighton P, Lawrence JS. Rheumatic disorders in the South African Negro. Osteoarthrosis. *S Afr Med J*. 1975; 49:1737-1740.

[30] Nevitt MC, Xu L, Zhang Y, et al. Very low prevalence of hip osteoarthritis among Chinese elderly in Beijing, China, compared with whites in the United States: the Beijing osteoarthritis study. *Arthritis Rheum*. 2002; 46:1773-1779.

[31] Herman JH. Musgrave CS, Koo KH, et al. Lymphokines: potential roll in the immunopathogenesis of osteoarthritis. *Semin Arthritis Rheum*. 1981; 11(Suppl 1):104-109.

[32] Engel A. *Osteoarthritis and body measurements*: *United States 1960-62*. Washington DC: PHS Publication; 1968.

[33] Walton M. Obesity as an etiological factor in the development of osteoarthrosis. Gerontology. 1979; 25:36-41.

[34] Marks R, Allegrante JP. Body mass indices in patients with disabling hip osteoarthritis. *Arthritis Res*. 2002; 4:112-116.

[35] Pope DP, Hunt IM, Birrell FN, Silman AJ, Macfarlane GJ. Hip pain onset in relation to cumulative workplace and leisure time mechanical load: a population based case-control study. *Ann Rheum Dis*. 2003; 62:322-326.

[36] Reikerås O, Høiseth A, Reigstad A. Femoral anteversion measured by the Dunlap/Rippstein and Norman methods. *Acta Radiologica Diagnosis*. 1985; 26:303-305.

[37] Vossinakis LC, Karnezis LA, Parry K, Learmonth ID. Radiographic associations for "primary" hip osteoarthrosis: a retrospective cohort study of 47 patients. *Acta Orthop Scand*. 2001; 72: 600-608.

[38] Dekker J, Tola P, Aufdemkampe G, Winckers M. Negative affect pain and disability in osteoarthritis patients: the mediating role of muscle weakness. *Behav Res Ther*. 1993; 31: 203-206.

[39] Dieppe P. Management of osteoarthritis of the hip and knee joints. *Curr Opin Rheumatol*. 1993; 5: 487-493.

[40] Wilson CH, Maier WP. Exercise and mobilization techniques. In: Leek JC, Gershwin ME, Fowler WM, eds. *Principles of physical medicine and rehabilitation in the musculoskeletal diseases*. Orlando: Grune Stratton, Inc; 1986:11-22.

[41] Gerber LH, Hicks JE. Rehabilitation in the management of patients with osteoarthritis. In: Moskowitz RW, Howell DS, Goldberg VM, Mankin HJ, eds. *Osteoarthritis: Diagnosis and management*. Philadelphia: WB Saunders, 1984:287-315.

[42] Beals CA, Lampman RM, Banwell BF, Braunstein EM, Albers JW, Castor CW. Measurement of exercise tolerance in patients with rheumatoid arthritis and osteoarthritis. *J Rheumatol.* 1985; 12: 458-461.

[43] Minor MA, Hewett JE, Webel RR, Anderson SK, Kay DR. Efficacy of physical conditioning exercise in patients with rheumatoid arthritis and osteoarthritis. *Arthritis Rheum.* 1989; 32:1396-1405.

[44] Nicholas JA, Strizak AM, Veras G. Study of thigh muscle weakness in different pathological states of the lower extremity. *Am J Sports Med.* 1976; 4:241-248.

[45] Sims KJ, Richardson CA, Brauer SG. Investigation of hip abductor activation in subjects with clinical unilateral hip osteoarthritis. *Ann Rheum Dis.* 2002; 61: 687-692.

[46] Hart DJ, Spector TD. The classification and assessment of osteoarthritis. *Bailliere's Clin Rheumatol.* 1995; 9:407-432.

[47] Hartofilakidis G, Karachalios T. Idiopathic osteoarthritis of the hip: incidence, classification, and natural history of 272 cases. *Orthopedics.* 2003; 26:161-166.

[48] Bellamy N. Instruments to assess osteoarthritis-current status and future needs. *Ann rheum Dis.* 1995; 54:692-693.

[49] Pendleton A, Arden N, Dougados M, et al. EULAR recommendations for the management of knee osteoarthritis: report of a task force of the Standing Committee for International Clinical Studies Including Therapeutic Trials (ESCISIT). *Ann Rheum Dis.* 2000; 59:936-944.

[50] Forman MD, Malamet R, Kaplan D. A survey of osteoarthritis of the knee in the elderly. *J Rheumatol.* 1983; 10:282-286.

[51] Davis MA, EttingerWH, Neuhaus JM, et al. Correlates of knee pain among US adults with and without radiographic knee osteoarthritis. *J Rheumatol.* 1992; 19:1943-1949.

[52] Dekker J, Tola P, Aufdemkampe G, Winckers M. Negative affect pain and disability in osteoarthritis patients: the mediating role of muscle weakness. *Behav Res Ther.* 1993; 31: 203-206.

[53] Muller EA. Influence of training and inactivity on muscle strength. *Arch Phys Med.* 1970; 51:449-462.

[54] Nicolakis P, Kollmitzer J, Crevenna R, Bittner C, Erdogmus CB, Nicolakis J. Pulsed magnetic field therapy for osteoarthritis of the knee--a double-blind sham-controlled trial. *Wien Klin Wochenschr.*2002;114:678-684.

[55] Perrot S, Menkes CJ. Nonpharmacological Approaches to Pain in Osteoarthritis. *Drugs.* 1996; 52 Suppl 3:21-26

[56] Taylor P, Hallet M, Flaherty L. Treatment of osteoarthritis of the knee with transcutaneous electrical nerve stimulation. *Pain.* 1981; 11:233-246.

[57] Bradley JD, Brandt KD, Katz BP, et al. Comparison of an antiinflammatory dose of ibuprofen, and analgesic dose of ibuprofen, and acetaminophen in the treatment of patients with osteoarthritis of the knee. *N Engl J Med.* 1991; 325: 87-91.

[58] Brooks PM, Day RO. Nonsteroidal anti-inflammatory drugs-differences and similarities. *N Engl J Med* .1991; 324:1716-1725.

[59] Makarowski W, Zhao WW, Bevirt T, Recker DP. Efficacy and safety of the COX-2 specific inhibitor valdecoxib in the management of osteoarthritis of the hip: a randomized, double-blind, placebo-controlled comparison with naproxen. *Osteoarthritis Cartilage.* 2002; 10: 290-296.

[60] Furst DE. Are there differences among nonsteroidal anti-inflammatory drugs? *Arthritis Rheum.* 1994; 37:1-9.

[61] Bolton W, Melo Gomes JA Stead H, et al. The gastroduodenal safety and efficacy of the fixed combination of diclofenac and misoprostol in the treatment of osteoarthritis. *Br J Rheumatol.* 1992; 31:753-758.

[62] Raynauld JP, Buckland-Wright C, Ward R, Choquette D, et al. Safety and efficacy of long-term intraarticular steroid injections in osteoarthritis of the knee: a randomized, double-blind, placebo-controlled trial. *Arthritis Rheum.* 2003; 48:370-377.

[63] Jensen EM, Ginsberg F. Tramadol versus dextropropoxyphene in the treatment of osteoarthritis. A short term double-blind study. *Drug Invest.* 1994; 8:211-218.

[64] Abatangelo G, Botti P, Del Bue M, et al. Intra-articular sodium hyaluronate injections in the Pond –Nuki experimental model of osteoarthritis in dogs. I. Biochemical results. *Clin Orthop.*1989; 241:278-283.

[65] Goa KL, Benfield P. Hyaluronic acid. A review of its pharmacology and use as a surgical aid in ophthalmology and its therapeutic potential in joint disease and wound healing. *Drugs.* 1994; 47:536-566.

[66] Provvedini D, Cohen P. Efficacy of diacerein on the symptoms and radiographic progression of osteoarthritis. *Presse Med.* 2002; 31:4S13-15.

[67] Nguyen M. Dougados M, Berdah L, et al. Diacerein in the treatment of osteoarthritis of the hip. *Arthritis Rheum.* 1994; 37: 529-536.

[68] Zupanets IA, Bezdetko NV, Dedukh NV, Otrishko IA. Experimental study of the effect of glucosamine hydrochloride on metabolic and repair processes in connective tissue structures. *Eksp Klin Farmakol.* 2002; 65: 67-69.

[69] Elkins R. SAMe: *The remarkable Substance that Promotes Detoxification, Relieves Arthritis and Fights Depression.* Pleasant Grove, UT: Woodland Publishing, 1999: 5-6.

[70] Konig B. A long-term (two years) clinical trial with S-adenosylmethionine for the treatment of osteoarthritis. *Am J Med.* 1987; 83:89-94.

[71] McAlindon T, Dieppe P. The medical management of osteoarthritis of the knee: an inflammatory issue? *Br J Rheumatol.* 1990; 29:471-473.

[72] Conrozier T, Flipo RM. Current management of osteoarthritis. Part 1: pharmacological strategies. *Rev Med Interne*. 2003; 24:183-188.

# Index

## Q



## R



## S



## T

## U



## V



## W